Biologically Active Peptides: Design, Synthesis, and Utilization

T0229723

VOLUME 1
Biologically Active Peptides: Design, Synthesis, and Utilization

EDITED BY

William V. Williams, M.D.
Director of Rheumatology Research
University of Pennsylvania

David B. Weiner, Ph.D.
Director of Biotechnology
The Wistar Institute

CRC PRESS

Boca Raton London New York Washington, D.C.

Library of Congress Cataloging-in-Publication Data

Main entry under title:
 Biologically Active Peptides: Design, Synthesis and Utilization

Full catalog record is available from the Library of Congress

Table of Contents

Introduction

THIS book marks the first in a series addressing the impact of the latest aspects of biotechnology on both clinical and experimental medicine. The biotechnology revolution currently underway has profoundly altered the approach of experimental biologists to their investigations. These changes are now reaching into clinical medicine with a barrage of novel diagnostic and therapeutic products. The pace of change has been both exhilarating and exhausting, as scientists and clinicians are challenged to keep abreast of developments which are more and more rapidly altering the study and practice of biology and medicine. The goal of this series is to acquaint the reader with some of the current approaches being taken in specific aspects of biotechnology as applied to experimental and clinical medicine.

The first book focuses on peptides, short strings of amino acids not large enough to warrant the term protein. This book is divided into three sections. The first section "Structural Approaches to Peptide Design" elaborates on theoretical aspects of peptide design for production of biologically active peptides and peptide mimetics. The second section "Chemical Synthetic Aspects of Peptide Production" explores the chemical synthetic strategies available for peptide production. The third section "Utilization of Bioactive Peptides" details several clinically relevant experimental systems where peptide use has led to either new therapeutic approaches or to important insights from the investigations. Thus, this book should lead the reader through the steps involved in development of biologically active peptides: design, synthesis, and evaluation.

Peptide design, as elaborated in the first section, has been greatly enhanced recently by the use of molecular structure analysis. These approaches are discussed in the first section. The chapter contributed by

Kieber-Emmons, "Strategies in Protein-Based Rational Drug Design," relates structural analysis of ligands and immunogens to rational peptide design. This chapter emphasizes structural homology for molecular modeling strategies related to peptide design. Recent advances in computational chemistry approaches with data base utilization are emphasized in a number of systems where bioactive peptides have been developed based on active site structures. While a peptide can exist in many conformations in solution, typically only a small set of conformations relate to the bioactive conformation of the peptide. Balaji and Ramnarayan explore their recent advances in biocomputational simulation of peptide energy minimization to determine the bioactive conformation of peptides and peptidomimetics. As discussed in "Computer Assisted Drug Design of Peptidomimetic Drugs," this approach has already led to the development of bioactive peptide analogs of relatively small size. Another aspect of peptide design of great interest is the development of small peptide analogs of larger molecules. This is aided by information relating to the active site of the molecule of interest. Von Feldt, Ugen, Kieber-Emmons, and Williams discuss the recently described approach of peptide design based on antibody structural analysis. This approach, as outlined in "Bioactive Peptide Design Based on Antibody Structure" capitalizes on the readily available information relating to antibody active sites. Critical information derived from peptide structural analysis can be applied to refinement of peptide structures. Shon and Opella, in "NMR Spectroscopy of Peptides and Proteins in Membrane Environments," discuss the principles of nuclear magnetic resonance spectroscopy as applied to the determination of peptide structure. They illustrate the use of two- and three-dimensional NMR to determine the structure of membrane associated peptides and proteins, including antibiotic magainin peptides and analogs as well as larger proteins. Thus, the first section elaborates on several approaches to molecular structural analysis as applied to bioactive peptide design.

The increasing utilization of peptides as both experimental tools and in drug design has been greatly facilitated by recent advances in synthetic strategies. The optimal synthetic approach for a particular peptide depends on several factors. This includes the amount desired, the length of the peptide, and the purpose for which it is intended. The synthetic strategies available include solid phase synthesis, liquid phase synthesis, and recombinant DNA approaches. These strategies are explored in depth in the chapter by Maria-Luisa Maccecchini, "Large Scale Peptide Production." The use of synthetic peptides as research tools has been greatly facilitated by solid-phase synthetic techniques. Pioneered by Merrienfeld, this approach has allowed short peptide synthesis to become a widely available experimental tool. Recent advances in this and related fields of peptide synthesis are discussed by Anwer and Kahn in "Advances in Peptide Synthesis." It has been appreciated for some time that proteins and peptides in nature are typically modified. Phosphorylation, glycosylation, and many other modifications are commonly encountered. Otvos, and Hollosi, in their chapter "Development of Chemically Modified Peptides" discuss several recently described strategies for developing stable chemically modified peptides which employ naturally occurring modifications. Peptides, while of great utility for many applications, suffer from poor stability when given *in vivo*. This has led to a great deal of interest in the development of more stable peptide analogs or peptidomimetics. In his chapter "Design and Synthesis of Biologically Active Peptide Mimics," Williams discusses some of the more successful approaches taken in recent years in peptidomimetic design. This has led to the development of a variety of pharmaceutical agents currently in use or under evaluation. This section of the book provides an overview of a number of synthetic strategies for peptide and peptidomimetic development.

The use of synthetic peptides has allowed basic insights into a large number of clinically relevant experimental systems. Peptides have been increasingly used in immunology to determine the molecular nature of immune responsiveness. Peptides can serve as antigens for both cellular and humoral immune responses directed toward a number of pathogens. This has been increasingly applied to vaccine development. The basic immunology of pathogen-derived peptides is discussed by Levy and Weiner in "Synthetic Peptide-Based Vaccines and Antiviral Agents, Including HIV/AIDS as a Model System." A related chapter, discussing the rewards and pitfalls of using peptides as immunogens, is provided by Heber-Katz and Ertl. In "Peptides as Molecular Probes of Immune Responses," they discuss the general and specific aspects of peptide immunogens in several viral systems. The recent elucidation of the molecular basis for cellular immune responses has allowed novel approaches for modulating immune responses. Cellular immunity arises from the ability of major histocompatibility complex (MHC) molecules to bind peptide fragments of antigens, and this peptide-MHC complex to then trigger specific T cells via their T cell antigen receptors. One approach for modulating immune responses centers on developing high-affinity peptide ligands for MHC molecules. This approach is discussed by Sette, Lamont, and Grey in "The Design of MHC Binding Peptides." This highlights the ability of peptides to serve as ligands for MHC molecules, influencing the nature and extent of the interaction of the peptide-MHC complex with T cell receptors. One of the most renowned successes of peptides as molecular probes lies in the field of cellular adhesion molecules. The famous RGD (Arg-Gly-Asp) motif of many cellular adhesion molecules has been exploited by the development of synthetic peptide analogs. This, and many less well-known adhesion-related peptides, are discussed by Robey in "Biology and Chemistry of Extracellular Matrix Cell Attachment Peptides." Peptides can serve as substitute substrates for enzymes, or as enzyme inhibitors. This can affect a wide variety of physiologic and pathophysiologic functions. Grant, Meek, Metcalf, and Petteway discuss the development of such peptides in "Design of Peptide Analog Inhibitors of Proteolytic Processes."

While many subjects related to biologically active peptides are not addressed in this book, the purpose was not to exhaustively cover the field. Instead, this book highlights some of the basic and advanced aspects of peptide design, synthesis, and utilization. The reader should come away with an appreciation for peptide development strategies that have been successfully employed by a number of investigators. While all of these may not apply to a particular experimental system, it is likely that aspects of the strategies discussed herein should have relevance to any given experimental system employing biologically active peptides.

VOLUME 1

Biologically Active Peptides: Design, Synthesis, and Utilization

STRUCTURAL APPROACHES TO PEPTIDE DESIGN

CHAPTER 1

Strategies in Protein-Based Rational Drug Design

THOMAS KIEBER-EMMONS[1,2]

INTRODUCTION

OF the strategies being considered for disease management, the use of native proteins as templates to develop therapeutic agents continues to be touted as one of the most powerful. This notion has grown from identification of many peptides with potent stimulatory and inhibitory effects on cell proliferation in the past ten years. Growth factors represented by interleukins are a good example. These polypeptides were first defined as signalling molecules controlling activities of cells in the immune system. However, it has now been shown that many of these peptides are multifunctional in that any one peptide in this set may exhibit proliferative effects, anti-proliferative effects, and effects unrelated to proliferation [1]. An appreciation of the ligand-receptor interactions underlying these functionalities can lead to a variety of synthetic chemical agents for medical applications.

More recently, protein-based drug design that uses the shape of pharmacologically active antibodies and other proteins to create new active drugs is increasing in popularity (see Chapter 3). Recent advances in genetic engineering coupled with immunoglobulin (Ig) sequence analysis and x-ray crystallography has made it possible to contemplate designing or building functionally better antibodies [2] for example. The design and synthesis of single-chain antigen binding proteins or polypeptides are expected to have advantages in some clinical applications because of their relatively small

[1]The Wistar Institute of Anatomy and Biology, 3601 Spruce Street, Philadelphia, PA 19104, U.S.A.
[2]Department of Medicine, University of Pennsylvania, Philadelphia, PA 19104, U.S.A.

size and fast serum clearance [3]. These molecules might have primary uses that parallel those applications for which monoclonal antibodies are in current use such as imaging, cancer therapy, and vaccine development.

Biological activities residing in the Fc region of Igs has contributed to the notion of using peptides derived from Igs to modulate immune responses [4]. The structural analysis of antibodies which are mimics of receptors and ligands, provides a further avenue for the development of novel drugs [5–7]. Conformational analysis of bioactive peptides can lead to suggestions for synthetic structures that lock in particular conformations that may enhance peptide efficacy [8–13]. Such ideas are consistent with medicinal chemistry practices spanning the last 20 years, but appear to be just discovered by immunologists and biologists alike [7]. From a structural standpoint, protein-based drug design may be viewed as a continuum in geometry, with the objective of mimicking the spatial positioning of reactive functional groups in large molecules by those of small molecules.

A multidisciplinary approach including knowledge-based systems involving crystallographic and sequence data bases, experimentally determined constraints and molecular modeling, provides a viable strategy for studying structure/function relationships necessary for protein-based drug design. In this chapter various strategies commonly used in molecular modeling and conformational analysis are briefly reviewed as an introduction to those uninitiated in the art. Practical aspects of the theory and practice of conformational energy analysis is first explored, followed by an overview of energy minimization strategies and design applications and approaches. Emphasis is placed upon structural design considerations and approaches for targeting effector molecules and cells, drawing upon available evidence for the value of antibodies and synthetic peptides in specific diseases.

THEORY AND METHODOLOGY

POTENTIAL ENERGY FUNCTIONS AND MINIMIZATION

Molecular simulation calculations have become a standard approach to describe the conformational properties of macromolecules and to test structural hypotheses of designed molecules. This approach coupled with Nuclear Magnetic Resonance (NMR) has become the *sine qua non* for studying peptide/protein and nucleic acid structure. From a biophysical perspective these combined approaches try to define the rules that determine macromolecular conformational properties. For example can we simulate how a linear amino acid sequence folds into a protein.

At the heart of such approaches is the mathematical description of the classical energy analog of quantum chemical treatments of a complex molecular system as a function of its coordinates [14,15]. In order to describe the classical energy, potential energy functions or force fields were formulated based upon physico-chemical descriptions of molecular interactions. The early molecular energy descriptions included classical energy functions for the electrostatic interactions, van der Waals interactions defined in terms of dispersion and repulsion components, and torsional terms about rotatable dihedral angles. Latter terms accounted for the Hookian behavior of a molecule's internal coordinates defined as bond lengths, bond angles, and dihedral angles. The potential energy of the system, as described by the various components is expressed as an analytical function and the internal coordinates of the molecule and the distances between atoms. The analytical function is also called a target function.

The potential energy of the system as a function of its coordinates describes the multidimensional energy hyperspace of the system [16]. By calculating the energy of the system at a particular set of coordinate values, one explores the multidimensional energy surface. An important method for exploring the energy surface is to find configurations for which the energy is a minimum. This method finds a point in configurational space where all the forces on an atom are balanced. By minimizing the energy of a molecule, stable molecular conformations can be identified. The analysis of minimized structures provides detailed structural information, while the calculated energy can be partitioned into contributions from specific interactions.

In the last thirty years force field descriptions have grown in their complexity. In general, the accuracy required in a force field depends on the properties of the system that are of interest. A force field may reproduce structural information compared to crystal structures very well, although the calculated energies may not be accurate enough for quantitative energy descriptions in terms of enthalpies. Several force fields are routinely used in molecular energy calculations. These include ECEPP [17], AMBER [18], CHARMM [19], CVFF [20] and MM2/3 [21]. ECEPP was one of the earliest force fields described for analysis of peptides and proteins [17]. The ECEPP force field did not include terms for evaluating strain energies resulting from bond stretching and angle deformations. The function was well parameterized based upon the physico-chemical information. A vast literature is available on the parameterization process of the force field by Scheraga and co-workers [17]. Like ECEPP, the MM2/3 force field is also well parameterized. This force field has been mainly used in conformational energy calculations of hydrocarbons. AMBER, CHARMM and CVFF force fields have become widely used due to the commercialization of software packages that contain these and derivatized versions of these force fields. CHARMM and CVFF have been principally used for peptide/protein studies, with AMBER also used in nucleic acid studies.

The development of potential energy functions is a discipline in its own right emphasizing the theoretical basis of force fields, their parameters, and the parameterization process. There are many limitations in the use of energy calculations and the work is incomplete. However, strategies involving conformational energy calculations can provide valuable information in probing conformations with the aim of developing novel molecules. There is a wealth of software and methods available for computer-assisted drug design (recently reviewed by Cohen et al. [22]) that is either the same or complementary to protein-based drug design.

DESIGN STRATEGIES USING MINIMIZATION AND DYNAMICS

At the heart of protein-based drug design is the description of the conformational properties of a protein or bioactive peptide. The essential difficulty in using potential energy approaches to study conformational properties is the multiple-minimum problem [16]. It is conceptually well noted that if a minimization is started from a conformation chosen at random, the probability of reaching its global minimum is essentially zero. Subsequently many computational chemists would agree that free space minimization, the process of starting with a random geometry and minimizing its free energy, would not necessarily lead to structures that would otherwise be observed by crystallography. However, this view is not universally shared (see Chapter 2). There are many applications in which the biasing of a target function is appropriate to test whether a particular conformation can be populated or to impose constraints on the molecular system so as to influence the energy pathway during the computing of conformational states. A target function is a term used to describe the function for which a minimum value is sought. Basically it is a customization of the function to address a specific modeling question. Such customization takes the form of constraints and restraints.

A constraint is the fixing of atoms in space. In examining the loop conformation of turn regions in antibodies for example, one popular constraint is to fix atoms at the base of the loop [23]. This fixing of atoms can be used to simulate the affect on the tertiary environment in preserving the beginning and the end of the turn region. In contrast, restraints can take many forms. Torsional restraints bias the harmonic torque about a bond to force it to adopt a new value. A good example of using such an approach is to study energy pathways across a barrier [24]. Another example of a restraint is the use of distances between atoms derived from NMR experiments or coupling constants used as torsional restraints [25].

One of the pioneering efforts in modifying potential functions is the strategy of template forcing [24]. In this approach one molecule is forced to adopt the conformation of another. This approach is useful in evaluating whether a particular peptide can adopt a binding mode conformation of a target peptide. This information is particularly useful in drug design applications. Atom pairs between the molecule under study are considered as flexible and the target molecule is assigned a Hookian type potential function, pulling the atoms in the flexible molecule toward the target molecule. The energy required to force the study molecule into the required conformation can be used to evaluate how easily an analog can adopt the conformation of a given template.

While strategies using energy minimization can lead to meaningful results, molecular dynamics approaches provide a means to simulate the motion of atoms. This approach allows for the study of the fluctuation in the relative positions of atoms in a macromolecule as a function of time. Molecular dynamics has been used to elucidate structures from NMR experiments, to refine x-ray crystallographic structures or molecular models from poor starting structures, and to calculate the free energy change resulting from mutations in proteins [26]. Molecular dynamics provides information on the accessibility of conformational states available to a molecule.

A combination of molecular dynamics simulations and minimization is useful to search for structural features that may be significant for the binding of peptides to receptors. Both low temperature (room temperature 300 K) and high temperature (900 K) dynamics is typically employed. High temperature dynamics greatly increases the efficiency of producing conformational transitions, however there are structural caveats that must be considered in such calculations. For example the omega or peptide bond typically deviates from its normal values under such conditions. Therefore caution is advised to the novice user in performing such calculations to be sure that there is geometrical consistency. In peptide design applications a good prototype example is provided by the identification of constrained analogs of gonotropin releasing hormone (GnRH) as antagonists using a combined strategy incorporating energy minimization, template forcing, molecular dynamics, and NMR information [10,27]. Again, numerous treatments have been presented on molecular dynamic simulations in biology [27–29].

While the solution conformation(s) of peptides is accessible for examination by physical techniques, interpretation of such observations is often difficult. Most peptides of interest like peptide hormones and neurotransmitters are small linear peptides and thereby have a considerable conformational flexibility in solution. Furthermore, the suggested conformer(s) can be dramatically affected by the environment [30]. Subsequently structures observed by physical techniques such as NMR or Circular Dichromism (CD) are relevant only to the condition under study—the physical properties of the solvent.

In contrast, theoretical calculations are typically performed *in vacuo*, where the influence of the solvent on the conformation(s) is largely ignored. The aim of these studies is nonetheless, to gain insight into the structure of a given peptide in a very particular milieu – that of the receptor where solvent is typically excluded. Subsequently such *in vacuo* type calculations are deemed as being representative of possible ligand binding modes for receptor binding. Nevertheless, the question still arises whether the conformation(s) determined in solutions or *in vacuo* have any relevance to the conformation of the peptide at the receptor in the bound state or even in the close vicinity of the receptor. However, in spite of these conceptual difficulties and the inherent limitations of available physical and theoretical methods, they could, particularly in conjunction with chemical modifications of the peptides, help to gain insight into the complex phenomena of ligand-receptor interaction. This information can then be further translated into testable synthetic compounds for evaluation that may lead to therapeutics.

COMPARATIVE MODELING TO DEFINE PROTEIN AND PEPTIDE STRUCTURES

The prediction of protein and peptide structure has a rich history. From the early work of Anfinsen showing that the inherent information for protein folding lies in the amino acid sequence of a protein [31], a large effort has been directed toward developing methods to predict structure [32]. The ability to predict structure has evolved to a state of heavy reliance on the use of data bases. The prediction of tertiary structure of proteins is cast in a knowledge-based approach depending on the identification of analogies in secondary structures, motifs, domains, or ligand interactions between a protein being modeled with structures already available [32,33]. The concept has evolved from early work on the prediction of protein structure based upon distance geometry relationships established from crystallographic data bases [34–38]. This approach is a topic called comparative model building or modeling by homology and discussed in various forms over the years [39–42].

The first step in this approach is to search structural data bases looking for sequence similarities between the protein or fragment being modeled with data base members. The prediction of an unknown protein structure by comparative modeling requires the correct correspondence between residues. Sequence alignments of proteins have become a standard approach to establishing both the family identity of a protein and as a method to define structural elements to be used in comparative model building ([43] and references therein). The approach however is not without caveats that can mislead the structural elucidation effort. Procedures such as those of Needleman and Wunsch [44] or Smith and Waterman [45], with scoring parameters expressed as mutation data matrix, correctly place proteins into phylogenetic families when the proteins are closely related. It has been long recognized that for distantly related proteins these procedures are not as accurate. One of the reasons attributed to this problem is that sequence alignment methods typically apply a gap penalty uniformly throughout a sequence [46]. When sequence alignments are compared with alignments based upon three-dimensional structures, insertion and deletions identified by sequence alignments alone have been observed to occur in the middle of structural elements that are important for protein structural organization. Sequence alignments with uniform gap penalties can change the pattern of residue relationships that affect packing organization, destroying the complementarity of occluded surfaces.

The use of variable gap penalties to improve the alignment of amino acid sequences of distantly related proteins has been proposed [46,47]. Such an approach to analyze relationships of distantly related proteins depends on the availability of three-dimensional structural information of family members. Three-dimensional information can be used to redistribute gap penalties, increasing penalties for insertions and deletions within definable secondary structural elements or motifs that are highly conserved among a protein family [48]. Family members can be of diverse structural nature. The Ig super-family is such a set of proteins with members that differ appreciably in the number of α helices and β strands. In addition, regions of secondary structure in related proteins do not always retain the same boundaries.

With the ever burgeoning number of available sequences, attention has been turned to the problem of multiple sequence alignment. The most common approach is based upon iterative pair wise alignment [49]. This method rests on linking a representation of a set of multiple aligned sequences as a profile, where the alignment column comprises the frequency of the amino acids at a given position with scoring based on this distribution. This approach is often relied upon to detect distantly related sequences. In general this approach has numerous caveats also associated with it [43,47–49].

Recently much effort has been directed to identifying structural relationships that may be utilized in relational data base schemes. Many approaches rely on pattern analysis of one form or another, such as neural network models [50], dot matrix methods [43], distance geometry [51], etc. Most of these approaches rely on searching for sequences that are similar to the sequence of a protein whose structure is known. This strategy works well for closely related structures but structural similarities can go undetected as the level of sequence identity drops. Alternative approaches have been presented that relate rules of 1D sequence information with 3D structure, by considering that nature preserves structure and not sequences [52]. Proteins that fold into similar structures can have large differences in their sizes and shapes of residues at equivalent residue positions.

The alignment of sequences based upon structural elements that are conserved within a family can be extended to include structural elements that are conserved across protein families. One such approach has been referred to as profile analysis [53]. Profile analysis can be used as a method for detecting secondary structure tendencies of protein regions. Such an approach could follow the general method outlined by Gribskov et al. [53] but reflects a knowledge-based strategy to identify the local structural order of a protein. This use of the profile method infers information on three-dimensional structure from primary sequence. The structural information can be contained in a database of structural motifs developed by considering differential geometry relationships among proteins containing the motifs [54,55]. The sequences of the geometrically similar motifs can then be aligned in order to establish a sequence profile that relates the motifs. Creation of a set of profiles for a variety of super-secondary structures offers a library of structural motifs that can be searched by typing in a sequence. Sequences that define a motif are related by assessing an evolutionary scoring matrix that considers the conservation of amino acids critical to maintaining the folding pattern of the motif.

Comparison of protein sequences with the library can yield information on structural motifs within a given protein. This approach is different from considering a sequence alignment of one member of a protein family with a given protein. Multiple sequences intrinsic to a particular fold define the alignment. Extensions of the multiple sequence alignment problem has been discussed [47,48]. Since there are usually insertions and deletions between sequences, it is difficult to match the backbone conformation of the unknown protein exactly with those of the known proteins and considerable care is required in order to correctly model the conformations of inserted loops as well as side chain conformations [56–61].

ANTIBODIES AS BIOSYNTHETIC TEMPLATES

A milieu of receptors have now been cloned that are potential targets for the development of pharmaceutics. Among the pharmaceutics are antibodies and compounds based upon the structural properties of antibodies. Antibodies serve as a well-characterized example of comparative modeling approaches with application to pharmaceutic and peptide design.

The therapeutic applications of Igs is continually increasing. However, a major limitation in the clinical use of rodent hybridomas in human therapy is the anti-globulin response during therapy. In addition to the anti-mouse response, another potential problem with these antibodies is the anti-idiotype (Id) response, blocking the binding of the antibodies to the target effector molecule. A partial solution to this problem is the construction of chimeric antibodies. Historically, such chimerics evolved by replacing the rodent constant domain with a human derived constant region [62]. This ability allowed for isotype tailoring to participate in antibody-dependent cellular cytotoxicity (ADCC) and complement-dependent cytotoxicity. However such antibodies can still induce anti-globulin affects that are directed toward the variable domain of antibodies [63].

The next level of designing chimerics involved transplanting complementary determining regions (CDRs) of rodent antibodies onto an antibody scaffold of human origin [64]. An example of this approach is most noted by the designing of CAMPATH-1 [65]. More recently this approach has been shown effective in the "humanizing" of a murine antibody to the interleukin-2 (IL-2) receptor as a potential immunosuppressive [66], a murine monoclonal directed toward the V3 domain of HIV-1 as a possible therapeutic [67], and a murine anti-CD4 antibody to be used as an immunosuppressive agent [68]. In all these studies three basic concepts were employed: (1) the human Frameworks (FRs) selected as the basis for designing the reshaped human antibodies should be as homologous as possible to the FRs of the rodent antibody; (2) the amino acid residues of the rodent antibody that are members of the canonical structures for CDR loops should be conserved; and (3) additional amino acid residues in the FRs that show nonconservative changes between the rodent and human sequences, particularly those in structurally relevant positions need to be examined for influence of antibody packing or combining site stabilization.

Ig TEMPLATE PROPERTIES

The structure of Igs is a topic much studied. Salient themes derived from these studies include the identification of residue side chains that are conserved in various regions of the V_L and the V_H primary structures as a means to preserve the geometry of the V_L-V_H interface [69], structural variability as it relates to sequence diversity [70,71], and the effect of packing of various side chains has on the conformational properties of CDR regions [72] and how in turn this affects antigen specificity. The variation in CDR topography which is dictated by the lengths of turn regions as well as the amino acid diversity of Igs [73,74], is fundamental to the antigen specificity of Igs. Proteins that express the Ig folding behavior may have different lengths associated with turn regions and exhibit a broader spectrum of amino acid variation within its sequence compared with other family members. Comparative modeling approaches are based upon defining structural elements that are transferable from members of a protein family to the unknown protein.

In comparative modeling approaches we first define structural elements that are conserved between members of the family. These structurally conserved regions define the basic template from which to build a structural perspective of the unknown protein. In Igs, the simplest structurally conserved regions are β strands that make up the scaffold. However, proteins can also be dissected into consensus micro-structures consisting of only several residues that are structurally discernable or dissected into consensus macro-structures which may span several secondary structural units. In a broader context consensus alignments can be utilized to engineer human antibodies from murine antibodies. For example, a generic template for antibodies can be generated by considering the average spatial position of $C\alpha$ backbone atoms under energy minimization constraints of superimposed structures. For β structures the spatial deviations are not large. We have recently extended this approach to develop consensus structures for turn regions including CDR domains.

In Figure 1.1 an illustrative example of sequence alignments involving a micro-definition of β type structures found in both heavy and light chains of Igs is presented. These regions are grouped based upon a least squares fitting procedure showing a minimum in the root-mean-square (RMS) deviations among the antibody crystal structures between heavy and light chains. Least squares fitting (superpositioning) is used as a measure to determine how close two structures are. $C\alpha$ crystal coordinates of respective structures are spatially positioned with respect to each other to determine whether the structures are superimposable. The lower the RMS the more alike are the two structures. The grouping in Figure 1.1 separates intervening secondary structural units such as CDR regions and Id determining regions (IDR) [70] or turn regions in the FR portion of the variable domains. The definition of consensus β structures define the beginnings and ends of loop or turn regions that may be of different lengths within antibodies and in molecules that belong to the Ig super-family.

An example of discordance between sequence alignment and structural alignment is observed in the consensus structure labeled A in Figure 1.1. In the comparison of 1REI and 1F19 structures which are of the same length, an insertion is observed in the TT tract of F19 V_L compared with the substance P (SP) tract found in REI V_L. Calculation of the RMS value for the homologous SSLSAS residue tract found in these two proteins is 1.8 A, compared with .74 A for the alignment shown in Figure 1.1. It is evident that the length of the turn region connecting structures A and B varies, being compensated by the consensus structures.

There is generally a structural distinction made between antibody heavy and light chains. From a comparative modeling perspective, these chains are structural analogs of each other. Analysis of crystallographically determined light chain dimers has shown that the light chain can adopt structural conformations that are similar to heavy chain conformations [75]. We have included structural consensus alignments in Figure 1.1 for heavy

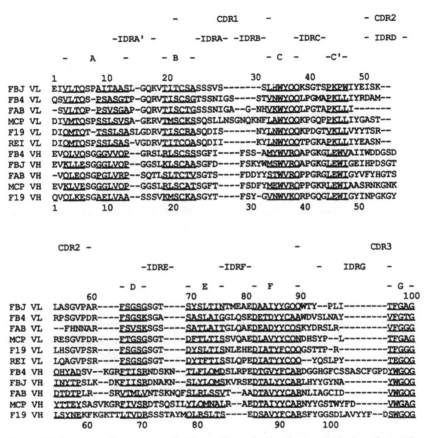

```
                           -         CDR1        -                    - CDR2

                 -IDRA' -          -IDRA- -IDRB-        -IDRC-         - IDRD -

          -      A     -       - B -                - C   -      -C'-

          1        10        20            30          40          50
FBJ  VL   EIVLTQSPAITAASL-GQKVTITCSASSSVS-------SLHWYQQKSGTSPKPWIYEISK--
FB4  VL   QSVLTQS-PSASGTP-GQRVTISCSGTSSNIGS----STVNWYQQLPGMAPKLLIYRDAM--
FAB  VL   -SVLTQP-PSVSGAP-GQRVTISCTGSSSNIGA--G-NHVKWYQQLPGTAPKLLI-------
MCP  VL   DIVMTQSPSSLSVSA-GERVTMSCKSSQSLLNSGNQKNFLAWYQQKPGQPPKLLIYGAST--
F19  VL   DIQMTQT-TSSLSASLGDRVTISCRASQDIS------NYLNWYQQKPDGTVKLLVYYTSR--
REI  VL   DIQMTQSPSSLSAS-VGDRVTITCQASQDII------KYLNWYQQTPGKAPKLLIYEASN--
FB4  VH   EVQLVQSGGGVVQP--GRSLRLSCSSSGFI----FSS-AMYWVRQAPGKGLEWVAIIWDDGSD
FBJ  VH   EVKLLESGGGLVQP--GGSLKLSCAASGFD----FSKYWMSWVRQAPGKGLEWIGEIHPDSGT
FAB  VH   -VQLEQSGPGLVRP--SQTLSLTCTVSGTS----FDDYYSTWVRQPPGRGLEWIGYVFYHGTS
MCP  VH   EVKLVESGGGLVQP--GRSLRLSCATSGFT----FSDFYMEWVRQPPGKRLEWIAASRNKGNK
F19  VH   QVQLKESGAELVAA--SSSVKMSCKASGYT----FSY-GVNWVKQRPGQGLEWIGYINPGKGY
          1        10        20            30          40          50


CDR2   -                                -                 CDR3

          -IDRE-            -IDRF-         -      IDRG    -

          - D -            - E -    - F -                    - G -
          60                70        80        90           100
FBJ  VL   LASGVPAR----FSGSGSGT----SYSLTINTMEAEDAAIYYGQQWTY--PLI--------TFGAG
FB4  VL   RPSGVPDR----FSGSKSGA----SASLAIGGLQSEDETDYYCAAWDVSLNAY--------VFGTG
FAB  VL   --FHNNAR----FSVSKSGS----SATLAITGLQAEDEADYYCQSKYDRSLR--------VFGGG
MCP  VL   RESGVPDR----FTGSGSGT----DFTLTISSVQAEDLAVYYCQNDHSYP--L--------TFGAG
F19  VL   LHSGVPSR----FSGSGSGT----DYSLTISNLEHEDIATYFCQQGSTTP-R--------TFGGG
REI  VL   LQAGVPSR----FSGSGSGT----DYTFTISSLQPEDIATYYCQQ--YQSLPY--------TFGQG
FB4  VH   OHYADSV--KGRFTISRNDSKN--TLFLQMDSLRPEDTGVYFCARDGGHGFCSSASCFGPDYWGQG
FBJ  VH   INYTPSLK--DKFIISRDNAKN--SLYLQMSKVRSEDTALYYCARLHYYGYNA--------YWGQG
FAB  VH   DTDTPLR---SRVTMLVNTSKNQFSLRLSSVT--AADTAVYYCARNLIAGCID--------VWGQG
MCP  VH   YTTEYSASVKGRFIVSRDTSQSILYLQMNALR--AEDTAIYYCARNYYGSTWYFD------VWGAG
F19  VH   LSYNEKFKGKTTLTVDRSSSTAYMQLRSLTS----EDSAVYFCARSFYGGSDLAVYYF--DSWGQG
          60                70        80        90           100
```

Figure 1.1 Sequence alignments implied by profile analysis and superpositioning of crystallographically known light and heavy chains. The following V_L and V_H sequences were extracted from the respective Brookhaven Protein Databank; KOL (1FB4), NEWM (3FAB), Bence-Jones protein REI (1REI), MCPC603 (2MCP), J539 (1FBJ), R19.9 (1F19). Underlined sequence fragments signify conserved β strands among the structures. Top numbering corresponds to established light chain scheme with bottom numbering corresponding to heavy chain scheme. Strands are conventionally labelled A–G and CDR regions illustrated. IDRs are labeled with the prefix IDR. Both CDR and IDR beginnings and ends are not to scale with respect to both heavy and light chains. CDRs and IDRs are variable in length between the chains.

chains with light chains. Such analysis contributes to our understanding of the molecular mechanisms involved in the generation of antibody diversity, extending the rules governing sequence-structure correlations of loop structures, and improving the accuracy of predicted Ig structures.

One of the more important features of examining residue substitutions in these structures is their effect on the conformational properties associated with CDR regions and turn packing [72]. Turns in general exhibit structural properties that can be both sequence-dependent and -independent [73]. It has been shown that relatively few residues through their packing, hydrogen bonding, or ability to assume unusual backbone angle conformations, are primarily responsible for the main-chain conformations of hypervariable regions [76]. These residues are found to occur within the hypervariable region and conserved β sheet FR [76]. The identification of conserved residues in multiple sequences of Igs suggest that these residues play an important role in preserving structure. It has been suggested that the repertoire of conformations appear to be limited to a relatively small number of discrete structural classes [76]. Chothia and Lesk [76] have referred to these commonly occurring main-chain conformations of the hypervariable region as "canonical structures."

Structural analysis of Igs indicates that FR residues play an important role in determining the conformational properties of hypervariable regions and are directly related to the class of chain [72]. For example, CDR2 loops in heavy chains are closely associated with the size of the residue at position 71. This association is also dependent upon the size of the CDR2 domain (loop length). Extending this original analysis [72], we find that there are 47 Ig sequences [77] that have CDR2 regions with three-residue lengths. Of these sequences there is either a Gly or Asp residue at position 55. This finding can be correlated with the subsequent identification of having an Arg or Lys residue at position 71 in 43 of these sequences and a Val or Leu residue at this position in the remaining four sequences. Based upon what we know about the role of position 71 in affecting the CDR2 conformation [72] the expected canonical conformation [76] for the majority of these three residue CDR2 regions would be that observed for the antibody NEWM and HY-HEL-10.

Continuing this type of analysis we find that there are 194 Ig sequences with CDR2 regions that are four residues in length. Of these there are 35 sequences with Arg or Lys at position 71, Gly, Asn, or Asp at position 54. The canonical conformation is expected to be like that found in KOL. Ninety-nine sequences have Pro at position 52a [77], Gly and in a few cases Asn or Asp at position 55. These sequences have Val or Leu at position 71. The expected conformation for these sequences is that observed for HY-HEL-5. There are 61 sequences with six residue CDR2 regions. All have Tyr at position 55, Arg at 71 and all but two have Gly, Asn, or Asp at position 54. The expected conformation for these CDRs would be that of MCPC603.

These aspects of CDR conformations and the role of packing residues may be transferable to light chains. One of the more notable effects would be the substitution of the highly conserved Gly residue at position 66 observed in human and murine light chain sequences [77]. Lys and Arg residues can be found in this position [77]. However, Gly substitution is likely to affect the hairpin turn at positions 68-69 and the conformational properties of CDR1 and CDR2 in light chains.

CDR LOOPS AS STRUCTURAL ANALOGUES

Competitive binding assays between analogous peptide ligands can be viewed in the context of identifying similarities in molecular structure between numbers of a congeneric series of drug compounds. Various atom types or functional group sites can be identified at particular relative geometrical positions to establish steric or electronic relationships between the molecular structures.

The molecular mimicry of one peptide by another can hinge on the ability of two analogues to adopt similar conformations, tantamount to illustrations of designing antagonists to peptide hormones [10,24]. It is also possible for two active analogues to have conformations that are relatively dissimilar with their activity the result of a shared configuration of functional reactive moieties. In other words, functional groups on amino acid side chains can be recognized independently of the backbone conformation. This result would be similar to that for active analogues of enkephalin where it was found that for several active conformers the backbone conformations were quite different, yet the spatial orientations of the side chains were similar [78].

Previous studies of the conformational properties of CDR loops indicate that loop conformations can be both sequence-dependent and -independent [73]. Those studies that have emphasized the sequence-independent nature of particular CDR loops have concluded that CDR length and base geometry are primary factors in determining CDR conformation [23,73,79–81]. Analysis of crystal structures of antibodies indicates that regions that are conserved in sequence are conserved in structure. Therefore, an analysis of CDR loops that are of similar length and share amino acid homology reduces to a study of the conformational attributes of structural analogues. However, analysis of CDR loops that are of the same length but lack sequence homology indicates that side-chain orientations are to a large extent preserved.

The superpositioning of CDR loops of equivalent length and varying sequence homology emphasizes the orientational importance of side chains in spite of differences in backbone conformation. This obviously indicates that packing considerations heavily influence the conformation of the backbone, with the conformations limited due to the constraints imposed by the antibody tertiary structure. If there is conservational pressure to preserve packing, and thus side-chain orientations, then the diversity in sequence within a hypervariable segment alone will not generate the topographical diversity required for anti-protein specificity. The increase in specificity will require CDRs of differing length as first suggested by Rees and co-workers [73], as well as some ability for local mobility within CDRs leading to a notion of inducible complementarity in antibody binding.

The importance of these observations has ramifications in understanding the structural and ultimately the evolutionary arrangement of CDRs within antibodies. An early assertion had been that the beta-barrel FR of antibodies constitutes a beta sheet scaffold onto which binding sites may be built, implying that the structure of CDRs is relatively independent of the FR context. However, this simple notion is not generally the case as cited in developing humanized antibodies. This observation reemphasizes that the packing arrangement of the FR with respect to the CDRs is an important determinator in directing the folding behavior of CDR turn regions.

BIOACTIVE PEPTIDE DESIGN AND ACTIVE SITE STRUCTURE

The identification of peptide forms having profound effects on the immune system has naturally led to strategies using peptides to modulate the immune response. Two early examples are peptides derived from Ig and complement. Peptides derived from Igs may provide a novel source of peptide-based drugs for the treatment of immunologically mediated diseases. The tetrapeptide tuftsin derived from the CH_2 domain of IgG (residues Thr-Lys-Pro-Arg) has a host of associated biological activities [82]. Structure/function and conformational studies of the tuftsin molecule predicted that another peptide, Gly-Gln-Pro-Arg, would mimic tuftsin activity. This peptide, called rigin, was synthesized and found to extend phagocytosis-stimulating activity towards heterologous erythrocytes and bacteria [83]. The immunomodulatory activity of these peptides is unrelated to their native parental form. Monomeric IgG does not stimulate phagocytosis, suggesting that peptides such as tuftsin are enzymatically released before expressing activity [84].

The agonist and antagonist activity of such immunoregulatory hormones may result from binding to a plethora of immunoregulatory receptors. The therapeutic activity of such peptides has been demonstrated *in vivo*. One Ig-derived peptide, human IgE pentapeptide (Asp-Ser-Asp-Pro-Arg) has been shown to have some therapeutic activity in humans [85]. The potential agonist/antagonist relation exhibited by these short peptides may be identified by considering the sequence similarities between peptides. The IgG-derived tuftsin resembles the N-terminus of Substance P (SP) (Arg-Pro-Lys-Pro-Gln-Gln-Phe-Phe-Gly-Leu-Met-NH_2) and has shown the ability to bind to SP receptors [84]. When injected intracerebroventricularly, tuftsin induces analgesia (SP antagonism). In turn, SP has similarly been demonstrated to have tuftsin-like phagocytosis-stimulatory activity.

SP is a neuropeptide that is a well-characterized member of the tachykinin family [86]. Sensory neuropeptide release by a sensory neuron may signal tissue damage in the spinal cord and participate in regulating the inflammation, immune response, and, ultimately, wound healing in the affected peripheral tissue [86]. Conformational analysis of tachykinins was first performed on the SP fragment [87]. Constrained agonists and antagonists of tachykinins have demonstrated the potential utility of cyclic peptides in modeling the interactions between a peptide and its binding site [88–90] as with GnRH [10,27]. Antibodies that mimic SP have been described [91]. The identification of sequence relationships between SP and these antibodies, coupled with comparative modeling and the conformational and analogue studies of SP as previously discussed, can lead to further design of SP and other tachykinin analogues [92,93].

Examples of similarity between Ig sequences and bioactive molecules have been demonstrated. Information derived from anti-receptor antibody sequences or related biologically significant proteins can lead to the development of peptides that bind the active sites of receptors, and possess biological activity. Such relationships suggest that Igs may serve as design templates for more classes of compounds for immunoregulation, thereby serving as potential therapeutic drugs. It is possible to produce or design fully synthetic peptides using essential sequence information obtained from anti-Id hybridomas. The conserved nature of antibody structures demonstrated by x-ray crystallography and amino acid sequence analysis is well suited to the process of comparative molecular model building. Since the structures of the light and heavy chains are known, FR region conformations can be used as constraints in performing energy minimization modeling of hypervariable regions. Therefore, comparative modeling of antibodies provide geometrical information that can be translated into designing therapeutic peptides by considering shape, charge distribution, and chemical functionality. Thus, in an antibody-directed approach to peptide and pharmacophore design, the amino acid sequences of the hypervariable region of antibodies that mimic agonist or antagonist properties can be used as starting points to develop peptide and nonpeptide agents.

ANTIBODY DERIVED PEPTIDES AS PROBES FOR RECEPTORS

In prior work, we have successfully developed receptor binding peptides based on analysis of antibody structure and protein loop structures (see Chapter 3). In one set of studies we utilized an experimental system involving a murine antibody mimic of a reovirus protein antigen that binds to specific receptors on murine neurons and lymphocytes [94–96]. Structural relationships were first established between the antibody and the reovirus antigen [94]. Peptides were developed to encompass reverse turn regions comprising the respective hypervariable loops that showed biological activity [95,96]. Implications of these studies include the ability to analyze antibody binding at a molecular level, the observation that antibodies and other ligands may utilize similar binding strategies for a common receptor site, and the ability to develop peptides with defined specificity directly from information on the molecular structure of the antibodies.

More recently, the design of peptide ligands based on antibody structure has progressed. These studies include the ability to apply analysis of the molecular structure of antibodies and structurally related proteins to the development of specific receptor binding peptides, even when these receptors are represented by chemically discrete, small molecules such as sialic acid. Variant peptides lacking specific side-chain hydroxyl groups postulated to be critical for binding to the reovirus receptor were deleted in these peptides, and their ability to interact with the receptor assessed [97]. Varying affinity for the receptor was displayed by these peptides, allowing us to assign a hierarchy for potential intermolecular interactions.

When coupled with prior studies implicating sialic acid as a potential reovirus receptor, it was possible to develop molecular models of the antibody-receptor interaction [97]. The models were useful in the subsequent development of peptides with higher affinity for receptor binding. Cyclic peptide analogs of the peptides were developed based on the molecular models [74]. This allowed determination of the optimal conformation for receptor interaction by the peptides. A cyclic peptide with an optimized conformation was demonstrated to possess $> 40 \times$ higher affinity for the receptor than the linear analog. The conformational properties of the cyclic peptide has been further defined by a constrained synthetic mimetic [7].

We have further utilized the notion of using antibody and protein structures as templates to develop antibodies and peptides with specific binding properties and biological activity in studies of the interaction of HIV-1 with specific cellular structures. The significance of these studies is that biologically active peptides were developed in the absence of direct crystallographic information but made use of structural templates to design the active peptides. These templates were chosen based upon sequence relationships with protein substructure data bases. Much like the reovirus system we have shown that regions of the envelope protein of HIV-1 and HIV-2 exhibit sequence homologies and folding properties with members of the Ig gene family [98]. Engineered peptides derived from these regions of the envelope protein were shown to modulate CD4 dependent cellular functions (block virus infectivity and are immuno-suppressive) and the respective anti-peptide antibodies recognize the native envelope protein [99-102]. Conformational calculations of the bioactive peptides were utilized in these studies to correlate peptide conformational properties with peptide biological activities and immunogenicity [99-102].

ANTIBODY DERIVED PEPTIDES AS PROBES OF FUNCTIONAL GROUPS

Monoclonal antibodies have been useful in the identification of reactive functional groups. In the studies of Taub et al. [103], analysis of antibody hypervariable loop structures of an anti-fibrinogen receptor monoclonal antibody referred to as PAC-1, resulted in identification of a sequence (RYDT) similar to the RGDS binding sequence of many adhesion molecules, and a peptide derived from that hypervariable loop sequence inhibited platelet aggregation in response to fibrinogen [103]. Adhesion receptors, principally integrins, play a prominent role in cellular and developmental biology. As a family, integrins promote cell attachment to fibronectin, vitronectin, laminin, collagen, fibrinogen, and von Willebrand factor [104]. The structural domains of integrins have been correlated with ligand binding by cross-linking to peptides containing the sequence Arg-Gly-Asp (RGD), a ligand recognition motif for several but not all integrins [104]. Presumably, recognition is influenced by the dipolar character of this motif.

Recent studies (unpublished) indicate that platelet activation can be achieved with certain monoclonal antibodies reactive with $\beta 3$ component of integrins. These antibodies termed OPG2 and CP3 activated the solubilized receptor, thus precluding a critical role for the membrane microenvironment, while the antibody PAC-1 does not. We have been modeling the antibodies OPG2, CP3, and PAC-1 to determine why they have different functionality in binding to platelets. All three antibodies contain an RYD tract in the CDR3 region of their heavy chain. In our effort to deduce possible conformations of the H3 domain shared by the respective antibodies, we have utilized a comparative modeling procedure previously used to model regions of antibodies and related molecules [74].

To develop possible models for the localized structural folds of the H3 domain we first examined the sequence and folding pattern of H3 regions of crystallographically known antibodies. These comparisons focused on identifying geometric constraints as defined by the spatial positions of the flanking invariant portions of the H3 region. The H3 domain of several antibodies of known crystal structure were least squares superimposed to define these residue positions (Table 1.1). The invariant positions define the amino-terminal beginning and the carboxy-terminal end that are shared among the putative H3 domains of varying lengths. Least squares fitting (superpositioning) of the Cα coordinates (positions) is used in this manner to determine the degree of similarity between the H3 structures. The systematic superpositioning of the H3 domain over short sequences defines a consensus region where the structure is conserved among the antibody templates. This consensus region defines the FR onto which a model can

TABLE 1.1. Comparison of Ig Templates Used to Define Starting Geometries.

X-Ray	N-Terminal	Putative Turn	C-Terminal
1F19	CARSF	YGGSDLAV	YYF–DSWG
2FB4	CARDG	GHGFCSSASCF	GPD–YWG
2MCP	CARNY	YGSTW	YFD–VWG
1FBJ	CARLH	YYGY	N–A–YWG
2FAB	CARNL	IAGC	I–D–VWG
Antibody			
OPG2	CTRHP	FYRYDGGN	YYAMDHWG
CP3	CARGR	NRNRYDGD	YYAMDYWG
PAC-1	CARRS	PSYYRYDGAGP	YYAMDYWG

VH sequences for the crystallographically known Igs were extracted from their respective Brookhaven Protein Databank entries; R19.9 (1F19), MCPC603 (2MCP), J539 (1FBJ), NEWM (3FAB), KOL (2FB4). Dashes in the sequence represent insertions identified by least squares fitting the N- and C-terminal structurally conserved regions. The fitting procedure allows for choosing an appropriate putative turn length for the target antibodies.

be built for the various loops. The procedure then is to search the crystallographic data base for loops of the same size as the putative loop to be modeled.

In this way we have defined the alignments in Table 1.1 to provide information on loop length of crystallographically known Igs compared with those of the antibodies under study. In this context the loop length of PAC-1 is that of the antibody FB4, while OPG2 and CP3 have loop lengths reflective of the F19 structure. The F19 template structure indicates that the alignment for CP3 and OPG2 are not in register, a result that has been previously discussed in comparative modeling procedures. In the search procedure, the spatially conserved Cα positions at the N- and C-terminal regions were held fixed. A Cα distance matrix was constructed for combinations of these positions and compared to precalculated Cα distance matrices made from high resolution protein structures. The 20 best matches were examined and an appropriate choice was made based upon similarities in chiralities of side-chains and at the junctures of the loops, and displayed sequence similarities between alternative loops and the H3 loop of the respective antibodies.

The strategy that we have employed was to test whether conformations for the H3 domain of OPG2 and CP3 could be shared between these antibodies. Our structural analysis indicates that the orientation of the RYD tract in PAC-1 is different from that of OPG2 and CP3 suggesting that the conformational properties of OPG2 and CP3 for the CDR3 region is more similar between these antibodies than that for PAC-1. This would suggest that the similar biological activity shared between OPG2 and CP3 might be directly related to the conformational properties of the CDR3 region of these two antibodies. It is also possible that the differences in activity between the antibodies is a function of the depth of the RGD binding pocket on GPIIb-IIIa accessible to the antigen binding surface of the antibodies. Recent studies of immobilized RGD peptides of varying lengths indicate that platelet interactions are sensitive to the length of the RGD presenting peptides.

Previous studies on the mimicking of haptens by antibodies suggested that RGD analogs such as KGD and KGGD might mimic the dipolar character of phosphorylcholine (PC) [105,106]. In fact recent analysis of the viper venom Barbourin shows that this integrin specific antagonist contains a KGD tract substituted for the RGD tract found in previous viper venoms [107]. The hapten, PC, is bound with high affinity and specificity by members of the Ig S107 germ line family. The crystal structure of one member of this family, MCPC603, has been well studied with its three-dimensional complex with PC known. Anti-Id antibodies have been developed that mimic the immunogenicity of PC containing formulations [106], that compete with PC for binding to the TEPC-15 myeloma protein. These anti-Id monoclonal antibodies were originally characterized as near-site specific (F6-3) and PC-binding site specific (4C11).

Sequence analysis of F6-3 and 4C11 [106] revealed several amino acid residues which might mimic the three-dimensional structure of PC in binding to S107 family members. The principal dipolar tract involved the sequence EKFKD [106]. Utilizing the information on the three-dimensional structure of the MCPC603-PC complex, *de novo* designed model synthetic peptides were developed of the form KGD and KGGD using molecular graphics and conformational energy analysis [105]. The tetramer KGGD was shown to inhibit 4C11 binding to TEPC-15 over the range of inhibitor used [105]. The tetramer was not however as effective as the hapten based upon the inhibitor molarity. Nevertheless, these studies were the first to indicate the feasibility of developing peptides from antibodies which mimic the structural and binding features of small chemical groups.

These studies were extended to identify peptides derived from anti-PC antibodies that would compete with PC for PC specific binding sites [108]. In these studies a 26 residue peptide derived from TEPC-15 was shown to be an effective inhibitor of PC. This peptide spanned the CDR2 region of TEPC-15 and part of the FR 3 region. This region shares discontinuous homology with human C-reactive protein (CRP) (Table 1.2). The PC-binding region of CRP appears to share an epitope with the mouse T-15 Id as shown by recognition of both the TEPC-15 myeloma protein and CRP by monoclonal antibody to the T-15 Id [109,110]. The TEPC-15 anti-Ids F6-3 and 4C11 have been shown to bind to CRP. The CRP1 derived peptide and the TEPC-15 derived peptide in Table 1.2 both inhibit anti-Id binding

TABLE 1.2. **Binding Domain Sequence Similarities.**

TEPC15	50	ASRNKANDYTTEYSASVKGRFIVSR	
CRP1	56	ATKRQDNEIL	
CRP2	83		SASGIVEFWV
β5	303	NEAN----EYTAS	
β3	302	GSDN----HYSAS	
β1	538	CRKRDNTNEIY	
β5	238	RVSRNDRDA	
β3	237	SVSRNRDA	

Regions of local residue similarity (bold face) between the T-15 Id self-binding region, CRP, and beta subunits. Residue numbering is at the left.

to TEPC-15 [109]. The CRP1 peptide is suggested to bind PC directly [109] and has been shown to bind both fibronectin and laminin presumably through phosphorylated amino acids. F6-3 binds to unconjugated CRP peptide directly while 4C11 apparently binds to conjugated (KLH) CRP peptide [109]. In this context the anti-Ids F6-3 and 4C11 act as surrogates for both fibronectin and laminin. Sequence homology is observed between these antibodies and integrin regions which needs to be examined further in a structural context.

We have shown that the TEPC-15 derived sequence is responsible for TEPC-15 self-binding and participates in defining the T-15 Id [108]. However our work also suggests that the binding properties of the TEPC-15 derived peptide defines a complementary hydropathy relationship required for protein recognition. The CRP1 peptide tract may contain an RGD analog defined as RQD. We have redesigned the T-15 derived 26 mer peptide to perturb the conformational properties of the CDR2 turn region by eliminating the KAN residues (Table 1.2, TEPC-15). This peptide is more effective than the 26 mer in inhibiting T15-PC binding (unpublished). In this redesigned peptide, the primary N-terminal sequence tract is AASRNDYTT. The RNDY tract might in turn be an analog of the RGDY peptide shown to be even more effective than RGD in inhibiting platelet aggregation. While our peptide was designed as a mimic for PC in binding to a PC specific binding site, it might be more representative of an alternative adhesion motif.

In Table 1.2 integrin sequences from β1, β3, and β5 subdomains are listed that exhibit sequence and hydropathic relationships similar to the TEPC-15 and CRP sequence. These sites have not been described in the literature as possible sites for association either to ligands or between respective integrin α and β chains. Initial studies of the conformational properties of the integrin sequences in Table 1.2 suggest that the β3 structures are more flexible. From a functional point of view, β3 structures are more promiscuous in their association with integrin subdomains.

The molecular basis for the self-binding characteristics of the T-15 Id has been shown to be associated with the charge spacing of a putative turn region involving the CDR2 region of T-15 (Table 1.2). Reverse turn regions of antibodies are typically associated with the immunoreactivity of monoclonal antibodies. This self-binding region has been implicated as a site of cross-reactivity between CRP and T-15 antibodies [110]. Subsets of charge spacings are also observed in suggested DNA binding antibodies [111]. This spacing is also observed in the β chain of T cell receptors (TCRs) associated with IL-2 receptor positive synovial T cells in rheumatoid arthritis patients [111]. This site has been implicated in binding to superantigen, suggesting a role for superantigen mediation in rheumatoid arthritis. In addition the relationships also suggest that the charge spacing may be inherent in the TCR lineage just as they are in antibody structures.

Adhesion motifs may be targets for complementary interactions involving autoantibodies and receptors. Adhesion motifs like that found in laminin may also be mimicked by antibodies. It is possible that the adhesion motif RGD found on a variety of integrins may be mimicked by autoantibodies. The analysis of such antibodies can provide information at several levels including information on how to target such autoantibodies to suppress their occurrence as well as learning the geometrical features required for binding such receptors. The geometrical information can be used to develop agents that block the fibrinogen receptor for example which could be useful in treating hypercoagulatable states and preventing myocardial infarctions. The study of antibody complexes with endothelium components may also lead to understanding how to develop small molecules that might interfere with immune complexes associated with some autoimmune diseases.

CONFORMATIONALLY CONSTRAINED PEPTIDES AND MIMETICS

Searching the protein sequence data base indicates a sampling of sequence homologies of varying degrees between viral, native host proteins and reverse turn regions of antibodies [111]. This type of analysis points out that viral sequences as well as native host proteins are readily encoded in the Ig repertoire. The homologies imply that local regions of sequence homology can be found principally due to the fact that there is a limited number of amino acid residues that form such turns. Turns as a recognition unit, are conserved evolutionarily among proteins of different types. The specificity of the recognition features are modulated by selecting amino acids that can change the conformational features of these turns, as well as selecting the appropriate contact residues.

In general terms, the topography of a binding site of a ligand can be viewed on the imprint of the general three-dimensional structure of the substrate. Elucidation of the conformation of a peptide should provide insights about the structural requirements of the binding receptor. A major problem, however, in structure-activity studies of linear peptides is the large degree of flexibility, not only of the side-chain residue, but also of the peptide backbone. Consequently, spectroscopic studies in solution, where a rapid equilibrium between numerous conformations is likely to occur, have had little impact on the design of linear peptide analogues.

For more rigid peptides like oxytocin [112] and somatostatin [113], the significance of taking the conformation into account has been demonstrated. The design of constrained cyclic analogues of a substrate that simulates predicted predominant conformers locking in turn or helical conformations for example is a decisive contribution for overcoming this problem [10,13,27,74,114]. By modifying various amide bonds in a peptide sequence [115] one would hope to maintain the geometry of the peptide backbone while investigating whether the nature of these bonds is essential for biological activity; either for binding to the receptor or perhaps more likely, for stabilizing a certain conformation by intramolecular hydrogen bonding. When active, such rigidified analogues provide a more accurate approach of the bioactive conformation and are valuable pharmacological probes, because generally they are more resistant to proteolytic degradation [13,116]. Methods for conformational constraints include head to tail, side chain to side chain, and side chain to backbone cyclization. Early work of this type is perhaps typified by the synthesis of cyclic enkephalin analogues [114].

Cyclic analogues are typically viewed as an attempt to mimic and lock the putative bioactive structure of a peptide. Peptide modifications can also avoid some of the problems encountered with peptide leads [117]. A host of chemistries have been suggested for this concept [118–121]. The notion of locking in the binding mode conformation to increase receptor binding can reduce the entropic contribution to binding. Cyclization reduces the conformational range available to a linear peptide. This possibility was observed in our own calculations of cyclic peptides derived from antibody structures ([74] and unpublished).

The ability to constrain peptides and cross-correlate the geometric properties of reactive functional groups with synthetic probes also allows for searching of organic data bases for possible alternative compounds. High speed search algorithms have been developed to identify pharmacophores [122,123] and approaches to identify recognition sites on proteins that can be used in the search criteria have been suggested [124–126]. In the development of substitutes for the peptide backbone as a pharmacophore for peptide receptors the benzodiazepine nucleus has emerged as a likely candidate. Many benzodiazepines have been previously found to interact with peptide receptors in binding assays: tifludom at the kappa opiate receptor

[127], midazolam at the TRH receptor [128] and alprazolam at the platelet activating factor (PAF) receptor [129]. These findings have led to the description of benzodiazepines as privileged structures for peptide receptors and suggested that more classical heterocyclic compounds could serve as templates for peptide receptor ligands [130]. It is instructive to reflect on one system in which an antibody was reduced to a peptide form and then to a mimetic [7]. The mimetic ultimately took 70 to 700 × molar excess to block antibody binding, indicating that the mimetic did not faithfully recapitulate all of the binding features of the antibody. Small organics do well when binding to cavities of receptors, but may not lend enough binding energy to other receptor binding site types.

FUTURE DIRECTIONS

Molecular modeling as an aid to drug design and discovery has been touted for some time [22,131]. A current problem in biotechnology is that biomolecular engineering is evolving far too slowly as a practical technological tool. This domain of expertise continues to reside with specialists and is commonly viewed by nonspecialists as being veiled in a mystique of exotic procedural knowledge. The true value of protein engineering and pharmacophore design cannot be fully realized until that technology is implemented for ready use by a wide spectrum of end users. Computer-assisted structural homology (CASH) is a concept that can help to make this implementation a reality. One approach we have been perusing is based on established artificial intelligence (AI) technology that provides for the integration of human expertise and interactive computer resources. The implementation of the CASH system is centered about four major components: a set of structural homology software tools, a consolidated data base of protein and nucleic acid information, a deductive/inductive inferencing engine, and a knowledge base of structural homology expertise.

The set of structural homology software tools in a CASH system performs traditional sequence-based analyses (e.g., hydropathic and structural profiling, codon usage frequency, motif searching, etc.). The resultant data generated by these tools is pooled for further use by the CASH system. In addition, this intermediate data is made available to the user in the form of a standardized report. The consolidated data base of structural information in a CASH system is derived from (but not limited to) existing data bases which provide data on nucleotide sequences, protein residue sequences, protein and motif structures, and nonprotein organic structures. This data base is automatically accessed by the system's software tools and may also be interactively interrogated by the user.

The deductive/inductive inferencing engine is the center of all AI operations and, along with the other components of a CASH system, forms a rule-based expert system. Drawing upon procedural rules contained in the knowledge base, this expert system can apply both deductive and inductive logic to any and all available data. Guided by the requests of the user, the system operates in an interactive goal-seeking manner, ultimately providing the user with high-order structural and physiochemical information extracted from user-specified primary residue and/or nucleotide sequences. Throughout this process, the user may interact with the system at practically any level, from step-to-step supervision to virtual hands-off operation requiring only minimal knowledge of structural homology. Resultant data generated by the expert system ranges in complexity from simple "yes or no" answers to complete tertiary structures. Where applicable, resultant data is provided in common formats for ready use by adjunct biomolecular engineering and graphics systems.

The final component of a CASH system, the knowledge base, acts as the system's repository of human expertise. The knowledge and art of structural homology (e.g., analytical relationships, working theoretical models, empirical rules-of-thumb, etc.) is translated into English-like conditional rules and stored in the knowledge base. It is these rules, and therein the inherent knowledge, that the inferencing engine applies in its deductive and inductive goal-seeking operation.

In order to accommodate the maturation of structural homology expertise, and in keeping with the philosophy of user interaction at every level of the system, the knowledge base is designed with the flexibility to be modified. Modification can be in the form of the alteration of existing rules, the deletion (or temporary suspension) of existing rules, or the addition of new rules. An important benefit of this approach is that it allows a CASH system to be used as an interactive structural homology workbench, allowing the user to readily evaluate and refine new rules and models.

In summary, a CASH system provides a practical path of migration, from art to technology, for current and future structural homology applications. The incorporation of human expertise permits the nonspecialist to utilize structural homology in an immediately productive fashion. The maintenance of a multilevel approach to user interaction provides the more sophisticated user with a convenient environment for furthering the state of structural homology art. Finally, when used in conjunction with molecular graphics systems, CASH becomes a valuable tool, for research and industry, in the application of biomolecular engineering in such domains as rational drug design, protein engineering, protein and nucleic acid structure folding problems, gene analysis, and molecular genetics.

REFERENCES

1 Robinson, B. E. and P. J. Quesenberry. 1990. "Hematopoietic Growth Factors: Overview and Clinical Applications, Part II," *Am. J. Med. Sci.*, 300:297.

2 Winter, G. and C. Milstein. 1991. "Man-Made Antibodies," *Nature*, 349:293.

3 Larson, S. M. 1990. "Improved Tumor Targeting with Radiolabeled, Recombinant, Single-Chain, Antigen-Binding Protein," *J. Natl. Cancer Inst.*, 82:1173.

4 Morgan, E. L. and W. O. Weigle. 1987. "Biological Activities in the Fc Region of Immunoglobulin," *Adv. Immunol.*, 40:61.

5 Williams, V. W., D. B. Weiner, J. C. Cohen and M. I. Greene. 1989. "Development and Use of Receptor Binding Peptides Derived from Anti-Receptor Antibodies," *Biotechnology*, 7:471.

6 Schick, M. R. and R. C. Kennedy. 1989. "Production and Characterization of Anti-Idiotypic Antibody Reagents," in *Methods in Enzymology, Antibodies, Antigens and Molecular Mimicry*, J. J. Langone, ed., 178:36.

7 Saragovi, H. U., D. Fitzpatrick, A. Raktabutr, H. Nakanishi, M. Kahn and M. I. Greene. 1991. "Design and Synthesis of a Mimetic from an Antibody Complementarity-Determining Region," *Science*, 253:792.

8 Gilon, C., D. Halle, M. Chorev, Z. Selinger and G. Byk. 1991. "Backbone Cyclization: A New Method for Conferring Conformational Constraint on Peptides," *Biopolymers*, 31:745.

9 Convert, O., H. Duplaa, S. Lavielle and G. Chassaing. 1991. "Influence of the Replacement of Amino Acid by Its D-Enantiomer in the Sequence of Substance P. 2. Conformational Analysis by NMR and Energy Calculations," *Neuropeptides*, 19:259.

10 Struthers, R. S., G. Tanaka, S. C. Koerber, T. Solmajer, E. L. Baniak, L. M. Gierasch, W. Vale, J. Rivier and A. T. Hagler. 1990. "Design of Biologically Active, Conformationally Constrained GnRH Antagonists," *Proteins*, 8:295.

11 DiMaio, J., B. Gibbs, D. Munn, J. Lefebvre, F. Ni and Y. Konishi. 1990. "Bifunctional Thrombin Inhibitors Based on the Sequence of Hirudin 45-65," *J. Biol. Chem.*, 265:21698.

12 DiMaio, J., J. Jaramillo, D. Wernic, L. Grenier, E. Welchner and J. Adams. 1990. "Synthesis and Biological Activity of Atrial Natriuretic Factor Analogues: Effect of Modifications to the Disulfide Bridge," *J. Med. Chem.*, 33:661.

13 Edwards, J. V., A. F. Spatola, C. Lemieux and P. W. Schiller. 1986. "*In vitro* Activity Profiles of Cyclic and Linear Enkephalin Pseudopeptide Analogs," *Biochem. Biophys. Res. Commun.*, 136:730.

14 Hagler, A. T., E. Huler and S. Lifson. 1974. "Energy Functions for Peptides and Proteins. I. Derivation of a Consistent Force Field Including the Hydrogen Bond from Amide Crystals," *J. Am. Chem. Soc.*, 96:5319.

15 Hagler, A. T. and A. Lapiccirella. 1975. "Conformational Calculations of Peptide Conformation: Synthesis of Quantum Mechanical and Empirical Approaches for Deriving Energy Functions," in *Peptides: Chemistry, Structure and Biology*, R. Walter and J. Meienhofer, eds., Ann Arbor: Ann Arbor Science Publishers, p. 279.

16 Meirovitch, H. and H. Scheraga. 1981. "An Approach to the Multiple-Minimum

Problem in Protein Folding, Involving a Long-Range Geometrical Restriction and Short-, Medium-, and Long-Range Interactions," *Macromolecules*, 14:1250.

17   Momany, F. A., R. F. McGuire, A. W. Burgess and H. Scheraga. 1975. "Energy Parameters in Polypeptides. VIII. Geometric Parameters, Partial Charges, Non-bonded Interactions, Hydrogen Bond Interactions, and Intrinsic Torsional Potentials for the Naturally Occurring Amino Acids," *J. Phys. Chem.*, 79:2361.

18   Weiner, S. J., P. A. Kollman and D. T. Nguyen. 1986. "An All Atom Forcefield for Simulations of Proteins and Nucleic Acids," *J. Comp. Chem.*, 7:230.

19   Brooks, B. R., R. E. Bruccoleri, B. D. Olafson, D. J. States, S. Swaminathan and M. Karplus. 1983. "CHARMM: A Program for Macromolecular Energy Minimization and Dynamics Calculations," *J. Comp. Chem.*, 4:187.

20   Hagler, A. T., S. Lifson and P. Dauber. 1979. "Consistent Force Field Studies of Intermolecular Forces in Hydrogen Bonded Crystals. II. A Benchmark for the Objective Comparisons of Alternative Force Fields," *J. Am. Chem. Soc.*, 101:5122.

21   Allinger, N. L., Y. H. Yuh and J.-H. Lii. 1989. "Molecular Mechanics. The MM3 Forcefield for Hydrocarbons," *J. Am. Chem. Soc.*, 111:8551.

22   Cohen, N. C., J. M. Blaney, C. Humblet, P. Gund and D. C. Barry. 1990. "Molecular Modeling Software and Methods for Medicinal Chemistry," *J. Am. Chem. Soc.*, 33:883.

23   Shenkin, P. S., D. L. Yarmush, R. M. Fine, H. Wang and C. Levinthal. 1987. "Predicting Antibody Hypervariable Loop Conformation. I. Ensembles of Random Conformations for Ringlike Structures," *Biopolymers*, 26:2053.

24   Struthers, R. S., J. Rivier and A. T. Hagler. 1984. "Design of Peptide Analogs: Theoretical Simulation of Conformation, Energetics and Dynamics," in *Conformationally Directed Drug Design: Peptides and Nucleic Acids as Templates or Targets*, J. A. Vida and M. Gordon, eds., Washington, DC: American Chemical Society, p. 239.

25   Wuthrich, K., C. Spitzfaden, K. Memmert, H. Widmer and G. Wider. 1991. "Protein Secondary Structure Determination by NMR Application with Recombinant Human Cyclophilin," *FEBS*, 285:237.

26   Karplus, M. and G. A. Petsko. 1990. "Molecular Dynamics Simulations in Biology," *Nature*, 347:631.

27   Baniak, E. I., J. E. Rivier, S. Struthers, A. T. Hagler and L. M. Gierasch. 1987. "Nuclear Magnetic Resonance Analysis and Conformational Characterization of a Cyclic Decapeptide Antagonist of GnRH," *Biochemistry*, 26:2642.

28   Hagler, A. T. 1985. "Theoretical Simulation of Conformation, Energetics and Dynamics of Peptides," in *Conformation in Biology and Drug Design, the Peptides*, J. Meienhofer, ed., New York: Academic Press, 7:213.

29   Levitt, M. and R. Sharon. 1988. "Accurate Simulation of Protein Dynamics in Solution," *Proc. Natl. Acad. Sci. USA*, 85:7557.

30   Daggett, V., P. A. Kollman and I. D. Kuntz. 1991. "Molecular Dynamics Simulations of Small Peptides: Dependence on Dielectric Model and pH," *Biopolymers*, 31:285.

31   Anfinsen, C. B., E. Haber, M. Sela and F. H. White. 1961. "The Kinetics of Formation of Native Ribonuclease During Oxidation of the Reduced Polypeptide Chain," *Proc. Natl. Acad. Sci. USA*, 47:1309.

32   Thornton, J. M. and S. P. Gardner. 1989. "Protein Motifs and Data-Base Searching," *TIBS*, 14:300.

33 Blundell, T. L., B. L. Sibanda, M. J. E. Sternberg and J. M. Thornton. 1987. "Knowledge-Based Prediction of Protein Structures and the Design of Novel Molecules," *Nature*, 326:347.

34 Crippen, G. M. 1979. "Distance Constraints on Macromolecular Conformation," *Int. J. Pept. Protein Res.*, 13:320.

35 Crippen, G. M. 1991. "Prediction of Protein Folding from Amino Acid Sequence Over Discrete Conformation Spaces," *Biochemistry*, 30:4232.

36 Kuntz, I. D., G. M. Crippen, P. A. Kollman and D. Kimelman. 1976. "Calculation of Protein Tertiary Structure," *J. Mol. Biol.*, 106:983.

37 Ycas, M., N. S. Goel and J. W. J. Jacobsen. 1978. "On the Computation of the Tertiary Structure of Globular Proteins," *J. Theor. Biol.*, 72:443.

38 Goel, N. S. and M. Ycas. 1979. "On the Computation of the Tertiary Structure of Globular Proteins II," *J. Theor. Biol.*, 77:253.

39 Havel, T. F. and M. E. Snow. 1991. "A New Method for Building Protein Conformations from Sequence Alignments with Homologues of Known Structure," *J. Mol. Biol.*, 217:1.

40 Blundell, T. L., D. Carney, S. Gardner, F. Hayes, B. Howlin, T. Hubbard, J. Overington, D. A. Singh, B. L. Sibana and M. Sutcliffe. 1988. "Knowledge-Based Protein Modelling and Design," *Eur. J. Biochem.*, 172:513.

41 Greer, J. 1981. "Comparative Model Building of the Mammalian Serine Proteases," *J. Mol. Biol.*, 153:1027.

42 Schiffer, C. A., J. W. Caldwell, P. A. Kollman and R. M. Stroud. 1990. "Prediction of Homologous Protein Structures Based on Conformational Searches and Energetics," *Proteins*, 8:30.

43 Vingron, M. and P. Argos. 1991. "Motif Recognition and Alignment for Many Sequences by Comparison of Dot-Matrices," *J. Mol. Biol.*, 218:33.

44 Needleman, S. B. and C. B. Wunsch. 1970. "A General Method Applicable to Search for Similarities in the Amino Acid Sequence of Two Proteins," *J. Mol. Biol.*, 48:443.

45 Smith, T. F. and M. S. Waterman. 1981. "Comparison of Biosequences," *Adv. Appl. Math.*, 2:482.

46 Lesk, A. M., M. Levitt and C. Chothia. 1986. "Alignment of the Amino Acid Sequences of Distantly Related Proteins Using Variable Gap Penalties," *Protein Engineering*, 1:77.

47 Sibbald, P. R. and P. Argos. 1990. "Weighting Aligned Protein or Nucleic Acid Sequences to Correct for Unequal Representation," *J. Mol. Biol.*, 216:813.

48 Subbiah, S. and S. C. Harrison. 1989. "A Method for Multiple Sequence Alignment with Gaps," *J. Mol. Biol.*, 209:539.

49 Doolittle, R. F. and D. F. Feng. 1990. "Nearest Neighbor Procedure for Relating Progressively Aligned Amino Acid Sequences," *Methods Enzymol.*, R. F. Doolittle, ed., 183:659.

50 Qian, N. and T. J. Sejnowski. 1988. "Predicting the Secondary Structure of Globular Proteins Using Neural Network Models," *J. Mol. Biol.*, 202:865.

51 Vriend, G. and C. Sander. 1991. "Detection of Common Three-Dimensional Substructures in Proteins," *Proteins: Structure, Function, and Genetics*, 11:52.

52 Bowie, J. U., R. Luthy and D. Eisenberg. 1991. "A Method to Identify Protein Sequences that Fold into a Known Three-Dimensional Structure," *Science*, 253:164.

53 Gribskov, M., A. D. McLachlan and D. Eisenberg. 1987. "Profile Analysis: Detection of Distantly Related Proteins," *Proc. Natl. Acad. Sci. USA*, 84:4355.

54 Rooman, M. J., J. Rodriquez and S. J. Wodak. 1990. "Automatic Definition of Recurrent Local Structure Motifs in Proteins," *J. Mol. Biol.*, 213:327.

55 Richards, F. M. and C. E. Kundrot. 1988. "Identification of Structural Motifs from Protein Coordinate Data: Secondary Structure and First-Level Supersecondary Structure," *Proteins: Structure, Function, and Genetics*, 3:71.

56 Lee, C. and S. Subbiah. 1991. "Prediction of Protein Side-Chain Conformation by Packing Optimization," *J. Mol. Biol.*, 217:373.

57 Bruccoleri, R. E. and M. Karplus. 1987. "Conformational Sampling," *Biopolymers*, 26:137.

58 Moult, J. and M. N. G. James. 1986. "An Algorithm for Determining the Conformations of Polypeptide Segments in Proteins by Systematic Search," *Proteins*, 1:146.

59 Holm, L. and C. Sander. 1991. "Database Algorithm for Generating Protein Backbone and Side Chain Co-Ordinates from the Cα Trace Application to Model Building and Detection of Co-Ordinate Errors," *J. Mol. Biol.*, 218:183.

60 Summers, N. L. and M. Karplus. 1990. "Modeling of Globular Proteins a Distance-Based Data Search Procedure for the Construction of Insertion/Deletion Regions and Pro-Non-Pro Mutations," *J. Mol. Biol.*, 216:991.

61 Hendlich, M., P. Lackner, S. Weitckus, H. Floeckner, R. Froschauer, K. Gottsbacher, G. Casari and M. J. Sippl. 1990. "Identification of Native Protein Folds amongst a Large Number of Incorrect Models the Calculation of Low Energy Conformations from Potentials of Mean Force," *J. Mol. Biol.*, 216:167.

62 Morrison, S. L., M. J. Johnson, L. A. Herzenberg and V. T. Oi. 1984. "Chimeric Human Antibody Molecules: Mouse Antigen-Binding Domains with Human Constant Region Domains," *Proc. Natl. Acad. Sci. USA*, 81:6851.

63 Jaffers, G. J., T. C. Fuller, A. B. Cosimi, P. S. Russell, H. J. Winn and R. B. Colvin. 1986. "Monoclonal Antibody Therapy. Anti-Idiotypic and Non-Anti-Idiotypic Antibodies to OKT3 Arising Despite Intense Immunosuppression," *Transplantation*, 41:572.

64 Jones, P. T., P. H. Dear, J. Foote, M. S. Neuberger and G. Winter. 1986. "Replacing the Complementary-Determining Regions in a Human Antibody with Those from a Mouse," *Nature*, 321:522.

65 Reichman, L., M. Clark, H. Waldmann and G. Winter. 1988. "Reshaping Human Antibodies for Therapy," *Nature*, 332:323.

66 Queen, C., W. P. Schneider, H. E. Selick, P. W. Payne, N. F. Landolfi, J. F. Duncan, N. M. Avdalovic, M. Levitt, R. P. Junghans and T. A. Waldman. 1989. "A Humanized Antibody that Binds to Il-2 Receptor," *Proc. Natl. Acad. Sci. USA*, 86:10029.

67 Maeda, H., S. Matsushita, Y. Eda, K. Kimachi, S. Tokiyoshi and M. M. Bending. 1991. "Construction of Reshaped Human Antibodies with HIV-Neutralizing Activity," *Human Antibodies Hybridomas*, 2:124.

68 Gorman, S. D., M. R. Clark, E. G. Routledge, S. P. Cobbold and H. Waldmann. 1991. "Reshaping a Therapeutic CD4 Antibody," *Proc. Natl. Acad. Sci. USA*, 88:4181.

69 Novotny, J., R. Bruccoleri, J. Newell, D. Murphy, E. Haber and M. Karplus.

1983. "Molecular Anatomy of the Antibody Binding Site," *J. Biol. Chem.*, 258:4433.

70 Kieber-Emmons, T. and H. Kohler. 1986. "Towards a Unified Theory of Immunoglobulin Structure-Function Relations," *Immunol. Rev.*, 90:29.

71 Davies, D. R., E. A. Padlan and S. Sheriff. 1990. "Antibody-Antigen Complexes," *Annu. Rev. Biochem.*, 59:439.

72 Tramontano, A., C. Chothia and A. M. Lesk. 1990. "Framework Residue 71 Is a Major Determinant of the Position and Conformation of the Second Hypervariable Region in the VH Domains of Immunoglobulins," *J. Mol. Biol.*, 215:175.

73 de la Paz, P., B. J. Sutton, M. J. Darsley and A. R. Rees. 1986. "Modelling of the Combining Sites of Three Anti-Lysozyme Monoclonal Antibodies and of the Complex between One of the Antibodies and Its Epitope," *EMBO J.*, 5:415.

74 Williams, V. W., T. Kieber-Emmons, J. Von Feldt, M. I. Greene and D. B. Weiner. 1991. "Design of Bioactive Peptides Based on Antibody Hypervariable Region Structures," *J. Biol. Chem.*, 266:5182.

75 Schiffer, M., R. L. Girling, K. R. Ely and A. B. Edmundson. 1973. "Structure of a Lambda-Type Bence-Jones Protein at 3.5-A Resolution," *Biochemistry*, 112:4620.

76 Chothia, C. and A. M. Lesk. 1987. "Canonical Structures for the Hypervariable Regions of Immunoglobulins," *J. Mol. Biol.*, 196:901.

77 Kabat, E. A., T. T. Wu, M. Reid-Miller, H. M. Perry and K. S. Gottesman. 1987. *Sequences of Proteins of Immunological Interest, 4th Ed.* Bethesda: National Institutes of Health.

78 Chew, C., H. O. Villar and G. H. Loew. 1991. "Theoretical Study of the Flexibility and Solution Conformation of the Cyclic Opioid Peptides [D-Pen2,D-Pen5]enkephalin and [D-Pen2,L-Pen5]enkephalin," *Mol. Pharmacol.*, 39:502.

79 Fine, R. M., H. Wang, P. S. Shenkin, D. L. Yarmush and C. Levinthal. 1986. "Predicting Antibody Hypervariable Loop Conformations. II: Minimization and Molecular Dynamics Studies of MCPC603 from Many Randomly Generated Loop Conformations," *Proteins*, 1:342.

80 Martin, A. C. R., J. C. Cheetham and A. R. Rees. 1989. "Modeling Antibody Hypervariable Loops: A Combined Algorithm," *Proc. Natl. Acad. Sci. USA*, 86:9268.

81 Bruccoleri, R. E., E. Haber and J. Novotny. 1988. "Structure of Antibody Hypervariable Loops Reproduced by a Conformational Search Algorithm," *Nature*, 335:564.

82 Najjar, V. A. and K. Nishioka. 1970. "Tuftsin: A Natural Phagocytosis Stimulating Peptide," *Nature*, 228:672.

83 Veretennikova, N. I., G. I. Chipens, G. V. Nikiforovich and Y. R. Betinsh. 1981. "Rigin, Another Phagocytosis-Stimulating Tetrapeptide Isolated from Human IgG. Confirmations of a Hypothesis," *Int. J. Pept. Protein Res.*, 17:430.

84 Spirer, Z., V. Zakuth, A. Golander, N. Bogair and M. Fridkin. 1975. "The Effect of Tuftsin on the Nitrous Blue Tetrazolium Reduction of Normal Human Polymorphonuclear Leukocytes," *J. Clin. Invest.*, 55:198.

85 Hahn, G. S. 1986. "Immunoglobulin-Derived Drugs," *Nature*, 324:283.

86 Jansen, I., C. Alafaci, J. McCulloch, R. Uddman and L. Edvinsson. 1991. "Tachykinins (Substance P, Neurokinin A, Neuropeptide K, and Neurokinin B) in

the Cerebral Circulation: Vasomotor Responses *in vitro* and *in Situ*," *J. Cereb. Blood Flow Metab.*, 11:567.

87 Manavalan, P. and F. A. Momany. 1982. "Conformational Energy Calculations on Substance P," *Int. J. Pept. Protein Res.*, 20:351.

88 Shenderovich, M. D., G. V. Nikiforovich, J. B. Saulitis and G. I. Chipens. 1988. "Determination of Cyclopeptide Conformations in Solution Using NMR Data and Conformational Energy Calculations," *Biophys. Chem.*, 31:163.

89 Sumner, S. C., K. S. Gallagher, D. G. Davis, D. G. Covell, R. L. Jernigan and J. A. Ferretti. 1990. "Conformational Analysis of the Tachykinins in Solution: Substance P and Physalaemin," *J. Biomol. Struct. Dyn.*, 8:687.

90 Kawaki, H., A. Otter, H. Beierbeck, G. Kotovych and J. M. Stewart. 1986. "The Conformational Analysis of Substance P Analogs Using High-Field NMR Techniques," *J. Biomol. Struct. Dyn.*, 3:795.

91 Pascual, D. W., J. E. Blalock and K. L. Bost. 1989. "Antipeptide Antibodies that Recognize a Lymphocyte Substance P Receptor," *J. Immunol.*, 143:3697.

92 Petitet, F., J. C. Beaujouan, M. Saffroy, Y. Torrens, G. Chassaing, S. Lavielle, J. Besseyre, C. Garrett, A. Carruette and J. Glowinski. 1991. "Further Demonstration that [Pro9]-Substance P Is a Potent and Selective Ligand of NK-1 Tachykinin Receptors," *J. Neurochem.*, 56:879.

93 Sakurada, T., T. Yamada, K. Tan-no, Y. Manome, S. Sakurada, K. Kisara and M. Ohba. 1991. "Differential Effects of Substance P Analogs on Neurokinin 1 Receptor Agonists in the Mouse Spinal Cord," *J. Pharmacol. Exp. Ther.*, 259:205.

94 Kieber-Emmons, T., E. Getzof and H. Kohler. 1987. "Perspectives on Idiotypes and Antigenicity," *Int. Rev. Immunol.*, 2:339.

95 Williams, W., R. H. Guy, D. Rubin, F. Robey, J. Myers, T. Kieber-Emmons, D. B. Weiner and M. I. Greene. 1988. "Sequence of the Cell Attachment Site of Reovirus Type 3 and Modeling of its Three-Dimensional Structure," *Proc. Natl. Acad. Sci. USA*, 85:6488.

96 Williams, W., D. Moss, T. Kieber-Emmons, J. Cohen, J. Myers, D. B. Weiner and M. I. Greene. 1989. "Development of Biologically Active Peptides Based on Antibody Structure," *Proc. Natl. Acad. Sci. USA*, 86:5537.

97 Williams, W. V., T. Kieber-Emmons, D. B. Weiner, D. H. Rubin and M. I. Greene. 1991. "Contact Residues and Predicted Structure of the Reovirus Type 3-Receptor Interactions," *J. Biol. Chem.*, 266:9241.

98 Kieber-Emmons, T., B. Jameson and W. J. W. Morrow. 1989. "The gp120-CD4 Interface: Structural, Immunological and Pathological Considerations," *Biochim. Biophys. Acta*, 989:281.

99 Kieber-Emmons, T., A. Whalley, W. M. Williams, T. Ryskamp, W. J. W. Morrow, J. Krowka, W. V. Williams, I. Schmid, J. V. Girogi, M. Merva and D. B. Weiner. 1990. "Biological Characteristics of an HIV-1 Envelope-Derived Synthetic Peptide," in *Vaccines '90: Modern Approaches to New Vaccines Including Prevention of AIDS*, F. Brown, R. M. Chanock, H. S. Ginsberg and R. A. Lerner, eds., New York: Cold Spring Harbor Laboratory Press, p. 321.

100 Kieber-Emmons, T., K. E. Ugen, M. Merva, A. Whalley, W. J. W. Morrow, W. V. Williams, P. L. Nara and D. B. Weiner. 1991. "Engineered Peptides That Mimic HIV-1 Neutralizing Envelope Structures," in *Vaccines '91: Modern Approaches to New Vaccines Including Prevention of AIDS*, R. M. Chanock, H. S. Ginsberg, F. Brown and R. A. Lerner, eds., New York: Cold Spring Harbor Laboratory Press, p. 165.

101 Kieber-Emmons, T., J. F. Krowka, J. Boyer, K. E. Ugen, V. W. Williams and D. B. Weiner. 1992. "Immunological Characteristics of the Putative CD4 Binding Site at the HIV-1 Envelope Protein," *Pathobiology*, in press.

102 Morrow, W. J. W., W. M. Williams, A. S. Whalley, T. Ryskamp, R. Newman, C.-Y. Kang, S. Chamut, H. Kohler and T. Kieber-Emmons. 1992. "Synthetic Peptides from a Conserved Region of the HIV Envelope Induce Broadly Reactive Anti-HIV Responses," *Immunology*, in press.

103 Taub, R., R. J. Gould, V. M. Garsky, T. M. Ciccarone, J. Hoxie, P. A. Friedman and S. J. Shattil. 1989. "A Monoclonal Antibody against the Platelet Fibrinogen Receptor Contains a Sequence That Mimics a Receptor Recognition Domain in Fibrinogen," *J. Biol. Chem.*, 264:259.

104 Springer, T. A. 1990. *Nature*, 346:425.

105 Kieber-Emmons, T., M. M. Ward, R. E. Ward and H. Kohler. 1987. "Structural Considerations in Idiotype Vaccine Design," *Monogr. Allergy*, 22:126.

106 Cheng, H.-L., A. K. Sood, R. E. Ward, T. Kieber-Emmons and H. Kohler. 1988. "Structural Basis of Stimulatory Anti-Idiotypic Antibodies," *Mol. Immunol.*, 25:33.

107 Scarborough, R. M., J. W. Rose, M. A. Hsu, D. R. Phillips, V. A. Fried, A. M. Campbell, L. Nannizzi and I. F. Charo. 1991. "Barbourin. A GPIIb-IIIa-Specific Integrin Antagonist from the Venom of *Sistrurus m. barbouri*," *J. Biol. Chem.*, 266:9359.

108 Kang, C.-Y., T. K. Brunck, T. Kieber-Emmons, J. E. Blalock and H. Kohler. 1988. "Inhibition of Self-Binding Antibodies (Autobodies) by a VH Derived Peptide," *Science*, 240:1034.

109 Swanson, S. J., B. F. Lin, M. C. Mullenix and R. F. Mortensen. 1991. "A Synthetic Peptide Corresponding to the Phosphorylcholine (PC)-Binding Region of Human C-Reactive Protein Possesses the TEPC-15 Myeloma PC-Idiotype," *J. Immunol.*, 146:1596.

110 Vasta, G. R., J. J. Marchalonis and H. Kohler. 1984. "Invertebrate Recognition Protein Cross-Reacts with an Immunoglobulin Idiotype," *J. Exp. Med.*, 159:1270.

111 Kieber-Emmons, T. 1992. "Structural Aspects of Recognition Motifs Contributing to Autoimmune Responses," *DNA and Cell Biology*, in press.

112 Husain, J., T. L. Blundell, S. Cooper, J. E. Pitts, I. J. Tickle, S. P. Wood, V. J. Hruby, A. Buku, A. J. Fischman and H. R. Wyssbrod, et al. 1990. "The Conformation of Deamino-Oxytocin: X-Ray Analysis of the 'Dry' and 'Wet' Forms," *Philos. Trans. R. Soc. Lond. (Biol.)*, 327:625 [published erratum appears in *Philos. Trans. R. Soc. Lond. (Biol.)*, 328:239.

113 Wynants, C., D. Tourwe, W. Kazmierski, V. J. Hruby and G. Van Binst. 1989. "Conformation of Two Somatostatin Analogues in Aqueous Solution. Study by NMR Methods and Circular Dichroism," *Eur. J. Biochem.*, 185:371.

114 DiMaio, J., T. M. Nguyen, C. Lemieux and P. W. Schiller. 1982. "Synthesis and Pharmacological Characterization *in vitro* of Cyclic Enkephalin Analogues: Effect of Conformational Constraints on Opiate Receptor Selectivity," *J. Med. Chem.*, 25:1432.

115 Sherman, D. B., A. F. Spatola, W. S. Wire, T. F. Burks, T. M. Nguyen and P. W. Schiller. 1989. "Biological Activities of Cyclic Enkephalin Pseudopeptides Containing Thioamides as Amide Bond Replacements," *Biochem. Biophys. Res. Commun.*, 162:1126.

116 Sandberg, B. E., C. M. Lee, M. R. Hanley and L. L. Iversen. 1981. "Synthesis

and Biological Properties of Enzyme-Resistant Analogues of Substance P," *Eur. J. Biochem.*, 114:329.

117 Plattner, J. J. and D. W. Norbeck. 1990. "Obstacles to Drug Development from Peptide Leads," in *Drug Discovery Technologies*, C. R. Clark and W. H. Moos, eds., Chichester, UK: Ellis Horwood, p. 92.

118 DiMaio, J., F. Ni, B. Gibbs and Y. Konishi. 1991. "A New Class of Potent Thrombin Inhibitors that Incorporates a Scissile Pseudopeptide Bond," *FEBS Lett.*, 282:47.

119 Anwer, M. K., D. B. Sherman and A. F. Spatola. 1990. "Backbone Modifications in Cyclic Peptides. Conformational Analysis of a Cyclic Pseudopentapeptide Containing a Thiomethylene Ether Amide Bond Replacement," *Int. J. Pept. Protein Res.*, 36:392.

120 Darlak, K., D. E. Benovitz, A. F. Spatola and Z. Grzonka. 1988. "Dermorphin Analogs: Resistance to *in vitro* Enzymatic Degradation Is Not Always Increased by Additional D-Amino Acid Substitutions," *Biochem. Biophys. Res. Commun.*, 156:125.

121 Gray, R. D., R. B. Miller and A. F. Spatola. 1986. "Inhibition of Mammalian Collagenases by Thiol-Containing Peptides," *J. Cell. Biochem.*, 32:71.

122 Smellie, A. S., G. M. Crippen and W. G. Richards. 1991. "Fast Drug-Receptor Mapping by Site-Directed Distances: A Novel Method of Predicting New Pharmacological Leads," *J. Chem. Inf. Comput. Sci.*, 31:386.

123 Sheridan, R. P., A. Rusinko, III, R. Nilakantan and R. Venkataraghavan. 1989. "Searching for Pharmacophores in Large Coordinate Data Bases and Its Use in Drug Design," *Proc. Natl. Acad. Sci. USA*, 86:8165.

124 Shoichet, B. K. and I. D. Kuntz. 1991. "Protein Docking and Complementarity," *J. Mol. Biol.*, 221:327.

125 DesJarlais, R. L., G. L. Seibel, I. D. Kuntz, P. S. Furth, J. C. Alvarez, P. R. Ortiz de Montellano, D. L. DeCamp, L. M. Babe and C. S. Craik. 1990. "Structure-Based Design of Nonpeptide Inhibitors Specific for the Human Immunodeficiency Virus 1 Protease," *Proc. Natl. Acad. Sci. USA*, 87:6644.

126 DesJarlais, R. L., R. P. Sheridan, G. L. Seibel, J. S. Dixon, I. D. Kuntz and R. Venkataraghavan. 1988. "Using Shape Complementarity as an Initial Screen in Designing Ligands for a Receptor Binding Site of Known Three-Dimensional Structure," *J. Med. Chem.*, 31:722.

127 Romer, D., H. H. Busher, R. C. Hill, R. Maurer, T. J. Petcher, H. Zuegner, W. Benson, E. Finner, W. Milkowski and P. W. Thies. 1982. "An Opioid Benzodiazepine," *Nature*, 198:759.

128 Sharif, N. and D. R. Burg. 1984. "Modulation of Receptors for Thyrotropin-Releasing Hormone by Benzodiazeprines: Brain Regional Differences," *J. Neurochem.*, 43:742.

129 Kornecki, E., Y. H. Ehrlich and R. H. Lennox. 1984. "Platelet-Activating Factor-Induced Aggregation of Human Platelets Specifically Inhibited by Triazolobenzodiazepines," *Science*, 226:1454.

130 Evans, B. E., K. E. Rittle, R. M. Di Pardo, R. M. Friedinger, W. L. Whittier, G. F. Lundell, D. F. Veber, P. S. Anderson, R. S. L. Chang, V. J. Lotti, D. J. Cerino, T. B. Chen, P. J. Kling, K. A. Kunkel, J. P. Springer and J. Hirschfield. 1988. "Methods for Drug Discovery: Development of Potent, Selective, Orally Effective, Cholecystokinin Antagonists," *J. Med. Chem.*, 31:2235.

131 Gund, P., A. Halgen and G. A. Smith. 1987. "Molecular Modeling as an Aid to Drug Design and Discovery," *Ann. Rep. Med. Chem.*, 22:269.

CHAPTER 2

Computer Assisted Design of Peptidomimetic Drugs

VIDUKUDI N. BALAJI[1]
KALYANARAMAN RAMNARAYAN[1]

SUMMARY

THERE is increased interest in the design of peptidomimetics of target oligopeptides to enhance metabolic stability, oral bioavailability, and to achieve lesser side effects. There is considerable success in the random trial methods in proposing peptidomimetics of oligopeptides. Hitherto, there are no reports in the literature of a rational procedure to design a peptidomimetic. In this chapter, we outline a rational strategy to arrive at a peptidomimetic of a target oligopeptide drug. The steps identified involve generation of probable conformations of the oligopeptide, design of specific rigid analogs including cyclic peptides using a data base of peptide mimics and identification of the bioactive conformation. We suggest the use of either the rigid bioactive analog itself as target peptidomimetic or use of the bioactive conformation to identify a lead peptidomimetic by searching a three dimensional data base of nonpeptide compounds. Further, the identified bioactive conformation of the oligopeptide will be used to construct other target peptidomimetics using interactive computer graphics and model building.

INTRODUCTION

Traditional drug design for many diseases involved identifying a chemical substance that interacts with either known or unknown receptor in

---

[1]ImmunoPharmaceutics, Inc., 11011 Via Frontera, San Diego, CA 92127, U.S.A.

some way showing therapeutic value. This mode of discovering a new drug by screening a large number of compounds has had a good deal of success, but it has drawbacks, including the random nature of screening. Recently, a novel family of peptide based drugs is becoming important as therapeutic agents. For example, a large number of mammalian and nonmammalian peptide hormones and neurotransmitters exhibiting a wide diversity of biological activities have been identified for therapy of several diseases [1,2]. Peptide based drugs are known to interact with specific receptors. For example, several specific membrane-bound protein receptors for peptide hormones exist in target organs [3]. Peptide based drug development has some disadvantages. The metabolic lability of the native peptides means that analogs with greater stability to proteases and longer duration of action would be very useful. Since many such agents also have potential utility in therapy, an additional desirable feature would be good oral bioavailability. In such an effort, considerable progress in obtaining peptides with improved properties has been achieved [4–7].

A peptidomimetic is a mimic of certain features of the original peptide of interest. The altered features can be in the main chain, the side chains, or the surface. In general a peptidomimetic is conceived which can provide enhanced biological activity and/or altered metabolic stability to systems of potential therapeutic interest. The identification and alteration of peptide linkages which can be replaced without sacrifice of activity can therefore be crucial for successful manipulation of biological response and pharmacokinetic behavior. Several peptide analogs resistant to proteolytic degradation have been synthesized by sequence truncation, incorporation of unnatural amino acids and cyclic amino acid derivatives, and preparation of cyclic peptides. In designing these analogs, consideration of possible receptor-bound "bioactive" conformations has played an important role. There are several successful examples of the development of such drugs. For example, synthetic analogs of somatostatin and luteining hormone-releasing hormone (LHRH) have recently become marketed drugs. Incorporation of partial nonpeptidal structures to produce pseudo-peptides, and C-terminal truncation have shown promise in certain cases [6]. Recently, an account of predicting the biologically active conformations of short polypeptides has been reviewed [8].

Some of the techniques to improve upon the drawbacks of peptides as drugs, is to replace the amide backbone by a novel amide-like moiety or to make suitable modifications to the side chains either to impart conformational rigidity or resistance to metabolic degradation to proteolytic enzymes (as in the case of D-residues or cyclic peptide analogs). In recent years increasing interest has been shown in the concept of isosteric replacement of amide bonds in biologically active peptides. The basic assumption for isosteric replacement is that it might be possible to modify one or more amide bonds in peptides such that conformation and binding are maintained, but enzymatic hydrolysis is prevented. Initial successes utilizing this concept have been reported with the use of methylenethio isostere, $[CH_2S]$, as an amide replacement in enkephalin analogues [9] and as renin inhibitors having both the methyleneamino, $[CH_2NH]$, and hydroxyethylene, $[CHOHCH_2]$, isosteres at the scissile Leu-Val amide bond in the 6–13 octapeptide derived from angiotensinogen [10]. Recently, synthesis of renin inhibitors in which amino acids are replaced with the hydroxyethylene dipeptide isosters which maintained activity and enhanced stability has been found [11]. Renin inhibitors containing 13 different isosteric replacements of the amide bond connecting the P_3 and P_2 positions of angiotensinogen including two most potent compounds containing hydroxyethylene $[CHOHCH_2]$ isosteres have been reported [12]. Modified di- and tripeptides derived from the C-terminal portion of oxytocin and vasopressin as possible cognition-activating agents have also been reported [13]. Another notable example of C-terminal modifications by different size lactam rings imposing conformational restriction is the design of angiotensin-converting enzyme (ACE) inhibitors [14]. Thus, the replacement of amide bonds by peptidomimetics has become a useful technique for imparting novel characteristics to bioactive peptides [9, 15,16]. A detailed account of conformation and biological activity relationships for receptor-selective, conformationally constrained opioid peptides has recently been presented [17]. Design of conformationally restricted cyclopeptides for the inhibition of cholate uptake of hepatocytes has also been reported [18]. In spite of considerable progress, the ideal goal of potent, orally bioavailable, long duration, selective peptide receptor ligands has remained largely elusive [5]. One potential solution is to search for completely nonpeptide ligands. Such compounds offer a much broader range of structure. One approach of finding nonpeptide ligands for peptide receptor system, is to find leads from natural sources or synthetic collections. A large number of extracts and compounds can be screened and once an active lead is established, medicinal chemists can design analogs with improved properties. For example, imidazole-5-acetic acid derivatives have been reported to be an angiotensin II (AII) antagonist by random screening [19]. Recently, based on this lead compound, highly potent, selective nonpeptide AII receptor antagonist which was designed to mimic the C-terminal region of AII has been reported [16]. The alternative approach is rational design based on the native peptide ligand. This strategy is an extension of the approaches already described for developing metabolically stable peptides. In this chapter, we will illustrate the salient features of the peptidomimetic design technology and present here an outline of a rational way of peptidomimetic design.

APPROACHES TO PEPTIDOMIMETIC DESIGN

The key for any rational drug design of a peptidomimetic is the bioactive conformation. The general protocol to identify the bioactive conformation for different cases can be summarized as follows.

Case (a): Once we know the three-dimensional structure of the target oligopeptide (through out our discussion "target oligopeptide" refers to the bioactive peptide for which we wish to design a smaller size peptide or a peptidomimetic) and the specific interaction of this oligopeptide with the target receptor, one can further establish the conformation by constrained analog design using a data base of constrained (and also, if needed, metabolically stable) peptide moieties. This is done by suggesting analogs at every residue level in a systematic fashion such that the main chain replacement does not disturb conformational features and the side chain substitutions are compatible to retain the receptor substrate interactions. Synthesis and biological evaluation of a series of compounds and iterative refinement of the peptidomimetic (in this case the constrained analog itself) can then be carried out. Another approach in this case is to search a three-dimensional data base of organic moieties to mimic the three-dimensional shape of the target oligopeptide (see later sections for details of peptidomimetic search).

Case (b): If we know the receptor geometry but lack the information as to how the target peptide interacts with the receptor, we can model build the peptide in the binding site of the receptor by computational methods and identify the bioactive or binding conformation. This can be further substantiated by designing rigid analogs of this initial binding conformation that we obtain using steps described in Case (a).

Case (c): In this case, we do not have *a priori* the knowledge of receptor geometry and we know only the target oligopeptide. The approach will be to simulate the most probable conformations by computational methods and to design constrained analogs. Such a design effort can be achieved by searching a data base of constrained peptide analogs which mimic the probable conformations at every residue. For these conformationally restricted analogs, using an iterative approach (using both activity and inactivity profile of rigid analogs) one can identify the bioactive conformation based on an evaluation of the biological activity. Such a bioactive conformation will then be used to design peptidomimetics or to search a three-dimensional data base of organic structures to suggest lead peptidomimetics. If we have structure activity relation (SAR) data on the target peptide and its analogs (this can be simple systematic amino acid substitutions), one can use such data to identify key amino acid residues for the bioactivity. The constrained analogs can then be designed at other residues to identify the bioactive conformation.

Thus, for a rational design of peptidomimetics, it is necessary to have data from different physico-chemical and theoretical techniques. Although these approaches have their own merits and limitations, the information gathered from these studies will help in the best possible design of the peptidomimetics. For the elucidation of the three-dimensional structure of target oligopeptide and or receptor, well established methods include x-ray crystallography, nuclear magnetic resonance (NMR), and computational techniques. We briefly review their applications in the following sections.

X-RAY CRYSTALLOGRAPHY

From x-ray crystallography one can determine a conformation of the target oligopeptide. The role of x-ray crystallography in drug design has proved to be invaluable [20]. Even though, this is the only known technique of getting a complete three-dimensional structure, since it is the structure in the solid state it may not truly reflect the biologically active conformation of the peptide being studied. However, it can be used as starting conformation for use in computer simulation.

One of the major contributions of x-ray crystallography towards oligo and cyclic peptide structures is the elucidation of the geometry of the peptide units as well as other rigid portions of the molecules, useful as starting geometries in computer simulations [21–28]. This type of geometry elucidation from available x-ray crystallographic data is very efficient in the absence of access to *ab initio* calculations for geometry optimization. Determination of receptor geometry to a high resolution, while possible by x-ray crystallography, is in many cases very difficult for several reasons—like unavailability of sufficient quantities of receptor, growing of good quality crystals suitable for x-ray diffraction [29]. The prediction of three-dimensional geometry of proteins (receptors) when amino acid sequence is known is still in its infancy. However, considerable success in model building the three-dimensional structure of homologous proteins has been achieved when the three-dimensional structure data of one of the proteins is known [30–34]. In particular, for antibodies, if we know the sequence of amino acids in the variable region one can construct three-dimensional models by using crystallographic data of other antibodies. Such models can be used to fit the identified mimotopes and hence arrive at the binding conformation (probably the bioactive conformation) of the mimotope [35] or peptide ligands resulting from a search of epitope library [36]. This approach gives us the so called bioactive conformation which can be used for design of peptidomimetics.

NUCLEAR MAGNETIC RESONANCE

Another spectroscopic technique that is a good source of information for peptidomimetic design is nuclear magnetic resonance (NMR). This technique has the advantage of elucidating the structure in both solid state and in solution [37–40]. This technology can give information on the structure of the free molecule in solution and when complexed with another macromolecule—possibly the receptor [40–43]. However, the major drawback of this technique is that the information for a rather complex molecule may not be very precise and also the refinement of the structural data becomes complicated for larger complexes. The use of NMR as a valuable tool in drug design has been recently reviewed [39] and its application to study of conformationally constrained peptides has been discussed [17]. NMR can complement the x-ray crystallographic techniques in several ways. Due to the fact that one can study the peptides in solution one can alter the conditions of experiments like varying pH, temperature, salt additions, etc. Thus, in principle, one can study the conformational changes, if any, over a wide range of conditions.

COMPUTATIONAL CHEMISTRY

By computational techniques one can determine the flexibility of these structures. The x-ray crystallography and NMR methods are complemented by theoretical computational techniques to lead to so called Computer Aided Drug Design (CADD) using a variety of computational chemistry techniques like steric fitting, molecular mechanics, molecular dynamics, Monte Carlo simulations, free energy perturbation, and quantum chemical calculations in combination with computer graphics. Using these techniques, one can arrive at a reasonable three-dimensional structure of the compound under investigation. In the next step, one can make suitable changes to the functional groups and visualize them on a graphics screen and study the interaction of a peptide or a peptidomimetic with a model receptor. The effectiveness of graphics tools in drug design has been discussed recently [14,44,45]. In a typical computer simulation, usually one starts with a reasonably good guess of the initial conformation of the peptide of interest. For example, this can be a good estimate of the conformation of the stable peptide having a known amino acid sequence. Such an estimate may be based on known data, e.g., as obtained using x-ray crystallography or as predicted using homology model building. Unfortunately, while such "starting points" do significantly shorten the amount of computer time required in such simulations, they also bias the final results. Frequently, such simulations end up identifying only a "local minimum" of the predicted peptide, with the most probable stable conformation of the peptide going undetected. What is clearly needed, therefore, is a method and technique of predicting the most probable stable peptide conformations using computer simulations that may be feasibly performed without bias to final results. In the next section we describe one such method being used by us in peptide simulations.

Our approach to designing a peptidomimetic of a target peptide based drug depends on available previous data on the drug. The strategies for designing of peptidomimetic of target peptide can be summarized as follows: (a) Receptor geometry and active conformation of the oligopeptide is known (that is, if the conformation of the target oligopeptide is known when it is bound to the receptor from methods like x-ray crystallography or NMR). (b) Receptor geometry is known but specific bioactive (or binding) conformation of the oligopeptide with the receptor is unknown. (c) Only the sequence of the oligopeptide is known and receptor geometry is unknown (this is the case with most of the oligopeptide based drugs).

SIMULATION OF THE THREE-DIMENSIONAL CONFORMATION OF OLIGOPEPTIDES

Even at the dipeptide level peptides show considerable flexibility [46]. The brute force method of arriving at the global minimum and other local minimum is to compute the energies of all possible conformations in a systematic search. To some extent such methods are now possible for small peptides. For large peptides such a method becomes computationally intensive and cannot be accessed even with the available super computer technology. However, there are other methods, like Monte Carlo type simulations wherein a random sample of starting geometries are selected for a given conformational angle and the energy minimized to obtain reasonable energy minima and study of such simulations can give a clue to the most probable conformation and other local minima. This technique also requires a reasonable amount of computer simulation time and works well with small oligopeptides (less than 10 residues long). The various techniques used are well documented [46,47].

The overall mobility and flexibility of an oligopeptide can be assessed by molecular dynamics approaches and the generated molecular dynamics trajectory depends on the starting conformation and the period of simulation. We have developed an *ab initio* technique to determine the probable conformation(s) of an oligopeptide [48,49]. The general protocol is given in Figure 2.1. In this chapter, we will not go into the details of this technology. However, we will outline the salient features of the method for the sake of completeness. The protocol starts with an input of amino acids which constitute the peptide to be analyzed. At this stage, one can also specify if cyclization is required, by indicating at what position we need the ring closure. In the next stage, a series of steps of minimization and dynamics are carried out in an iterative fashion. The final step in the process is the analysis of the peptide conformation. We have simulated a number of linear and cyclic homo and hetero peptides by this protocol. Preliminary tests suggest that if there are constraints, as in the case of cyclic peptides and oligopeptides containing disulfide bridges, the struc-

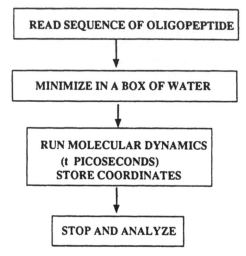

Figure 2.1 Flow chart of simulation of oligopeptides.

ture simulated corresponds to well characterized most probable conformation [48,49].

SURFACE FEATURE MIMICRY

If we are interested in accessing the information about the key residues of a given bioactive oligopeptide or polypeptide, several biochemical techniques such as systematic alanine scan are available. If we know the three-dimensional structure of the polypeptide, the first step will be to construct a surface feature mimic to establish the bioactive portion. Such mimicry may be possible in the case of antagonist design. For rapid evaluation and elucidation of the bioactive surface itself, it is of interest to design molecules similar to the surface features. This can be accomplished by the design of cyclic peptides.

The methods to mimic the surface feature of a given three-dimensional structure of a polypeptide have been worked out in our laboratory [50] and is schematically illustrated in Figure 2.2. This involves the creation of a data base of cyclic peptide library by *ab initio* methods. We have simulated a large number of cyclic peptides (5 to 10 mers) having permutation and combination of L and D amino acid residues and conformationally restricted unnatural amino acids. We have included selected monomer residues in the cyclic peptide data such that, a linear oligopeptide can be easily synthesized using automated amino acid synthesizer and in most of the cases the cyclization can be achieved externally.

INCORPORATION OF CONFORMATIONAL CONSTRAINTS

This can be done in many ways for a target oligopeptide. It can be a cyclization of the oligopeptides or main chain modification of the peptide moiety or side chain modifications at the residue level. The different options for constraining an oligopeptide is shown schematically in Figure 2.3.

Main Chain Modifications

Many main chain modifications leading to different degree of constraints (or flexibility) are well used in previous design work of peptidomimetics. A list of peptide bond isosteres is given in Table 2.1. Incidentally, these isosteres exhibit different degree of metabolic stability. Appropriate use of them can lead to peptide analogs of higher or lower metabolic stability.

Side Chain Modifications

Several simple modifications of the side chain can impart conformational rigidity for a given oligopeptide at the residue level. The simpler ones are the so called α-amino isobutyric acid residue and the dehydro amino acid substitutions. The other interesting substitutions are the cyclic side chains illustrated in Figure 2.4. These side chains not only constrain

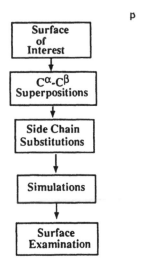

Figure 2.2 Scheme for identifying peptides to mimic three-dimensional surface features of an oligopeptide.

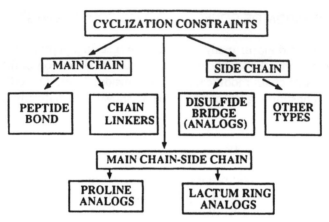

Figure 2.3 Scheme of introduction of constraints by cyclization.

the main chain to specific angles (one can restrict the main chain conformational angles by further substitution of methyl groups on the C^β hydrogens) but provide different bulk to mimic the volume and surface area of the parent amino acids. Charge characteristics can also be incorporated on these cyclic moieties to replace specific amino acid moieties. A set of typical aromatic and heteroaromatic substituted amino acid analogs [51] which restricts the main chain conformational freedom are illustrated in Figure 2.5.

TABLE 2.1. **Peptide Bond Isosteres.**

N-methyl peptide
Thioamide (thiopeptide)
N-methyl thioamide
[CH(OH)CH₂] Hydroxyethylene Isosteres
[CH=CH] Double Bond Isosteres
[CHCHO] Epoxide Isosteres
[CH₂CH₂] Dimethylene Isosteres
[CHOHCHOH] Diol Isosteres
[CHOHCH=CHCO] Hydroxy Double Bond Isosteres
[CHOHCHOHCHOHOHCO] Trihydroxy Isostere
[CHOHCH₂] Hydroxyethylene Isosteres
[COCH₂] Ketomethylene Isosteres
[CH₂NH] Methyleneamino Isosteres (Methyleneamine)
[CH₂NOH] Methylenehydroxyamino Isosteres
[CH₂S] Methylenethio Isosteres
[CH₂SO] Methylenethio Isosteres
[CH₂SO₂] Methylenethio Isosteres

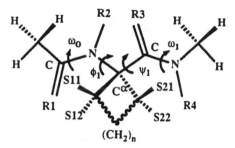

Figure 2.4 Side chain modifications: Cyclic propyl (n = 0), butyl (n = 1), pentyl (n = 3), hexyl (n = 4), heptyl (n = 5), octyl (n = 6) moieties within a dipeptide model [R1 = R3 = 0, R2 = R4 = H].

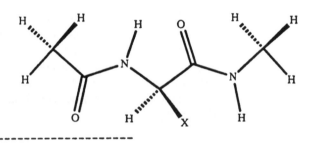

X

C_6H_5
$4-C_6H_4OH$
$4-C_6H_4OCH_3$
$2OOH-5-CH_3C_6H_3$
$2-C_{10}H_7$
2-furnyl
$5-CH_3-2-pyrrolyl$
$1-CH_3-2-pyrrolyl$
2-thienyl
3-thienyl
beonzo[b]furan-2yl
indo-3-yl
benzo[b]thien-2-yl

[Note: The substitution at C^α can be in either R or S configuration]

Figure 2.5 Aromatic and heteroaromatic substituted amino acid derivatives.

Main Chain–Main Chain Cyclization Constraints

The regular peptide bond formation of the main chain can lead to the cyclic peptides which leads to reasonable constraint on the flexibility of such molecules. Such cyclic peptides can also have other types of chain linkers like − (CH_2) − moieties. It is also possible to incorporate appropriate linker formation between one peptide unit to the other. For example, one can force α-helical conformation by replacing the hydrogen bonds by linkers of the type $-C=C-$. Similar linkers can constrain a dipeptide to 2_7 conformation or β-turn formation.

Side Chain–Side Chain Cyclization Constraints

Cyclization via side chains can lead to conformational restrictions. Conformational freedom can also be restricted by the use of disulfide bridge like linkages (see Table 2.2). Other miscellaneous types of bridges between side chains are also possible. For example, if the side chain involved in the oligopeptide is HIS and is of importance to the biological activity of the peptide, L-2-thiolhistidine residue (HisS) can be used leading to the formation of HisS-$(CH_2)_3$-HisS bridge.

Main Chain–Side Chain Cyclization Constraints

The naturally occurring imino acid proline is an example of the main chain side chain cyclization constraint which imparts conformational rigidity around ϕ which is restricted to $-60°$ to $-80°$. Several prolyl like analogs (Figure 2.6) are possible with similar rigidity about ϕ angle, for example, in the case of Dtc (5,5-dimethylthiazolidine-4-carboxylic acid) it is restricted to $-60°$. Another example is 2′-methylphenylalanine moiety. One should note that incorporation of such constraints can lead to the possibility of both *trans* and *cis* peptide bonds. To restrict the freedom of ψ angle main chain − side chain cyclization constraints that can be used are lactam rings of different sizes (Figure 2.7). Similarly ring constraints with

TABLE 2.2. A List of Disulfide Bridge (—S—S—) Analogs.

[Disulfide	—S—S—]
Thiomethly	—S—CH$_2$—
Thioether	—S—O—
Ethylene	—CH$_2$—CH$_2$—
Thioselenyl	—S—Se—
Diselenide	—Se—Se—
Selenomethyl	—Se—CH$_2$—

$(CH_2)_n$

Figure 2.6 Side chain–main chain ring constraints: n = 1 or 2. Prolyl analogs (note n = 1 corresponds to prolyl-dipeptide).

succinyl (Asu) and glutaryl (Agl) groups (Figure 2.8) impose restriction not only on ψ angle but also forcing specific turns to the oligopeptides (Balaji et al. unpublished results).

CONFORMATIONAL FEATURES OF MODEL PEPTIDE ANALOGS

A rational approach to peptidomimetic design has greater chances of success only when one has a thorough knowledge about the conformational space that a given oligopeptide can span. There is an abundance of literature on the theoretical conformational analysis of oligo- and cyclic peptides [46,52–56]. In addition to this, we have computed the conformational features of several model constrained peptide analogs by molecular mechanics methods at the dipeptide level [57].

METHOD USED TO COMPUTE CONFORMATIONAL ENERGY MAPS OF CONSTRAINED PEPTIDE ANALOGS

Conformational energies were computed using the AMBER molecular mechanics program [58] in the (θ_1, θ_2) plane at 10° intervals (θ_1, θ_2 are the

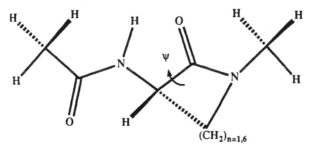

$(CH_2)_{n=1,6}$

Figure 2.7 Side chain–main chain ring constraints: lactam dipeptide analogs.

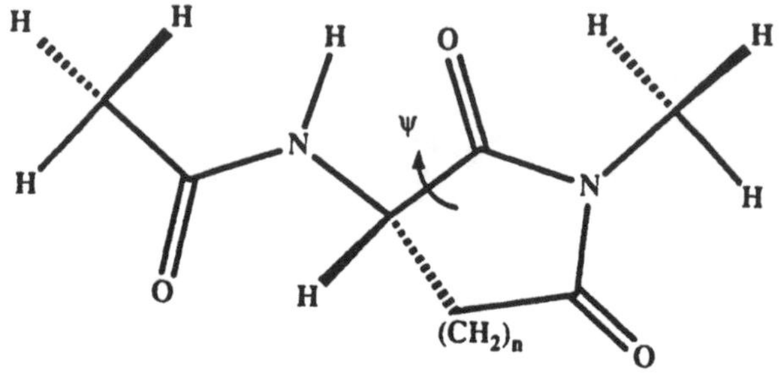

Figure 2.8 Example of main chain–side chain ring constraint. Succinyl (Asu) [n = 1] and gly-taryl (Alu) [n = 2] dipeptide moieties.

dihedral angles of interest in the model compounds—for example for the case of alanyl dipeptide this corresponds to the Ramachandran ϕ,ψ angles). The parameters used were those published previously [59] or derived by fitting to the experimental and *ab initio* [60,61] derived structures, dipole moments and conformational energies of model compounds. All AMBER calculations were performed using monopole charges and a dielectric constant of 4.0. For each (θ_1,θ_2) angle frozen, the energy was minimized with convergence criteria of 0.1 kcal/mole. The conformational energy contour maps (with *trans* peptide and thiopeptide units) were drawn in the (θ_1,θ_2) plane at 1 kcal/mole intervals with respect to the global minimum for each of the model compounds shown in Figures 2.4 and 2.5. Contours greater than 5 kcal/mole have been omitted. The percentage availability of the conformational space with 1, 2, 3, 4, and 5 kcal/mole from the global minimum for each conformational energy map were computed. Probability maps were computed at 300°K.

Typical conformational energy map we obtain for a model compound like Aib-dipeptide is presented in Figure 2.9. In this figure we have also prefixed a table containing the key conformational features (the position of global and local minima, the overall flexibility of the molecule which is obtainable by the percent occupation of 1 to 5 kcal/mole contours). Also, to assess the relative population of each minima we can use the data from probability information. We have similar data for several hundred model dipeptide analogs and computation and compilation for several new analogs are under continuous development.

CONFORMATIONAL FEATURE DATA BASE OF PEPTIDE ANALOGS

At present we have computed and compiled conformational features of several peptide analogs at the dipeptide level. The moieties include several main chain peptide mimics and side chain substitutions. Our goal is the compilation and establishment of a data base of the conformational features on several model compounds. The data base is used to search and suggest conformationally restricted analog of a target oligopeptide. As and when some new peptide moieties appear in literature, they will be appended to the data base.

PEPTIDOMIMETIC SEARCH

The constrained analog approach detailed (schematically summarized in Figure 2.10) so far can itself lead in some cases to the peptidomimetic of interest. This is mainly so, since some of the ingredients which make up the constrained analog contains subtle modifications leading to more proteolytic and metabolic stability. If the bioactivity of such an analog is to be fine tuned, made cost effective, as well as improve metabolic profile and bioavailability, one can use the derived bioactive conformation as a starting point for further peptidomimetic design. In such an effort design of other molecules which mimic the essential bioactive conformation and features of the oligopeptide, one searches a three-dimensional data base of nonpeptide (organic and other) structures for three-dimensional similarity. The three-dimensional data base for such a search can be either Cambridge Crystal Structure Data Base [62,63] or three-dimensional structures

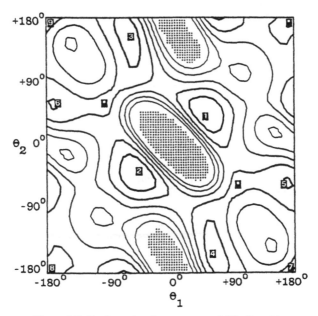

Figure 2.9 Conformational energy map of Aib-dipeptide.

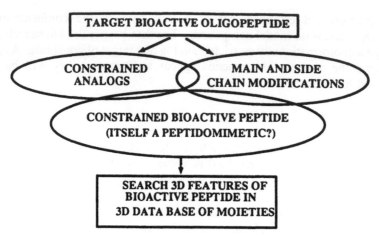

Figure 2.10 General steps involved in peptidomimetic design.

generated for organic structures by other means [64]. The search algorithm for three- dimensional data base comparison is available in literature and can be implemented for such searches [65–68]. Also, software for such searches are available commercially [69,70].

ACKNOWLEDGEMENTS

We thank Drs. M. E. Wolff and U. C. Singh for useful discussions.

REFERENCES

1 Krieger, D. T. 1983. "Brain Peptides: What, Where, and Why?" *Science*, 222:975–985.

2 Dutta, A. S. 1989. "Small Peptides–New Targets for Drug Research," *Chemistry in Britain*, pp. 159–162.

3 Kalimi, M. Y. and J. R. Hubbard, eds. 1987. *Peptide Hormone Receptors*. Berlin, Fed. Rep. Ger.: de Gruyter, p. 720.

4 Farmer, P. S. and E. J. Ariëns. 1982. "Speculations on the Design of Nonpeptidic Peptidomimetics," *Trends Pharmacol. Sci.*, 3:362–365.

5 Verber, D. F. and R. M. Fredinger. 1985. "The Design of Metabolically-Stable Peptide Analogs," *Trends Neurosci.*, 8:392–396.

6 Freidinger, R. M. 1989. "Non-Peptide Ligands for Peptide Receptors," *Trends Pharmacol. Sci.*, 10:270–274.

7 Morgan, B. A. and J. A. Gainor. 1990. "Approaches to the Discovery of Non-Peptide Ligands for Peptide Receptors and Peptidases," *Ann. Rep. Med. Chem.*, 24:243–252.

8 Milner-White, E. J. 1989. "Predicting the Biologically Active Conformations of Short Polypeptides," *Trends Pharmacol. Sci.*, 10:70–73.

9 Spatola, A. F. 1983. "Peptide Backbone Modifications: A Structure-Activity Analysis of Peptides Containing Amide Bond Surrogates, Conformational Constraints, and Related," in *Chemistry and Biochemistry of Amino Acids, Peptides, and Proteins Vol. 7*, B. Weistein, ed., New York: Marcell Dekker, pp. 257–267.

10 Szelke, M., D. M. Jones, B. Atrash, A. Hallet and B. Leckie. 1983. "Novel Transition-State Analog Inhibitors of Renin," *Peptides: Structure and Function, Proceedings of the Eighth American Peptide Symposium*, V. J. Hruby and D. H. Rich, eds., Rockford, IL: Pierce Chemical Co., pp. 579–582.

11 Kempf, D. J., E. de Lara, H. H. Stein, J. Cohen, D. A. Egan and J. J. Plattner. 1990. "Renin Inhibitors Based on Dipeptide Analogues. Incorporation of the Hydroxyethylene Isostere at the P2/P3 Sites," *J. Med. Chem.*, 33:371–374.

12 Kaltenbronn, J. S., J. P. Hudspeth, E. A. Lunney, B. M. Michniewicz, E. D. Nicolaides, J. T. Repine, W. H. Roark, M. A. Stier, F. J. Tinney and P. K. W. Woo. 1990. "Renin Inhibitors Containing Isosteric Replacements of the Amide Bond Connecting the P3 and P2 Sites," *J. Med. Chem.*, 33:838–845.

13 Nicolaides, E. D., F. J. Tinney, J. S. Kaltenbronn, J. T. Repine, D. E. DeJohn, E. A. Lunney, W. H. Roark, J. G. Marriott, R. E. Davis and R. E. Voigtman. 1986. "Modified Di- and Tripeptides of C-Terminal Portion of Oxytocin and Vasopressin as Possible Cognition Activation Agents," *J. Med. Chem.*, 29:959–971.

14 Hangauer, D. G. 1989. "Computer-Aided Design and Evaluation of Angiotensin-Coverting Enzyme Inhibitors," in *Computer-Aided Drug Design (Methods and Applications)*, T. J. Perun and C. L. Propst, eds., New York: Marcel Dekker, Inc., pp. 253–295.

15 Tourwe, D. 1985. "The Synthesis of Peptide Analogs with a Modified Peptide Bond," *Janssen Chim. Acta*, 3:3–15.

16 Weinstock, R. M., J. Keenan, J. Samanen, J. A. Hempel, R. G. Finkelstein, D. E. Franz, G. R. Gaitanopoulos, J. G. Girard, D. T. Gleason, T. M. Hill, C. E. Morgan, N. Peishoff, D. P. Aiyar, T. A. Brooks, E. H. Fredrickson, R. R. Ohlstein, E. J. Ruffolo, Jr., A. C. Stack, E. F. Sulpizio, R. M. Weldley and J. O. Edwards. 1991. "1-(Carboxybenzyl) Imidazole-5-Acrylic Acids: Potent and Selective Angiotensin II Receptor Antagonists," *J. Med. Chem.*, 34:1514–1517.

17 Hruby, V. H. and B. M. Pettitt. 1989. "Conformation Biological Activity Relationships for Receptor-Selective, Conformationally Constrained Opioid Peptides," in *Computer-Aided Drug Design (Methods and Applications)*, T. J. Perun and C. L. Propst, eds., New York: Marcel Dekker, Inc., pp. 405–460.

18 Kessler, H., A. Haupt and M. Will. 1989. "Design of Conformationally Restricted Cyclopeptides for the Inhibition of Cholate Uptake of Hepatocytes," in *Computer-Aided Drug Design (Methods and Applications)*, T. J. Perun and C. L. Propst, eds., New York: Marcel Dekker, Inc., pp. 461–484.

19 Furukawa, Y., S. Kishimoto and K. Nishikawa. Hypotensive Imidazole-5-Acetic Acid Derivatives: US Patent 4355040.

20 Abraham, D. J. 1989. "X-Ray Crystallography and Drug Design," in *Computer-Aided Drug Design (Methods and Applications)*, T. J. Perun and C. L. Propst, eds., New York: Marcel Dekker, Inc., pp. 93–132.

21 Corey, R. B. and L. Pauling. 1953. "Fundamental Dimensions of Polypeptide Chains," *Proc. Roy. Soc. Lond.*, B1412:10–20.

22 Ramachandran, G. N. and C. M. Venkatachalam. 1968. "Stereochemical Criteria

for Polypeptides and Proteins. IV. Standard Dimensions for the cis-Peptide Unit and Conformation of cis-Polypeptides," *Biopolymers*, pp. 1255–1262.

23 Ramachandran, G. N., A. S. Kolaskar, C. Ramakrishnan and V. Sasisekharan. 1974. "Mean Geometry of the Peptide Unit from Crystal Structure Data," *Biochim. Biophys. Acta*, 359:298–302.

24 Benedetti, E. 1977. "Structure and Conformation of Peptides: A Critical Analysis of Crystallographic Data," *Pept. Proc. Am. Pept. Symp.*, *5th*, M. Goodman and J. Meinhofer, eds., New York: John Wiley & Sons, pp. 257–273.

25 Jayati, M. and C. Ramakrishnan. 1981. "Studies on Hydrogen Bonds. Part IV. Proposed Working Criteria for Assessing Qualitative Strength of Hydrogen Bonds," *Int. J. Pept. Prot. Res.*, 17:401–411.

26 Balaji, V. N., M. J. Rao, S. N. Rao, S. W. Dietrich and V. Sasisekharan. 1986. "Geometry of Proline and Hydroxyproline. I: An Analysis of X-Ray Crystal Structure Data," *Biochem. Biophys. Res. Commun.*, 140:895–900.

27 Singh, T. P., P. Narula and H. C. Patel. 1990. "a,b-Dehydro Residues in the Design of Peptide and Protein Structures," *Acta Cryst.*, B46:539–545.

28 Ramnarayan, K. and C. Ramakrishnan. 1987. "Standard Dimensions for cis N-Methyl Peptide Unit and Flexibility of cis Peptide Units," *J. Biosci.*, 12:331–347.

29 McPherson, A. 1989. "Macromolecular Crystals," *Scientific American*, pp. 62–69.

30 Greer, J. 1981. "Comparative Model-Building of the Mammalian Serine Proteases," *J. Mol. Biol.*, 153:1027–1042.

31 Ponder, J. W. and F. M. Richards. 1987. "Tertiary Templates for Proteins. Use of Packing Criteria in the Enumeration of Allowed Sequences for Different Structural Classes," *J. Mol. Biol.*, 193:775–791.

32 Sutcliffe, M. J., F. R. F. Hayes and T. L. Blundell. 1987. "Knowledge Based Modeling of Homologous Proteins. Part II: Rules for the Conformations of Substituted Side Chains," *Protein Engg.*, 1:385–392.

33 Summers, N. L. and M. Karplus. 1989. "Construction of Side-Chains in Homology Modelling. Application to the C-Terminal Lobe of Rhizopuspepsin," *J. Mol. Biol.*, 210:785–811.

34 Correa, P. E. 1990. "The Building of Protein Structures from α-Carbon Coordinates," *Proteins: Struct. Funct. Genet.*, 7:366–377.

35 Geysen, H. M., S. J. Rodda and T. J. Mason. 1986. "The Delineation of Peptides Able to Mimic Assembled Epitopes," *Ciba Foundation Symposium (Synth. Pept. Antigens)*, 119:130–149.

36 Scott, J. K. and G. P. Smith. 1990. "Searching for Peptide Ligands with an Epitope Library," *Science*, 249:386–390.

37 Kessler, H., W. Bermel and A. Muller. 1985. "Modern Nuclear Magnetic Resonance Spectroscopy of Peptides," *Peptides (NY)*, 7:437–473.

38 Opella, S. J. and L. M. Gierasch. 1985. "Solid-State Nuclear Magnetic Resonance of Peptides," *Peptides (NY)*, 7:405–436.

39 Wuthrich, K. 1988. "Three-Dimensional Protein Structures in Solution Viewed by NMR," *NMR Spectroscopy in Drug Research, Alfred Benzon Symposium 1987, Vol. 26*, J. W. Jaroszewski, K. Schaumburg and H. Kofod, eds., Copenhagen: Munksgaard, pp. 194–208.

40 Braun, W., G. Wider, K. H. Lee and K. Wuthrich. 1983. "Conformation of

Glucagon in a Lipid-Water Interphase by Proton Nuclear Magnetic Resonance," *J. Mol. Biol.*, 169:921–948.

41 Brown, L. R., W. Braun, G. Anil-Kumar and K. Wuthrich. 1982. "High Resolution Nuclear Magnetic Resonance Studies of the Conformation and Orientation of Melittin Bound to a Lipid-Water Interface," *Biophys. J.*, 37:319–328.

42 Deber, C. M., M. K. Lutek, E. P. Heimer and A. M. Felix. 1990. "A Possible β-Sheet/β-Turn Structure in Resin-Bound Segments of a Human GRF Analog: Conformational Origin of a Difficult Coupling," *Peptide: Chemistry, Structure and Biology, Proc. Amer. Pept. Symp., 11th, 1989*, J. E. Rivier and G. R. Marshall, eds., Leiden, Netherlands: ESCOM Sci. Pub, pp. 223–225.

43 Lee, K. H., J. E. Fitton and K. Wuthrich. 1987. "Nuclear Magnetic Resonance Investigation of the Conformation of δ-Hemolysin Bound to Dodecylphosphocholine Micelles," *Biochim. Biophys. Acta*, 911:144–153.

44 O'Donnel, T. J. 1989. "Uses of Computer Graphics in Computer-Assisted Drug Design," in *Computer-Aided Drug Design (Methods and Applications)*, T. J. Perun and C. L. Propst, eds., New York: Marcel Dekker, Inc., pp. 19–54.

45 Bolis, G. and J. Greer. 1989. "Role of Computer-Aided Molecular Modeling in the Design of Novel Inhibitors of Renin," in *Computer-Aided Drug Design (Methods and Applications)*, T. J. Perun and C. L. Propst, eds., New York: Marcel Dekker, Inc., pp. 297–326.

46 Ramachandran, G. N. and V. Sasisekharan. 1968. "Conformation of Polypeptides," *Adv. Prot. Chem.*, 23:283–437.

47 Nemethy, G. and H. A. Scheraga. 1977. "Protein Folding," *Quart. Rev. Biophys.*, 10:239–352.

48 Balaji, V. N., K. Ramnarayan and U. C. Singh. 1991. "Simulation of Probable Conformations of Oligopeptides," *Programs and Abstracts, Twelfth American Peptide Symposium, June 16–21, Cambridge, MA*, p. 106.

49 Balaji, V. N., K. Ramnarayan and U. C. Singh. 1991. "Simulation of Probable Conformations of Cyclicpeptides," *Program and Abstracts, Twelfth American Peptide Symposium, June 16–21, Cambridge, MA*, p. 107.

50 Balaji, V. N. Unpublished results.

51 Kohn, H., K. N. Sawhney, P. LeGall, J. D. Conley, D. W. Robertson, J. D. Leander. 1990. "Separation," *J. Med. Chem.*, 33:919–926.

52 Ramakrishnan, C. and K. P. Sarathy. 1968. "Stereochemical Studies on Cyclic Peptides. III. Conformational Analysis of Cyclotetrapeptides," *Biochim. Biophys. Acta*, 168:402–410.

53 Venkatachalam, C. M. 1968. "Stereochemical Studies on Cyclic Peptides. II. Molecular Structure of Cyclotriprolyl," *Biochim. Biophys. Acta*, 168:397–401.

54 Ramakrishnan, C. and B. N. N. Rao. 1980. "Stereochemical Studies on Cyclic Peptides. Part XI. Conformation of Cyclic Pentapeptides Having Intramolecular 3->1 Hydrogen Bonds," *Int. J. Pept. Protein Res.*, 15:81–95.

55 Paul, P. K. C. and C. Ramakrishnan. 1987. "Stereochemical Studies on Cyclic Peptides. XIII. Energy Minimization Studies on Cyclic Hexapeptides Having Hydrogen Bonds," *Int. J. Pept. Protein Res.*, 29:433–454.

56 Paul, P. K. C., P. A. Burney, M. M. Campbell and D. J. Osguthorpe. 1990. "The Conformational Preferences of γ-Lactam and its Role in Constraining Peptide Structure," *Jou. Comput.-Aided Mol. Des.*, 4:239–253.

57 Balaji, V. N. Unpublished data.

58 Singh, U. C., P. K. Weiner, J. W. Caldwell and P. A. Kollman. 1986. *AMBER-Assisted Model Building with Energy Refinement (Version 3.3) Is a Fully Vectorized Version of AMBER (Version 3.0)*, San Francisco: The University of California.

59 Weiner, S. J., P. A. Kollman, D. A. Case, U. C. Singh, C. Ghio, G. Algona, S. Profeta, Jr. and P. Weiner. 1984. "A New Force Field for Molecular Mechanical Simulation of Nucleic Acids and Proteins," *J. Am. Chem. Soc.*, 106:765–784.

60 Singh, U. C. and P. A. Kollman. 1984. "An Approach to Computing Electrostatic Charges of Molecules," *J. Comput. Chem.*, 5:129–145.

61 Singh, U. C. and P. A. Kollman. 1986. *QUEST (Version 1.1)*. San Francisco: University of California.

62 Allen, F. H., S. Bellard, M. D. Brice, B. A. Cartwright, A. Doubleday, H. Higgs, T. Hummelink, B. G. Hummelink-Peters, O. Kennard and W. D. S. Motherwell. 1979. "The Cambridge Crystallographic Data Centre: Computer-Based Search, Retrieval, Analysis and Display of Information," *Acta Crystallogr.*, B35:2331–2339.

63 Cambridge Crystallographic Database System, Cambridge Crystallographic Data Centre, Univ. Chem. Lab., Lensfield Rd., Cambridge CB2 1EW, England, UK.

64 Rusinko, III, A., J. M. Skell, R. Balducci, C. M. McGarity and R. S. Pearlman. 1988. *CONCORD, a Program for the Rapid Generation of High Quality Approximate 3-Dimensional Molecular Structures.* Austin, Texas: The University of Texas at Austin, and St. Louis, Missouri: Tripos Associates.

65 Sheridan, R. P., R. Nilakantan, A. Rusinko, III, N. Bauman, K. S. Haraki and R. Venkataraghavan. 1989. "3DSEARCH, a System for Three-Dimensional Substructure Searching," *J. Chem. Inf. Comput. Sci.*, 29:251–255.

66 Nilakantan, R., N. Bauman and R. Venkataraghavan. 1991. "A Method for Automatic Generation of Novel Chemical Structures and its Potential Applications to Drug Discovery," *J. Chem. Inf. Comput. Sci.*, 31:527–530.

67 Van Drie, J. H., D. Weininger and Y. C. Martin. 1989. "ALADDIN: An Integrated Tool for Computer-Assisted Molecular Design and Pharmacophore Recognition from Geometric, Steric, and Substructure Searching of 3-Dimensional Molecular Structures," *J. Comput.-Aided Mol. Des.*, 3:225–251.

68 Martin, Y. C., M. G. Bures and P. Willett. 1990. "Searching Databases of Three-Dimensional Structures," in *Reviews in Computational Chemistry*, K. B. Lipkowitz and D. B. Boyd, eds., New York: VCH Publishers, Inc., pp. 213–263.

69 Daylight Chemical Information Systems, Inc., P.O. Box 17821, Irvine, CA 92713.

70 MACCS-3D software product from Molecular Design, Ltd., San Leandro, CA 94577.

CHAPTER 3

Bioactive Peptide Design Based on Antibody Structure

JOAN M. VON FELDT[1]
KENNETH E. UGEN[1,2]
THOMAS KIEBER-EMMONS[1,2]
WILLIAM V. WILLIAMS[1,3]

ANTIBODIES: A NATURAL PHARMACOLOGIC MODEL

ANTIBODIES are the molecules of the humoral immune system which possess exquisite specificity and selectivity for millions of antigenic targets in the environment. The landmark studies of Kohler and Milstein [1] allowed the development of monoclonal antibodies and ushered in a new era of molecular biology. Monoclonal antibodies have been developed that have a wide range of biological activities including stimulation [2] and inhibition of cell growth [3,4], binding to specific cell receptors [5–8], modulation of enzyme activity [9,10] as well as enzyme activity itself [11–13]. Despite the tremendous therapeutic potential of monoclonal antibodies and their ease of manufacture, widespread use has been restricted by technologic difficulties. For example, most monoclonal antibodies are of mouse origin, and therefore elicit human immune responses which can neutralize their activity, and which may produce deleterious side effects. The development of human monoclonal antibodies has been hampered by poor hybridoma stability, and low antibody productivity. Additionally, the requirement for parenteral administration and high cost for widespread use further limit monoclonal antibodies as pharmacologic agents [14]. Smaller, less immunogenic compounds (such as short peptides and peptidomimetics) have distinct advantages as pharmacophores. Thus, there are

This work was supported by grants from the NIH and the Lupus Foundation of America.

[1]Department of Medicine, University of Pennsylvania, Philadelphia, PA 19104, U.S.A.
[2]Biotechnology Center, The Wistar Institute, Philadelphia, PA 19104, U.S.A.
[3]Childrens Hospital of Philadelphia, Philadelphia, PA 19104, U.S.A.

obvious biotechnological and therapeutic applications if the specificity of monoclonal antibodies can be translated into peptide design.

Bioactive antibodies can serve as excellent models from which to derive peptide sequences for study. The nature of the antibody binding site has been extensively studied for several decades. These studies indicate that the specificity with which antibodies can target an enzyme or receptor arises from the primary, secondary, and tertiary structure of the antibody binding site. As the structure of many antibody binding sites has been elucidated, peptide modeling from these binding sites is an excellent means for the development of specific pharmacological agents. This chapter will summarize several approaches which utilize the structural information contained within antibody binding sites for peptide design. These all stem from an understanding of the structural aspects of antibody binding.

IMMUNOGLOBULIN GENETICS AND STRUCTURE

THE GENETIC BASIS FOR THE GENERATION OF ANTIBODY DIVERSITY

A tremendous level of antibody diversity is evident by noting that noncovalent peptide binding between small portions of an immunoglobulin molecule and a target receptor can stimulate a diverse cascade of immunologic and biologic phenomena. These antibody proteins generate a sufficient number of combining sites to recognize billions of antigenic shapes encountered in the environment. In order to understand the architecture of antibody combining sites and antibody complementarity, it is useful to appreciate the genetic basis for the generation of antibody diversity. This is aided by the evaluation of large numbers of sequences of light and heavy chains of immunoglobulins of different species. The ability to locate residues in the site-making contact with antigenic determinants and to predict the structures of antibody combining sites depends heavily on such sequence analyses.

Antibody binding to antigenic determinants on a target molecule is dependent on the three-dimensional structure of the combining site and the variability of the amino acids within that site. This variability in amino acid sequence is generated by a number of mechanisms. If the diversity of antibodies were only due to a multiplicity of genes coding for the variable regions of antibodies, the amount of cellular DNA present in mammalian cells would be insufficient to code for the observed number of antibody combining sites. Therefore, genetic mechanisms have evolved to increase diversity without inordinate use of genetic material. Each immunoglobulin molecule is composed of heavy and light chains. The heavy chain can belong to several classes (IgM, IgG, IgA, IgE, IgD), which in turn are comprised of subclasses (i.e., IgG1, IgG2, IgG3, and IgG4). The light chain in turn derives from two classes either x (kappa) or λ (lambda). Since either light chain can combine with any heavy chain, part of the variability of antibody structure is derived from the interaction of these separate polypeptide chains. This phenomenon is known as isotypic variation. When the sequences of light and heavy chains from different antibodies are compared, each chain can also be divided into a constant region and a variable region. The constant regions are identical between antibodies of the same subclass, while the variable regions differ between individual antibodies. Idiotypic variation is a term which refers to the differences between variable regions from different antibodies, and is attributed to hypervariable segments of the antibody binding site. Allotypic variation describes differences in conserved regions which vary between different individuals in a species.

Hypervariable regions within antibody variable regions were described by Kabat and Wu who analyzed the amino acid sequences of many light and heavy chains [15]. When the variable regions from several light chains derived from myeloma proteins were compared, it was clear that the variability in amino acid sequence was concentrated in three different stretches separated by relatively invariant framework regions [15]. These hypervariable regions were postulated to be the areas which made contact with antigen. Three hypervariable segments of the light chain variable region were delineated from a statistical examination of sequences of human V_K and V_L and mouse V_K light chains aligned for maximum homology. The hypervariable regions of light and heavy chains containing certain residues were accessible to affinity labeling [16–23]. These studies suggested that the three light chain hypervariable regions, and the corresponding segments of the heavy chain, were the segments containing the residues which make contact with various antigenic determinants. Subsequently this was verified by x-ray diffraction studies at high resolution. The hypervariable regions are also referred to as complementarity determining regions, or CDRs. (They are also abbreviated hv for hypervariable region). Each light and heavy chain has three CDRs, termed CDR-1_L, CDR-2_L, CDR-3_L; and CDR-1_H, CDR-2_H and CDR-3_H. These assignments are the basis of organization of the CDR regions in the Kabat data base [24].

Framework regions are also present in the variable regions. The framework regions are relatively constant within each variable region family, although there is some variation within each subgroup. These framework regions and the CDR-1 and CDR-2 regions are coded for by the V genes, of which there are a large number (V_1 thru V_n). The CDR-3 regions are coded for by genes that have undergone gene rearrangement. Table 3.1 outlines these segments and their position on the light and heavy chains of immunoglobulin variable regions.

TABLE 3.1. **Organization of Immunoglobulin Variable Regions.**

Segment	Residue Number	
	Light Chain	Heavy Chain
FR1	1–23 (occasionally with a residue at 0, and a deletion at 10 in λ light chains)	1–30 (occasionally with a residue at 0)
CDR1	24–34 (occasionally with up to 6 insertions at position 27)	31–35 (occasionally with up to 2 insertions at position 35)
FR2	35–49	36–49
CDR2	50–56	50–65 (occasionally with up to 3 insertions at position 52)
FR3	57–88	66–94 (occasionally with up to 3 insertions at position 82)
CDR3	89–97 (occasionally with up to 6 insertions at position 95)	95–102 (occasionally with up to 11 insertions at position 100)
FR4	98–107 (occasionally with an insertion at position 106)	103–113

Modified from Reference [24].

The process of immunoglobulin gene rearrangement was first elucidated by Tonegawa [25], and subsequently confirmed by others [26,27]. The immunoglobulins are products of genes organized into three discrete families, each located on a separate chromosome. In man the kappa gene family has been localized to chromosome 2, the lambda chain is to chromosome 22, and the heavy chain locus is on chromosome 14. One of the most valuable insights into the structure and diversity of the immunoglobulin genes was the demonstration that the elements coding for the variable and constant regions of the light and heavy chains were not contiguous on their respective chromosomes. There is a 1500 base pair separation between the V gene (V = variable region) and the C gene (C = constant region). In this intervening stretch there are further codon motifs for the immunoglobulin that multiply its diversity. In the light chain there is an intervening segment of DNA known as the J (J = joining region) segment, and in the heavy chain there is the V, C, J and a D (D = diversity) segment gene. Genetic rearrangement occurs at the level of somatic cell DNA. While the precise mechanism of gene recombination is unknown, specific base sequences that appear to act as joining signals have been identified. On the 3' or downstream side of each V and D segment (i.e., in the direction of the J gene) are found two signal sequences each of which is highly conserved. The first is composed of seven nucleotides, a heptamer CACAGTG (or its analog) followed by a spacer of nonconserved sequence and then a nonamer ACAAAAACC (or its analog). Immediately 5' (or upstream) of all germ line D and J segments are again two signal sequences, first a nonamer and then a heptamer, again separated by an non-conserved sequence, and these are complementary to the heptamer and nonamer motifs downstream from the V and D segments. It is thus presumed that recombination is brought about by a recombinase enzyme containing two DNA binding proteins, that recognize the heptamer and nonamer with the intervening spacers. Such a protein has recently been cloned, [28]. Simplistically, the complementary pairing of the heptamer/nonamer motifs forms a lasso wherein the loop of intervening DNA is flanked by a set of paired heptamers and nonamers which form the knot. Only the main rope is eventually transcribed and translated, and the loop is discarded. The lasso formation and length is somewhat random, so that any given V region can pair with any given D or J region, and this logarithmically increases the diversity of that gene segment. The overall scheme of immunoglobulin gene rearrangement leading to functional messenger RNA encoding intact immunoglobulin chains is schematized in Figure 3.1. To multiply this diversity, there can be imprecision in joining causing variability in subsequent amino acid sequence and in fact, occasionally nonfunctional chains and nonfunctional lymphocytes are formed. Additionally there is evidence of somatic mutation in the V region genes [29-35] resulting in further diversification of the antibody combining site. This appears concentrated in the hypervariable regions. Therefore, there are at least three different methods by which antibody diversity is achieved: a large number of V genes, somatic recombination, and somatic mutation. Each of these contribute to the tremendous accomplishment of creating a selective and specific humoral immunity. This information becomes of great importance when selecting strategies for sequencing the variable regions of interest.

ANTIBODY STRUCTURE

Structural and functional information on antibodies continues to be utilized in the development of molecular probes for many biological systems. Antibodies consist of four polypeptide chains linked together by covalent and noncovalent forces, two light chains and two heavy chains. The two classes of light chains (x and λ) have a molecular weight of 25,000 each and are common to all five classes of immunoglobulins. The light chains consist of two distinct regions: the carboxy terminal half is constant (constant light = C_L) and varies only between immunoglobulin light chain classes; and the amino terminal half (variable light = V_L) which exhibits extensive sequence variability. The heavy chain has a molecular weight of 50,000 to 75,000 and the structure of this chain determines the class or subclass of the immunoglobulin molecule. It also has an amino terminal region of sequence variability (variable heavy = V_H) and a carboxy ter-

IMMUNOGLOBULIN HEAVY CHAIN GENE REARRANGEMENT

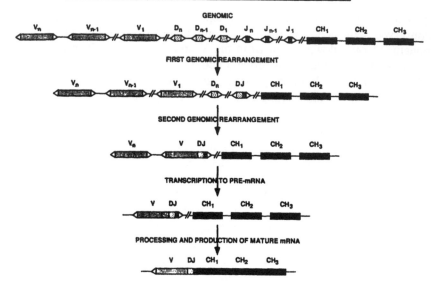

IMMUNOGLOBULIN LIGHT CHAIN GENE REARRANGEMENT

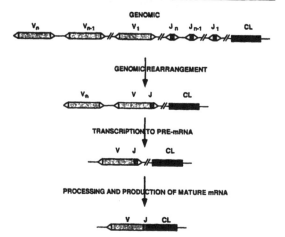

Figure 3.1 Immunoglobulin gene rearrangement—germ line DNA is spliced and arranged to produce a VDJ combination for the heavy chain (top) and a VJ combination for the light chain (bottom). This is transcribed and processed to form a mature VDJC or VJC mRNA, which is in turn translated into the mature protein. The small triangles ($\triangleleft$ $\triangleright$) represent the heptamer/nonamer motif involved in splicing (see text). Introns are represented by straight lines, and exons by rectangles. This method of rearrangement of different gene segments provides the diversity of the antibody molecule, and specificity of its binding site.

minal half that is constant (constant heavy $= C_H$). A proteolytic enzyme (papain) splits IgG into three fragments which retain biologic activity: two Fab (Fab = antigen binding fragment) and one Fc (Fc = crystallizable fragment). Each Fab fragment contains one antigen-combining site consisting of one intact light chain, and the amino terminal half of the heavy chain. The remaining carboxy terminal halves of the two heavy chains, including the inter-heavy chain disulfide bonds (or hinge region) are the Fc fragment, which contains the sites responsible for most biologic functions. These biologic functions include complement fixation, and binding to Fc receptors on host tissue cells, especially phagocytic cells. The relevant regions of antibodies are depicted in Figure 3.2.

The IgG molecule, serving as a prototypic immunoglobulin, has twelve intrachain disulfide bonds, one in each variable and constant region of the light chain and four in each heavy chain. These disulfide bonds, encompassing 60–70 amino acid residues, define the antibody "domains," and these domains possess a striking degree of homology in secondary and tertiary structure. The domains correspond to the V_L and C_L regions of the light chain, and the V_H, C_H1, C_H2, and C_H3 regions of the heavy chain. Variation in the variable domain, especially in the highly variable segments known as hypervariable regions, produce different idiotypes. The term idiotype was first used to describe an antigenic epitope on an antibody that was idiosyncratic to that particular antibody [36,37]. Idiotype, isotype, and allotype (conserved regions which vary between different individuals in a species) were all initially characterized by making antibodies against antibodies (anti-antibodies). It was found that certain epitopes were common between all antibodies of a given class (isotype), varied between different individuals within a species (allotype), or were specific for a given antibody clone (idiotype). Idiotypes are thus a characteristic of the individual antibody clone. The idiotype of an antibody often correlates with binding of the antibodies to unique antigens.

Idiotypes can be further subdivided into idiotopes. This corresponds with the subdivision of an antigen into a collection of epitopes, with an epitope comprising the minimal determinant on an antigen that can be bound by one antibody molecule. An idiotype is similarly a collection of idiotopes. An idiotope is an epitope within an idiotype that is recognized by a single anti-antibody directed against the antibody [38]. Although idiotopes exist throughout the immunoglobulin molecule, the hypervariable region produces unique motifs that can specify a binding site, both chemically and immunologically. The idiotopes that are responsible for binding to a particular antigen are referred to as the paratope. The paratope of an antibody is complementary to the epitope of the antigen bound. It is the idiotype motifs created by the hypervariable regions which comprise the paratope that we will concentrate on in the design of peptides.

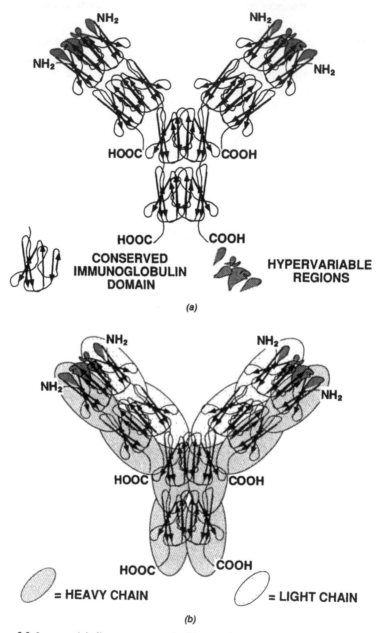

Figure 3.2 Immunoglobulin structure: (a) in this wire frame model the conserved and hypervariable domains of the immunoglobulin variable region are depicted; (b) the shading superimposed on the wire model depicts the portions of the immunoglobulin molecule contributed by the light and heavy chains. (Note: This is an artist's depiction, not an actual antibody structure.)

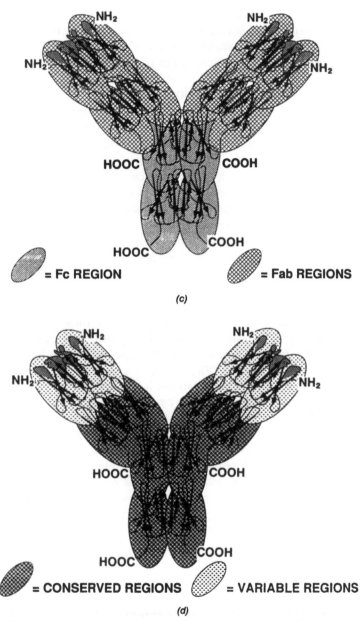

(c)

(d)

Figure 3.2 (continued) Immunoglobulin structure: (c) the cross-hatched Fab fragment contains one antigenic binding site at the amino terminus of the heavy and light chains, and the striped Fc fragment is important for biologic function of the immunoglobulin molecule; (d) the immunoglobulin variable regions are differentially shaded. (Note: This is an artist's depiction, not an actual antibody structure.)

The structure of antibody binding sites is determined by the characteristic folding of the immunoglobulin molecule. Crystallographic studies have confirmed the domain type organization of the IgG molecule previously deduced from amino acid sequence analysis. The domains are ovoid or cylindrical, measuring between 20–40 Å. All domains, regardless of their origin, have essentially the same three-dimensional organization. In each domain, the polypeptide chain is folded in a characteristic way, called the *immunoglobulin fold*. More than 50% of the chain forms short straight stretches that bend in a hairpin fashion. Nearly all the hairpin bends contain glycine, often flanked on the N-terminal side by proline, serine or threonine. The straight strands are organized into two parallel planes: one containing three and the other four straight stretches. These parallel sections are arranged in two layers running in opposite directions (antiparallel β sheets) with many hydrophobic amino acid chains between the layers. The entire arrangement is stabilized by hydrogen bonds between adjacent strands. Within an intact variable region, this folding causes the formation of six loops, three from the light and three from the heavy chain. These loops are often reverse turn stretches and encompass the hypervariable regions which are exposed within these peptide loops (Figures 3.2 and 3.3). The hypervariable regions designated as complementarity determining regions, or CDRs, are involved in binding antigen. The framework regions (FR) are the intervening peptide segments within the peptide loops, adjacent to the hypervariable regions [39].

The overall avidity of an antibody is a measure of antigen:antibody binding strength. This binding depends on the affinity of the epitope:paratope reaction and the effective binding valency. The conformation and chemical composition of the hypervariable loops implicates them as critical in determining antibody specificity and affinity for binding. Studies of antigen:antibody complexes cocrystallized, as well as with synthetic peptides derived from antibody CDRs, confirm that these structures are involved in contacting antigen. The chemical properties of specific amino acids and the tertiary structure of the CDRs are crucial in determining binding selectivity and affinity.

ANTIBODY:ANTIGEN INTERACTIONS

X-ray crystallographic studies have aided in the elucidation of interactions between antibody and antigen. In general, antibody binding sites (paratopes) are topographically described as concave and complementary antigenic sites (epitopes) as predominantly convex. This generalization is gradually being altered as more antigen:antibody complexes are studied by x-ray crystallography. Perhaps a more accurate analogy for the tongue and

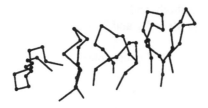

NEWM VARIABLE REGION COMBINED CDRs

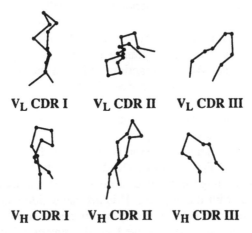

V_L CDR I V_L CDR II V_L CDR III

V_H CDR I V_H CDR II V_H CDR III

Figure 3.3 Immunoglobulin fold—the amino terminus of the immunoglobulin molecule has a characteristic pattern of folding that forms six loops, three each from the heavy and light chains. It is within these loops that antigenic binding occurs. An artist's depiction of the alpha carbon backbone of the immunoglobulin NEWM [80] is shown (top), with the structure of each individual hypervariable loop shown below.

groove interactions of the amino acid side chains would be the perfect fit of a set of upper and lower molars in a closed bite.

An antibody specific for a protein antigen binds noncovalently to a region of the protein surface that is antigenic. A crystallographic study of a lysozyme:antibody interaction [40] showed the epitope area to be 2–3 nanometers in size, confirming previous deductions that about six amino acids or monosaccharide units can fit into the antibody binding site. High resolution crystallography revealed that contact between the lysozyme and the Fab fragment of monoclonal antilysozyme D1.3 occurs on a rather flat surface with the interactions largely due to protuberances and depressions formed by the amino acid side chains, producing a tightly packed region of interaction. The epitope on the lysozyme molecule involves two non-contiguous areas, residues 18–27 and 116–119 of its polypeptide chain [40].

All six CDRs of the antibody and two residues outside the CDRs but adjacent to the CDRs, (Tyr 49 in V_L and Thr 30 in V_H) make contact with the lysozyme.

The crystal structure of the complex hen egg white lysozyme and another monoclonal Fab, derived from the antilysozyme antibody HyHEL-10, was determined to a resolution of 3 Å [10]. The combining site of the antibody is mostly flat, with a protuberance made of two tyrosines that penetrate the cleft. The lysozyme epitope crosses the active site cleft including a tryptophan that penetrates the cleft. It consists of the exposed residues of an α-helix together with surrounding amino acids. The contacting residues on the antibody contain a disproportionate number of aromatic side chains. The antibody:antigen contact mainly involves hydrogen bonds and van der Waals interactions. Most of the contact residues of the lysozyme epitope are polar and five of them are charged. The surface of HyHEL-10 that interacts with lysozyme is unusual in that it is not noticeably concave and contains no pronounced grooves or cavities. On the contrary, the surface has a large protrusion which fits into the active site cleft of the lysozyme. This protrusion is formed by the side chains of Tyr-33 from CDR-1_H and Tyr-53 from CDR-2_H. The interacting surface of the antibody contains a large number of aromatic side chains that point outward and interact with the antigen. This aromatic side chain phenomena has been observed with the previously mentioned monoclonal antibodies D1.3, the antibody McPc603, as well as the presumed binding site of another member of the immunoglobulin supergene family, the human class 1 major histocompatibility antigen A2. The complementarity of the contacting surfaces of HyHEL-10 and the lysozyme is so great that there are no cavities in the interface large enough to add a water molecule. The contact of the two proteins consist of polar and apolar interactions; of the 126 pairwise atomic contacts, 111 are van der Waals and 14 are hydrogen bonding [10]. These crystallographic studies help us in designing peptides based on these antibody:antigen interactions. They emphasize the presumption that the side chain functional group orientations may be more important than backbone geometry. From the backbone figures however, strategies of design could evolve. Figure 3.4 (see insert) depicts the lysozyme-antilysozyme complex, showing the region of interaction. In the backbone wire frame model the protruding CDRs appear as simple loops that with few modifications could be designed into ideal peptides for inhibition of the active site of the molecule.

More recently, the crystallographically determined structure of an antibody with a synthetic peptide has been reported [41]. The antigen was a synthetic 19 amino acid peptide homolog of the C helix of myohemerythrin (Mhr). This study was important not only because a synthetic peptide was utilized, but also because comparison could be made between the crystallographic structure of the peptide epitope in its native form ver-

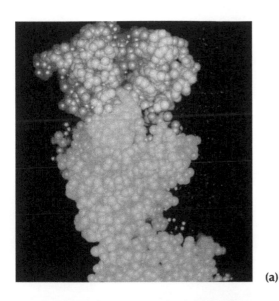

(a)

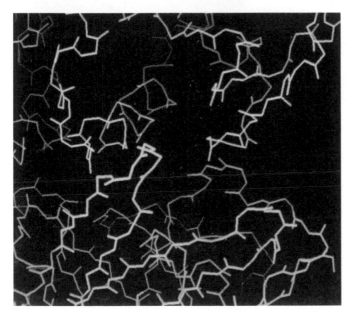

(b)

FIGURE 3.4 Antibody antigen interactions at the binding site — interaction of Fab fragment of HyHEL-10 with its antigenic target, hen egg lysozyme. (a) Space-filling model of HyHEL-10 (green) demonstrating the protrusion of the CDR2 (blue) and CDRI (red) into the active site cleft of the lysozyme (purple). In the space-filling model, the side chains are depicted, and the penetrance of the tyrosine of CDR2 into the cleft of the lysozyme is evident. (b) Demonstrates the backbone structure of the CDRs in a wire frame model (same color codes). In this depiction, the CDRs appear as simple loops upon which peptide modelling could be performed.

sus its complexed form. Interestingly, the peptide underwent a conformational change when binding with the monoclonal antibody. Five of the six CDRs of the Fab' fragment were found to contact with the peptide. The free and peptide bound Fab' structures share the same immunoglobulin fold found in all known Fab' structures. The Fab' amino acid residues directly involved in hydrogen bonding or charge:charge interactions with the peptide came from the CDR's as well as from the framework regions. The buried surface area on the Fab' is 540 Å^2 and the peptide buried surface covers 460 Å^2, an indication that the surfaces are highly complementary, although the fit is not exact. The binding pocket includes a large percentage of hydrophobic residues. While no major changes were seen in the antibody structure, there were small but significant side chain and main chain rearrangements to produce the binding mode. The amino-terminal portion of the peptide sequence (NH$_2$-Glu-Val-Val-Pro-His-Lys-Lys) adopts a well defined type 2 β turn in the concave antigen pocket. This same peptide amino acid sequence in native myohemerythrin is α-helical.

Although the peptide conformation that is recognized by the antibody differs from that in the native protein, the antibody binds to the peptide in a well-defined secondary structure found in proteins. Immunologic mapping had previously identified this sequence as the peptide epitope, and its fine specificity correlated well with the structural analysis. Since the peptide conformation when bound to the monoclonal antibody Fab fragment is inconsistent with binding of the Fab to native Mhr, this may suggest that binding can only occur to conformationally altered forms of the Mhr. Efforts are now in progress to cocrystallize the antibody while bound to native Mhr to elucidate this point.

These crystallographic studies on the surface are daunting with regard to the prospects for peptide design based on antibody variable region structure. However, on closer inspection several points indicate the feasibility of this approach. The generalization that antibody binding surfaces are concave would seem to prohibit peptide design based on a single region of the surface. However, this is not invariably the case as demonstrated by Padlan's studies [10]. Their studies of the binding of an antibody to the active site of an enzyme may resemble the binding of an antibody to the active site of a receptor. This suggests that convex surfaces can be adapted by antibodies, and when the site bound is concave, the complementary antibody surface may adopt a convex configuration. In general, a large surface area (about 400 Å^2) is involved in the contacting surfaces. This suggests that large surfaces must come in opposition for adequate binding energies to develop. However, in some instances energetically important contacts stemming from one or two CDRs can be identified. Thus, for appropriately selected antibodies, peptide design to develop bioactive analogs is possible. Specific strategies are outlined in the following sections.

STRATEGIES FOR ANTIBODY-BASED PEPTIDE DESIGN

SELECTING A MONOCLONAL ANTIBODY FOR PEPTIDE SEQUENCE ANALYSIS

Monoclonal antibodies have been developed that evidence a wide range of biological activities. These range from stimulation or inhibition of cell growth [3,4,42], binding to specific receptors [2,8,43], modulating enzyme activity [9,44], and possessing enzyme activity [11–13]. In selecting a monoclonal antibody for peptide design, a biologically or enzymatically active antibody would be desirable. Activity can be demonstrated by interference with enzyme activity, such as preventing proteolytic degradation by a site-specific protease, inhibition of metabolic conversion of a precursor molecule to its final form, or inhibition of a biosynthetic pathway. For an anti-receptor antibody, inhibition of ligand binding in a competitive binding assay is a relatively straightforward method. Alternatively, a monoclonal antibody that binds a receptor or its ligand and modulates cellular activity in functional assays would also be a candidate for hypervariable loop analysis. Two examples will be described further, the monoclonal antibody 87.92.6 that binds to the reovirus type 3 receptor on a number of cell types [45], and a monoclonal antibody PAC1, which binds to the platelet fibrinogen receptor [5].

In characterizing the monoclonal antibody 87.92.6, this antibody was developed to bind reovirus type 3 receptors on cells [46–49], and is able to competitively inhibit binding of reovirus type 3 particles to these cells [50,51]. 87.92.6 was also found to inhibit DNA synthesis in fibroblasts, neuronal cells, and lymphocytes [50–52]. These effects mimic the biological properties of reovirus type 3, as well as replication defective reovirus particles (i.e., virions that are not competent to infect) suggesting that these effects are due to binding of a common receptor.

Similarly, the monoclonal antibody PAC1 was selected for sequencing. This antibody binds to the platelet fibrinogen receptor, inhibits fibrinogen binding, and blocks fibrinogen-induced platelet aggregation [5]. These two antibodies have been successfully utilized for the development of biologically active peptides.

SEQUENCING THE HYPERVARIABLE REGION OF THE MONOCLONAL OF INTEREST

Several strategies exist for determining hv sequences. The first V regions sequenced were by enzyme degradation of purified myeloma proteins [15]. Subsequently, cDNA cloning and sequencing methods became available and were broadly utilized [53]. Currently, DNA amplification utilizing the polymerase chain reaction is the technique of choice for cloning V regions and sequencing is by the Sanger method [54].

The ability to amplify specific segments of DNA has been made possible by the polymerase chain reaction (PCR). PCR is an *in vitro* method for the enzymatic synthesis of specific DNA sequences, using two oligonucleotide primers that hybridize to opposite strands and flank the region of interest in the target DNA. A sequential and repetitive series of cycles involving template denaturation, primer annealing and the extension of the annealed primers by DNA polymerase results in the exponential accumulation of the specific fragment whose termini are defined by the five prime ends of the primers. Since the primer extension products synthesized in one cycle can serve as a template in the next, the number of target DNA copies approximately doubles at every cycle. Therefore, twenty cycles of PCR yields about a million fold amplification. Initially, PCR used the Klenow fragment of *E. coli* DNA polymerase I to extend the annealed primers. This enzyme was inactivated by the high temperature required to separate the two DNA strands at the outset of each synthetic cycle. The introduction of the thermostable DNA polymerase (Taq polymerase) isolated from *Thermus aquaticus* solved this problem, allowing the PCR reaction to become automated by a thermal cycling device.

Utilizing PCR to amplify and sequence variable domains of murine immunoglobulins is the most efficient way to sequence a particular monoclonal antibody of interest. This has now been done by a number of research investigators. As an example, Winter's group cloned and sequenced the variable domains of five hybridoma antibodies [55]. The first step was to identify conserved regions at each end of the nucleotide sequences encoding V domains of murine immunoglobulin heavy chain (V_H) and K light chains (V_K). This was done using the Kabat data base [24]. The amplification primers were selected on the basis of a computer program that calculated the frequency of the most common nucleotide by a score for each site. The cDNA was then amplified and cloned, and the amplified cDNA was expressed in vectors. These vectors were bacterial phages that carried the immunoglobulin heavy chain gene promoter, signal sequence and leader peptide. They were then able to express the cloned, variable region gene as a chimeric mouse-human antibody that bound to a human mammary carcinoma cell line.

This technique also can be applied to cloning isolated variable domains. Once these isolated single domains are incorporated into a vector that expresses them joined to an immunoglobulin heavy chain, a single domain immunoglobulin protein is produced. These have been coined "dAbs" (single domain antibodies), and they can compete with monoclonal antibodies for binding in selected biologic systems [56]. Peptide sequences may be more easily derived from biologically active dAbs, as they can employ a single variable region with three (versus six) CDRs. However, this awaits demonstration.

Once the sequence of the variable region is known, and the isotype of the immunoglobulin has been determined, the subgroup of the variable region light chain and heavy chain sequences can be deduced. This is done by comparing framework and CDR regions and looking for homology between the amino acids of the subgroups published in the Kabat data base [24] and the monoclonal of interest.

SELECTING A PEPTIDE FROM THE SEQUENCED HYPERVARIABLE REGION

In selecting a peptide from the traditional hypervariable amino acid sequences (not dAbs), several strategies can be used. To select and test peptides based on all six hypervariable loops can be costly and time consuming, but with improvements in peptide synthesis this remains a viable strategy. Clues that could focus the selection and subsequent testing of the various peptides can be sought by evaluating the amino acid sequences of the domains, and concentrating on the loops that appear to be the most likely key loops, based on secondary and tertiary structure.

If the monoclonal antibody mimics a specific biologic entity (such as a receptor ligand), then the sequences of the six hypervariable loops of the monoclonal can be compared with the sequence of the ligand, and the CDR that evidences the most sequence similarity with the ligand can be determined. As an example, in the reovirus system previously described, the molecule that was suspected of initiating binding of reovirus particles to target cells was the reovirus type 3 hemagglutinin. Therefore after the amino acid sequences of V_H and V_L of the monoclonal antibody 87.92.6 were deduced, a computer analysis was utilized that compared the hemagglutinin of reovirus type 3 (HA3) to these hypervariable regions [57]. Sequence similarity was found between the amino acids 317–332 of the HA3 and a combined determinant composed of the second complementarity determining regions (CDR2s) of both V_H and V_L. Therefore, these sequences were used to develop peptides [45]. Similarly, for the monoclonal antibody PAC-1 directed to the platelet fibrinogen receptor, the hypervariable region sequences were compared to fibrinogen, the biologic substance that binds to the platelet fibrinogen receptor. Five of the six CDRs demonstrated no regions of significant sequence similarity to fibrinogen. However, the CDR3 of the PAC1 heavy chain contained a sequence Arg-Tyr-Asp Thr that if present in proper conformation could behave like Arg-Gly-Asp Ser which was present in the fibrinogen Aμ-chain and felt to be the sequence mediating binding to the platelet fibrinogen receptor. This information was also utilized to design peptides with specific receptor binding properties [5].

The reovirus system just described, utilized anti-receptor antibodies which were also anti-idiotypes. Specifically, 87.92.6 binds to both the reovirus type 3 receptor and a neutralizing monoclonal antibody 9B.G5, and is anti-idiotypic to 9B.G5 [50,51] (see Figure 3.5 for interactions). An anti-idiotypic antibody that binds to the paratope of the idiotype, thereby mimicking the original antigen, is often referred to as an "internal image" anti-idiotype. A paratope is an antigen binding site. While peptide design

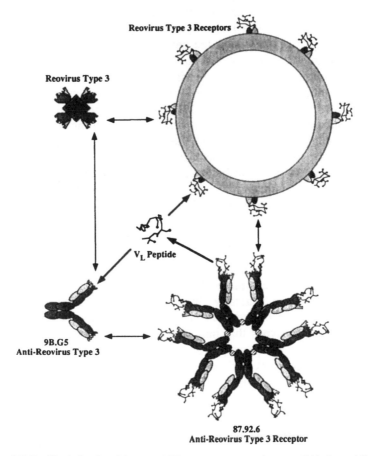

Figure 3.5 Peptide design based in an anti-idiotype system – reovirus type 3 binds to sialic acid residues on cell membrane receptors [81,82]. This binding is inhibited by monoclonal antibody 9B.G5 [83]. An anti-idiotype (87.92.6) raised against 9B.G5 also binds to reovirus receptors [50, 51]. The hypervariable region 2 of the 87.92.6 light chain was predicted to interact with the reovirus receptor [57]. A peptide derived from this sequence (V_L peptide) binds to 9B.G5, and the reovirus type 3 receptor on cells [45,58,70].

in these systems does not depend on anti-idiotypic mimicry, the principles involved in idiotype:anti-idiotype interactions are useful to consider as they illustrate potential binding interactions implicit in the design process. These principles are reviewed in the following section.

THE USE OF ANTI-IDIOTYPES AS MODELS OF RECEPTOR:LIGAND INTERACTIONS

The network hypothesis of Jerne [36] offers us the use of antibodies as antigens themselves. By analogy, antibodies can serve as both ligands and receptors. Anti-idiotypes can be developed by immunizing animals with antibodies that have been raised against a specific antigen. These anti-idiotypes may therefore mimic the antigen, and the mimicry is typically localized to the variable regions of the immunoglobulin. Each unique configuration within the idiotype comprises an idiotope. It has been possible to develop anti-idiotypic antibodies in several systems which simulate the properties of the original antigen [38,58]. The hypervariable loops of a monoclonal antibody not only create the antigen binding site, but can also be the antigenic surfaces involved in developing anti-idiotypes. Thus there is considerable overlap in the definition of antibody recognition sites and idiotypic sites. Antigens which have been used to develop anti-idiotypes include chemical haptens [59–62], carbohydrates [63,64], and proteins [6,7,46,65–70]. Anti-idiotypic antibodies that mimic antigen are said to bear the "internal image" of the antigen. While most of the idiotypic sites of an antibody reside within the hypervariable regions, some idiotypic sites have been predicted to include residues within framework regions. This suggests that a distinction may be made between the hypervariable regions per se and the complementarity determining regions [38].

Anti-idiotypes are generally characterized by their ability to bind a specific antibody in a manner unrelated to the isotype and allotype of the antibody. Anti-idiotypes that inhibit antigen binding to the idiotype are said to recognize the paratope, or antigen binding site. When an anti-idiotype does not block antigen binding, it does not recognize the paratope, but instead binds a distinct idiotope. If antigen binding is blocked by the anti-idiotype, it does not necessarily imply that the anti-idiotype binds in the same manner or even to the same site the antigen binds. Thus, if an anti-idiotype binds to an idiotope on a site near or overlapping with the same site the antigen binds, it may block antigen binding but not completely mimic the antigen. While such an anti-idiotype may have unique chemical properties, it may not utilize the same intermolecular attractive forces that are used by the antigen. Figure 3.5 illustrates the way that an anti-idiotype can bind to the hypervariable region of the antibody. To establish that an anti-idiotype mimics the same binding interactions as the antigen, binding to additional molecular structures is investigated.

The determination of secondary and tertiary structure of the hypervariable regions of an immunoglobulin can be of tremendous assistance in selecting a peptide for study. In considering different models of antibody structure, Chothia et al. [72] describe a canonical structure model presuming that antibodies have only a few main chain conformations for each hypervariable region and that sequence variations only modify the surface provided by the side chains on a main chain structure. Data to support this theory include conserved residues within certain sets of hypervariable regions, and experimental evidence showing that some of the hypervariable regions in immunoglobulins of known structure have the same central chain conformation despite several differences in sequence. Chothia was able to identify residues primarily responsible for central chain conformation by evaluation of packing, hydrogen bonding, and ability to assume unusual values of the torsion angles, ϕ, φ, ω, in the structures of the then known hypervariable regions. Extending this concept further, once the hypervariable region of interest is identified, the tertiary structure can be predicted. The peptide selected could then be designed to predictably fold in a conformation similar to that of the presumed architecture of the hypervariable region being studied.

Computer modelling has made this task easier. Using hydrophilicity, surface probability, chain flexibility scores, and antigenicity indices, software packages can help predict the secondary structure of specific peptide sequences [73,74]. Such structural analyses can be performed on the variable region of interest, and subsequently on proposed peptides. The analyses for the peptides can then be compared to the original antibody molecule to assure structural consistency.

SPECIFIC DESIGN PRINCIPLES

Once the CDRs to be evaluated are identified, it is often tempting to synthesize only the region of interest, excluding regions that do not play a role as contact residues. However, it needs to be emphasized that several factors are important for binding interactions to occur. Chief among these is the ability to orient the contact residues in a "binding mode," whereby they will be geometrically positioned in a manner complementary to the receptor bound. The shorter a peptide sequence, the less likely it is to fold into an ordered secondary structure. This makes it energetically costly to assume the binding mode, thereby decreasing the net binding energy. In addition, side chain interactions with neighboring amino acids can be important in orienting contact residues in a favorable geometry. Thus, initial peptide synthesis should employ a sufficient number of residues to preserve some of these interactions.

In the reovirus system, a specific region of sequence similarity was identified [57]. The region of most significant homology was contained within a 9 amino acid sequence, matching the V_L CDR2 and amino acids 323–332 of the hemagglutinin. The entire CDR was synthesized, as opposed to the regions of sequence similarity alone, as these were more likely to fold into a three-dimensional structure similar to that present in the variable region. While this peptide had activity in multiple assays, the binding affinity was quite low (μM range) [45]. When peptides comprising only the region of sequence similarity were evaluated, the affinity was even lower, and these failed to work at all in several assays [71]. However, when cyclic peptides were developed in an effort to stabilize the binding mode conformation, the affinity was markedly improved [58]. When substitutions were made in the peptide sequences, some were found to lower affinity while others improved affinity [71]. This suggests that multiple interactions need to be assessed in the design process.

In the example of the reovirus system described above, monoclonal antibody 9B.G5 was used as the antigen to which 87.92.6 was raised. This monoclonal antibody (87.92.6) was shown to be the internal image antibody by showing that it recognized the receptor, down modulated the receptor and mimicked the reovirus HA3 by inhibiting cellular proliferation [46,47,50,51]. It was from these anti-idiotypic antibody hypervariable loops that the peptides described above were derived.

The ability of antibodies to serve as both idiotypes and anti-idiotypes has been exploited to investigate many receptor:ligand interactions (reviewed in Reference [67]). These studies confirm the ability of antibodies to uniquely mimic both a given receptor and the ligand for the receptor. Since antibodies are all derived from similar structural motifs, this suggests that antibody shape is quite adaptable to the binding constraints implicit in receptor:ligand interactions. Binding trajectory may play a role, as this is a characteristic of the particular surface of the antibody recognized. The trajectory of the interaction takes into account not only secondary structure of the binding site but the "angle of approach" at which the interaction occurs (see Figure 3.6). As an example, if a variable region is comprised of six hypervariable loops, and these combine to form a relatively flat or concave surface, the "corner" of the flat surface may still have the characteristics of a convex, or even a protuberant surface. Binding to such a site by an anti-idiotype can be easily visualized. In addition, a certain degree of deformability may be present within a variable region upon antigen:antibody binding. By considering idiotype:anti-idiotype interactions and visualizing the possible trajectories and surfaces involved, the versatility of antibody binding can be understood. Such considerations have contributed to the development of peptide design based on antibody structural analysis. By seeking amino acid sequence similarity between antigens and anti-idiotypes, critical contact residues for binding to the idiotype have been identified (reviewed in Reference [71]). The relatively few amino acids typically identified in such interactions led to the initial

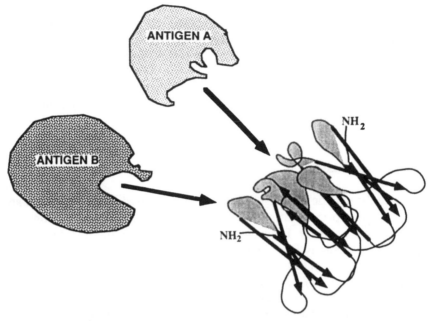

Figure 3.6 Binding trajectories to antibody variable regions – peptide design depends on the binding trajectory of the antigen:antibody interaction. In some antigen:antibody interactions, the antigen binds to a relatively flat surface (i.e., the HyHEL-5-lysozyme complex [40]), making peptide design conceptually more difficult. Other antigens which bind to the "edge" of the variable region (i.e., the HyHEL-10-lysozyme complex [10]), recognize a reverse turn structure, facilitating peptide design.

use of peptides derived from such sequences as binding moieties. By exploiting similar observations made in the study of anti-idiotype mimics of receptor ligands, receptor binding peptides were subsequently derived.

THE USE OF COMPUTER MODELING TO PREDICT THE BIOACTIVE PEPTIDE

While amino acid sequence similarity between an antibody and a ligand or a substrate can help identify contact residues critical for peptide design, such analyses are not always available. Another way of selecting a peptide is to predict ligand receptor interactions. If the receptor is known, the CDR regions can be evaluated on the basis of likely amino acids that would bind with the receptor site. Again using the reovirus system as an example, the suspected receptor for the hemagglutinin of reovirus type 3 on some cells is sialic acid. The peptide which bound the receptor was chosen from the V_L CDR2 of the monoclonal antibody 87.92.6. This hypervariable region could have been predicted to be the one responsible for binding the reovirus receptor, sialic acid, by analysis for complementarity. When evaluated in tertiary structure, there is comfortable and tight hydrogen bonding between spatially compatible amino acid side chains of the V_L CDR2 of 87.92.6 and hydroxy, amino, and carboxy groups of the sialic acid moiety [71]. With currently available biocomputational capabilities, this site could be predicted based on complementarity analysis of each hypervariable region.

PEPTIDE EVALUATION

Once the peptide has been defined and synthesized it is necessary to apply the same principles in evaluating its bioactivity as in evaluating the monoclonal antibody. However, one must keep in mind that an isolated peptide (particularly in the initial stages of the design process) will likely have lower affinity than the intact antibody from which it was derived. Thus, failure on any one assay might be anticipated, and multiple assays for binding and/or activity are preferable. In addition, assay conditions can be adjusted to favor detection of peptide binding by lowering the stringency of buffers, adjusting incubation times, etc. With these caveats in mind, the peptide should demonstrate the ability to mimic the monoclonal antibody from which it was derived. For example, binding to the antigen on solid phase assays may be demonstrable, but may require protracted incubation periods and mild washing conditions. Appropriate controls are essential to rule out nonspecific binding. A more sensitive assay is to test the ability of the peptide to successfully inhibit binding of the monoclonal antibody (from which it was derived) to the antigen in a competitive inhibition assay. This typically allows pre-incubation with the peptide, providing an opportunity for folding into a binding conformation. Once pre-bound, inhibition of subsequent binding by a second ligand (such as the parent monoclonal antibody) is more likely to be detected. If the parent monoclonal antibody inhibits enzymatic activity, modulation of enzyme function by the peptide might be demonstrable. Similarly, if the parent monoclonal binds a cellular receptor, thereby altering cellular physiology, the peptide may either reproduce this effect or inhibit the effect of the monoclonal by competing for binding to the receptor.

Peptides derived from the variable region of an anti-idiotypic antibody have additional assays available for evaluation. For example, the peptide should inhibit binding of the anti-idiotypic antibody to the idiotypic monoclonal antibody to which the anti-idiotypic antibody was raised. Additionally, since the anti-idiotype may mimic the original antigen, the peptide should inhibit binding of the antigen to the idiotypic monoclonal antibody. Again in the reovirus system described, peptides were developed based on the sequences of two hypervariable loops (Figure 3.5). The peptides that were selected were synthesized by solid phase synthetic techniques, using a model 430A Applied Biosystems peptide synthesizer, (Applied Biosystems, Foster City, CA) and called V_H and V_L peptides. These peptides were utilized in a series of experiments to determine their ability to bind and interact with the reovirus type 3 receptor. A complex peptide was also formed by coupling V_H to V_L peptide using amino-terminal cysteine residues. Interactions with the monoclonal antibody 9B.G5 (which is bound by 87.92.6 and reovirus type 3 similarly to the reovirus type 3 receptor) were exploited, with 9B.G5 serving as a surrogate reovirus type 3 receptor. Both V_L peptide and the coupled V_H-V_L peptide were found to be bound specifically by 9B.G5 [45]. V_H peptide alone and several other control peptides were not bound by 9B.G5. V_L and the complex V_H-V_L peptides were able to inhibit the interactions of 9B.G5 with both the reovirus type 3 and 87.92.6. Binding of V_L peptide to the reovirus type 3 receptor was evidenced by its ability to inhibit binding of both reovirus type 3 and 87.92.6 to cells [45,75–77]. This data supported the hypothesis that V_L CDR2 of 87.92.6 mimicked the epitope of the reovirus HA3 that bound to the monoclonal Ab 9B.G5 and represents an important site of receptor interaction.

In addition to evaluating peptide binding it would be useful to evaluate the ability of the peptide to be used as an immunogen. This can provide information independent of the function of the peptide alone. For example, the ability of a peptide to elicit antibodies that also bind the native protein supports the ability of the peptide to fold into a conformation similar to that present in the native protein. The antibodies that recognize such a cross-reactive determinant can be utilized in additional assays to determine their biological activity, or ability to block the activity of the original antigen. In the reovirus system immunization of BALB/c mice with V_L peptide coupled to a protein carrier elicited antibodies which bound specifically to reovirus type 3 and neutralized reovirus type 3 reactivity in a serotype specific manner. Interestingly, the peptide derived from the corresponding region of the reovirus type 3 hemagglutinin was an effective immunogen by itself, but free V_L peptide was unable to elicit antibodies unless linked to a carrier protein. This phenomenon is a common property of immune responses to short peptides. The development of an immune response that mimics immunization with whole antigen may provide useful information in further stages of peptide design.

If the monoclonal antibody from which the peptide was derived has bioactivity, it would be useful to demonstrate reproduction of this activity with a peptide, or inhibition of the parent antibody's activity by the peptide. For example if there is a bioassay that demonstrates monoclonal antibody stimulation of cellular proliferation, the inhibition of such mono-clonal antibody induced proliferation in the presence of the peptide would be useful in demonstrating bioactivity. If a stimulatory peptide is desired, additional modifications may be necessary to alter the state of aggregation of the peptide, or to add additional functional groups.

REDESIGNING THE PEPTIDE TO ENHANCE ACTIVITY

In the initial peptide design phase, linear peptides corresponding exactly to the sequences of individual CDRs are typically evaluated. Once these results are known, the peptide may be redesigned to enhance activity. This may occur in several cycles, employing several strategies. Both the shape and chemical composition of the peptides can be altered to produce specific effects. Each phase of redesign should lead to retesting and further refinement. By repeating the cycle of redesign and retesting for several iterations, peptide ligands with high affinity and specificity may eventually be produced.

One of the initial modifications often evaluated is the minimal length of peptide sequence necessary for binding/activity. Peptides of decreasing length are synthesized and tested. This helps in the identification of critical contact residues, as well as providing information relevant to the geometry of the binding conformation. While in many systems very short peptides are effective (i.e., the Arg Gly Asp Ser (RGDS) peptides which are impor-tant in adhesion phenomena), in others a longer peptide is needed for ac-tivity. In some studies, peptides less than 10 amino acids in length were unable to bind effectively, with optimal binding seen only for much longer (17 residue) peptides [71]. This needs to be assessed for each system and peptide sequence.

While peptide length provides some information regarding active site residues, the identification of the contact residues should be evaluated by several strategies. Deletion mutants, wherein single amino acid deletions are made throughout the peptide sequence, may help delineate the contact residues in a crude fashion [78]. However, deletions may alter local sec-ondary structure so that residues adjacent to the contact residues may be incorrectly identified as contact residues. Another approach is to use con-servative substitutions of suspected contact residues. This may include "alanine scans" where alanine is systematically substituted for each suspected contact residue. This method preserves the secondary structure of the peptide, and does not introduce side chains that may alter conforma-tion. Other more conservative substitutions such as phenylalanine for tyro-sine, glutamine or asparginine for the corresponding carboxylic acids, or serine for cysteine can also provide important information by altering the side chains without greatly affecting the peptide conformation. These approaches have been utilized to develop peptides with both enhanced and reduced activity [5,58,71,79]. The nature of such substitutions provides insights into critical intermolecular contacts.

Conformational issues can still confound the analysis of even the most conservative amino acid substitutions. This issue may be addressed by conformationally stabilizing the peptides with disulfide bridges. Hypervariable region-derived peptides are particularly suited to this approach, as in the native antibody structure they typically fold into reverse turns. By constraining the peptide shapes with disulfide bridges, a similar reverse turn geometry can be obtained. This should enhance the affinity of the peptide, and stabilize the shape so that the effect of substitutions on conformation may be minimized. This approach was utilized in the reovirus system with an optimal geometry arrived at through the use of several different constrained peptides [58]. The optimal cyclic peptide was ~40 fold higher in affinity than the linear peptide from which it was derived. This raises the potential to derive high affinity binding peptides by similar cyclic designs. The clinical use of cyclic peptides such as cyclosporin and gramicidin suggests that peptides designed in this fashion may be derived.

SUMMARY

Biologically active peptides have been developed in several systems based on analysis of the active sites of biomolecules. In order to develop such biologically active peptides, the active site of the biomolecule under consideration must be known. Antibodies which possess biological activity are uniquely suited to the definition of their active site structures, as the hypervariable regions are known to contain the major binding determinants. A strategy has been developed to utilize the primary structural information contained in the amino acid sequences of antibody hypervariable regions to develop biologically active peptides. This strategy depends on the availability of biologically active monoclonal or recombinant antibodies with well characterized binding characteristics. Through analysis of the hypervariable region sequences, potential contact residues are identified. Synthetic peptides are designed based on this information which are likely to fold into conformations similar to that of the native antibody. The peptides are evaluated for their binding characteristics and biological activity. This information is subsequently utilized to redesign the peptides, allowing more precise analysis of the contact residues and optimal conformations for binding.

This strategy has been applied to several anti-receptor antibodies to date. Peptides have been developed which inhibit viral binding and platelet aggregation. Enzyme inhibitors and other biologically active peptides can be developed by these techniques. With progress in antibody technology, biologically active antibodies will continue to be developed. Crystallographic analysis has elucidated the structure of many antibodies and several antigen:antibody complexes. This facilitates structural analysis of new antibody variable regions. Structural information contained in the variable regions of these antibodies should be useful for peptide design in many systems. This technology offers a direct strategy for developing bioactive peptides, as well as starting geometries which can be utilized for the development of peptidomimetic drugs.

ACKNOWLEDGEMENTS

We would like to thank C. E. Laine and J. Leo for their helpful comments. This work was supported by an NIH First Award, and grants from the Lupus Foundations of Philadelphia and Pennsylvania, and the Center for the Study of Aging to William V. Williams; a Foundation for AIDS Research Scholars award to Kenneth E. Ugen; a grant from the American Foundation for AIDS Research to Thomas Kieber-Emmons; and an NIH post-doctoral fellowship to Joan M. Von Feldt.

REFERENCES

1 Kohler, G. and C. Milstein. 1975. "Continuous Cultures of Fused Cells Secreting Antibody of Predefined Specificity," *Nature*, 256:52.

2 Yarden, Y. 1990. "Agonistic Antibodies Stimulate the Kinase Encoded by the Neu Protooncogene in Living Cells but the Oncogenic Mutant Is Constitutively Active," *Proc. Natl. Acad. Sci. USA*, 87:2569.

3 Drebin, J. A., D. F. Stern, V. C. Link, R. A. Weinberg and M. I. Greene. 1984. "Monoclonal Antibodies Identify a Cell-Surface Antigen Associated with an Activated Cellular Oncogene," *Nature*, 312:545.

4 Drebin, J., V. Link and M. Greene. 1988. "Monoclonal Antibodies Specific for the Neu Oncogene Product Directly Mediate Anti-Tumor Effects *in Vivo*," *Oncogene*, 4:387.

5 Taub, R., R. J. Gould, V. M. Garsky, T. M. Ciccarone, J. Hoxie, P. A. Friedman and S. J. Shattil. 1989. "A Monoclonal Antibody against the Platelet Fibrinogen Receptor Contains a Sequence that Mimics a Receptor Recognition Domain in Fibrinogen," *J. Biol. Chem.*, 264:25.

6 Shechter, Y., R. Maron, D. Elias and I. Cohen. 1982. "Autoantibodies to Insulin Receptor Spontaneously Develop as Anti-Idiotypes in Mice Immunized with Insulin," *Science*, 216:542.

7 Shechter, Y., D. Elias, R. Maron and I. Cohen. 1984. "Mouse Antibodies to the Insulin Receptor Developing Spontaneously as Anti-Idiotypes. I. Characterization of the Antibodies," *J. Biol. Chem.*, 259:6411.

8 Steele-Perkins, G. and R. A. Roth. 1990. "Insulin-Mimetic Anti-Insulin Receptor Monoclonal Antibodies Stimulate Receptor Kinase Activity in Intact Cells," *J. Biol. Chem.*, 265:9458.

9 Suzuki, K., J. Nishioka and T. Hayashi. 1990. "Localization of Thrombomodulin-Binding Site within Human Thrombin," *J. Biol. Chem.*, 265:13263.

10 Padlan, E., E. Silverton, S. Sheriff, G. Cohen, S. Smith-Gill and D. Davies. 1989. "Structure of an Antibody-Antigen Complex: Crystal Structure of the HyHEL-10 Fab-Lysozyme Complex," *Proc. Natl. Acad. Sci. USA*, 86:5938.

11 Cochran, A. G. and P. G. Schultz. 1990. "Antibody-Catalyzed Porphyrin Metallation," *Science*, 249:781.

12 Shokat, K. M., C. J. Leumann, R. Sugasawara and P. G. Schultz. 1989. "A New Strategy for the Generation of Catalytic Antibodies," *Nature*, 338:269.

13 Shokat, K. M. and P. C. Schultz. 1990. "Catalytic Antibodies," *Annu. Rev. Immunol.*, 8:335.

14 Borrebaeck, C. A. K. and J. W. Larrick. 1990. *Therapeutic Monoclonal Antibodies*. New York: Stockton Press.

15 Wu, T. and E. Kabat. 1970. "An Analysis of the Variable Regions of Bence Jones Proteins and Myeloma Light Chains and Their Implications for Antibody Diversity," *J. Exp. Med.*, 132:211.

16 Goetzl, E. and H. Metzger. 1970. "Affinity Labeling of a Mouse Myeloma Protein Which Binds to Nitrophenyl Ligands. Kinetics of Labeling and Isolation of a Labeled Peptide," *Biochemistry*, 9:1267.

17 Fleet, G., J. Knowles and R. Porter. 1972. "The Antibody Binding Site. Labeling of a Specific Antibody against the Photoprecursor of Aryl Nitrene," *Biochem. J.*, 128:499.

18 Thorpe, N. and S. Singer. 1969. "The Affinity-Labeled Residues in Antibody Active Sites. II. Nearest-Neighbor Analysis," *Biochemistry*, 8:4523.

19 Ray, A. and J. Cebra. 1972. "Localization of Affinity-Labeled Residues in the Primary Structure of Antidinitrophenyl Antibody Raised in Strain 13 Guinea Pigs,"*Biochemistry*, 11:3647.

20 Fisher, C. and E. Press. 1974. "Affinity Labeling of the Binding Site of Rabbit Antibody. Evidence for the Involvement of the Hypervariable Regions of the Heavy Chain," *Biochem. J.*, 139:135.

21 Cheseboro, B., N. Hadler and H. Metzger. 1973. "Affinity Labeling Studies on Five Mouse Myeloma Proteins Which Bind Phosphocholine," *3rd Int. Convoc. Immunol.*, 205.

22 Cebra, J., P. Koo and A. Ray. 1974. "Specificity of Antibodies: Primary Structural Basis of Antibody Binding," *Science*, 186:263.

23 Givol, D. 1974. "Affinity Labeling and Topology of the Antibody Combining Site," *Essays in Biochemistry*, 10:1.

24 Kabat, E. A., T. T. Wu, M. Reid-Miller and K. S. Gottesman. 1987. "Sequences of Proteins of Immunological Interest," *Sequences of Proteins of Immunologic Interest*.

25 Brack, C., M. Hirama, R. Lenhard-Schuller and S. Tonegawa. 1978. "A Complete Immunoglobulin Genen Is Created by Somatic Recombination," *Cell.*, 15:1.

26 Tonegawa, S. 1983. "Somatic Generation of Antibody Diversity," *Nature*, 302:573.

27 Baltimore, D. 1981. "Somatic Mutation Gains Its Place among the Generators of Diversity," *Cell.*, 26:295.

28 Oettinger, M. A., D. G. Schatz, C. Gorka and D. Baltimore. 1990. "RAG-1 and RAG-2, Adjacent Genes that Synergistically Activate V(D)J Recombination," *Science*, 248:1517.

29 Eisen, H. and E. Reilly. 1985. *Ann. Rev. Immunol.*, 3:337.

30 Wysocki, L., T. Manser and M. Gefter. 1986. "Somatic Evolution of Variable Region Structures during an Immune Response," *Proc. Natl. Acad. Sci. USA*, 83:1847.

31 Manser, T. and M. Gefter. 1986. "The Molecular Evolution of the Immune Response: Idiotope-Specific Suppression Indicates that B Cells Express Germ-Line–Encoded V Genes Prior to Antigenic Stimulation," *Eur. J. Immunol.*, 16:1439.

32 Manser, T., L. Wysocki, M. Margolies and M. Gefter. 1987. "Evolution of Antibody Variable Region Structure during the Immune Response," *Immunol. Rev.*, 96:141.

33 Manser, T., B. Parhami-Seren, M. Margolies and M. Gefter. 1987. "Somatically Mutated Forms of a Major Anti-*p*-Azophenylarsonate Antibody Variable Region with Drastically Reduced Affinity for *p*-Azophenylarsonate. By-Products of an Antigen-Driven Immune Response?" *J. Exp. Med.*, 166:1456.

34 Manser, T. 1990. "The Efficiency of Antibody Affinity Maturation: Can the Rate of B-Cell Division Be Limiting?" *Immunol. Today*, 11:305.

35 Manser, T. 1990. "Limits on Heavy Chain Junctional Diversity Contribute to the Recurrence of an Antibody Variable Region," *Mol. Immunol.*, 27:503.

36 Jerne, N. 1974. "Towards a Network Theory of the Immune System," *Ann. Immunol.*, 125C:373.

37 Jerne, N., J. Roland and P.-A. Cazenave. 1982. "Recurrent Idiotopes and Internal Images," *EMBO J.*, 1:243.

38 Kieber-Emmons, T., E. Getzoff and H. Kohler. 1987. "Perspectives on Antigenicity and Idiotypy," *Intern. Rev. Immunol.*, 2:339.

39 Kieber-Emmons, T. and H. Kohler. 1986. "Towards a Unified Theory of Immunoglobulin Structure-Function Relations," *Imm. Rev.*, 90:29.

40 Amit, A., R. Mariuzza, S. Phillips and R. Poljak. 1986. "Three-Dimensional Structure of an Antigen-Antibody Complex at 2.8 Å Resolution," *Science*, 233:747.

41 Stanfield, R., T. Fieser, R. Lerner and I. Wilson. 1990. "Crystal Structures of an Antibody to a Peptide and Its Complex with Peptide Antigen at 2.8 Å," *Science*, 248:712.

42 Beyers, A. D., A. N. Barclay, D. A. Law, Q. He and A. F. Williams. 1989. "Activation of T Lymphocytes via Monoclonal Antibodies against Rat Cell Surface Antigens with Particular Reference to CD2 Antigen," *Immunol. Rev.*, 111:59.

43 Seaman, W. E. and D. Wofsy. 1988. "Selective Manipulation of the Immune Response *in vivo* Monoclonal Antibodies," *Annu. Rev. Med.*, 39:231.

44 Birkedal-Hansen, B., W. G. Moore, R. E. Taylor, A. S. Bhown and H. Birkedal-Hansen. 1988. "Monoclonal Antibodies to Human Fibroblast Procollagenase. Inhibition of Enzymatic Activity, Affinity Purification of the Enzyme, and Evidence for Clustering of Epitopes in the NH2-Terminal End of the Activated Enzyme," *Biochemistry*, 27:6751.

45 Williams, W., H. Guy, D. Rubin, F. Robey, J. Myers, T. Kieber-Emmons, D. Weiner and M. Greene. 1988. "Sequences of the Cell-Attachment Sites of Reovirus Type 3 and Its Anti-Idiotypic/Antireceptor Antibody: Modelling of Their Three-Dimensional Structures," *Proc. Natl. Acad. Sci. USA*, 85:6488.

46 Gaulton, G., M. Co, H.-D. Royer and M. Greene. 1985. "Anti-Idiotypic Antibodies as Probes of Cell Surface Receptors," *Mol. Cell. Biochem.*, 65:5.

47 Gaulton, G., M. Co, and M. Greene. 1985. "Anti-Idiotypic Antibody Identifies the Cellular Receptor of Reovirus Type 3," *J. Cell. Biochem.*, 28:69.

48 Nepom, J., H. Weiner, M. Dichter, M. Tardieu, D. Spriggs, C. Gramm, M. Powers, B. Fields and M. Greene. 1982. "Identification of a Hemagglutinin-Specific Idiotype Associated with Reovirus Recognition Shared by Lymphoid and Neural Cells," *J. Exp. Med.*, 155:155.

49 Nepom, J., M. Tardieu, R. Epstein, J. Noseworthy, H. Weiner, J. Gentsch, B. Fields and M. Greene. 1982. "Virus-Binding Receptors: Similarities to Immune Receptors as Determined by Anti-Idiotypic Antibodies," *Surv. Immunol. Res.*, 1:255.

50 Noseworthy, J., B. Fields, M. Dichter, C. Sobotka, E. Pizer, L. Perry, J. Nepom and M. Greene. 1983. "Cell Receptors for the Mammalina Reovirus. I. Syngeneic Monoclonal Anti-Idiotypic Antibody Identifies a Cell Surface Receptor for Reovirus," *J. Immunol.*, 131:2533.

51 Kauffman, R., J. Noseworthy, J. Nepom, R. Finberg, B. Fields and M. Greene. 1983. "Cell Receptors for the Mammalian Reovirus. II. Monoclonal Anti-Idiotypic Antibody Blocks Viral Binding to Cells," *J. Immunol.*, 131:2539.

52 Gaulton, G. and M. Greene. 1989. "Inhibition of Cellular DNA Synthesis by Reovirus Occurs through a Receptor-Linked Signaling Pathway That Is Mimicked by Antiidiotypic Antireceptor Antibody," *J. Exp. Med.*, 169:197.

53 Sambrook, J., E. F. Fritsch and T. Maniatis. 1989. "Molecular Cloning," *A Laboratory Manual*.

54 Sanger, F., S. Nicklen and A. Coulsen. 1977. "DNA Sequencing with Chain Terminating Inhibitors," *PNAS*, 74:5463.

55 Orlandi, R., D. H. Güssow, P. T. Jones and G. Winter. 1989. "Cloning Immunoglobulin Variable Domains for Expression by the Polymerase Chain Reaction," *Proc. Natl. Acad. Sci. USA*, 86:3833.

56 Ward, E. S., D. Güssow, A. D. Griffiths, P. T. Jones and G. Winter. 1989. "Binding Activities of a Repertoire of Single Immunoglobulin Variable Domains Secreted from *Escherichia coli*," *Nature*, 341:544.

57 Bruck, C., M. Co, M. Slaoui, G. Gaulton, T. Smith, B. Fields, J. Mullins and M. Greene. 1986. "Nucleic Acid Sequence of an Internal Image-Bearing Monoclonal Anti-Idiotype and Its Comparison to the Sequence of the External Antigen," *Proc. Natl. Acad. Sci. USA*, 83:6578.

58 Williams, W. V., T. Kieber-Emmons, J. M. Von Feldt, M. I. Greene and D. B. Weiner. 1991. "Design of Bioactive Peptides Based on Antibody Hypervariable Region Structures: Development of Conformationally Constrained and Dimeric Peptides with Enhanced Affinity," *J. Biol. Chem.*, 266:5182.

59 Kearney, J., R. Barletta, Z. Quan and J. Quintans. 1981. "Monoclonal vs Heterogeneous Anti H-8 Antibodies in the Analysis of the Anti-Phosphrylcoline Response in BALB/c Mice," *Eur. J. Immunol.*, 11:877.

60 Meek, K., C. Hasemann, B. Pollok, S. Alkan, M. Brait, J. Slaoui, J. Urbain

and J. Capra. 1989. "Structural Characterization of Antiidiotypic Antibodies," *J. Exp. Med.*, 169:519.

61 Moser, M., O. Leo, J. Hiernaux and J. Urbain. 1983. "Recurrent Idiotypes and Internal Images," *Proc. Natl. Acad. Sci. USA*, 80:4474.

62 Cheng, H., A. Sood, R. Ward, T. Kieber-Emmons and H. Kohler. 1988. "Structural Basis of Stimulatory Anti-Idiotypic Antibodies," *Mol. Immunol.*, 25:33.

63 Stohrer, R. and J. F. Kearney. 1983. "Fine Idiotype Analysis of B Cell Precursors in the T-Dependent and T-Independent Responses to Alpha 1–>3 Dextran in BALB/c Mice," *J. Exp. Med.*, 158:2081.

64 Umeda, M., I. Diega and D. Marcus. 1986. "The Occurrence of Anti-3-Fucosyl Lactosamine Antibodies and Their Cross Reactive Idiotypes in Preimmune and Immune Mouse Sera," *J. Immunol.*, 137:3263.

65 Van Cleave, V., C. W. Naeve and D. W. Metzger. 1988. "Do Antibodies Recognize Amino Acid Side Chains of Protein Antigens Independently of the Carbon Backbone?" *J. Exp. Med.*, 167:1841.

66 Ollier, P., J. Rocca-Serra, G. Somme, J. Theze and M. Fougereau. 1985. "The Idiotypic Network and the Internal Image: Possible Regulation of a Germ-Line Network by Paucigene Encoded Ab2 (Anti-Idiotypic) Antibodies in the GAT System," *EMBO*, 4:3681.

67 Gaulton, G. and M. Greene. 1986. "Idiotypic Mimicry of Biological Receptors," *Ann. Rev. Immunol.*, 4:253.

68 Sege, K. and P. Peterson. 1978. "Anti-Idiotypic Antibodies against Anti-Vitamin A Transporting Protein React with Prealbumin," *Nature*, 271:167.

69 Sege, K. and P. Peterson. 1978. "Use of Anti-Idiotypic Antibodies as Cell-Surface Receptor Probes," *Proc. Natl. Acad. Sci. USA*, 75:2443.

70 Homcy, C., S. Rockson and E. Haber. 1982. "An Antiidiotype Antibody that Recognizes the β-Adrenergic Receptor," *J. Clin. Invest.*, 69:1147.

71 Williams, W. V., T. Kieber-Emmons, D. B. Weiner, D. H. Rubin and M. I. Greene. 1991. "Contact Residues and Predicted Structure of the Reovirus Type 3–Receptor Interaction," *J. Biol. Chem.*, 266:9241.

72 Chothia, C., A. Lesk, M. Levitt, A. Amit, R. Mariuzza, S. Phillips and R. Poljak. 1986. "The Predicted Structure of Immunoglobulin D1.3 and Its Comparison with the Crystal Structure," *Science*, 233:755.

73 Devereux, J., P. Haeberli and O. Smithies. 1984. "A Comprehensive Set of Sequence Analysis Programs for the VAX," *Nucleic Acids Res.*, 12:387.

74 Gribskov, M., R. R. Burgess and J. Devereux. 1986. "PEPPLOT, a Protein Secondary Structure Analysis Program for the UWGCG Sequence Analysis Software Package," *Nucleic Acids Res.*, 14:327.

75 Williams, W. V., D. B. Weiner and M. I. Greene. 1989. "Development and Use of Antireceptor Antibodies to Study Interaction of Mammalian Reovirus Type 3 with its Cell Surface Receptor," *Methods Enzymol.*, 178:321.

76 Williams, W. V., H. R. Guy, D. B. Weiner and M. I. Greene. 1989. "Three Dimensional Structure of a Functional Internal Image," *Viral Immunol.*, 2:239.

77 Williams, W. V., D. B. Weiner, J. C. Cohen and M. I. Greene. 1989. "Development and Use of Receptor Binding Peptides Derived from Antireceptor Antibodies," *Biotechnology*, 7:471.

78 Houghten, R., J. Appel and C. Pinilla. 1988. "Use of Multiple Peptide Analogs in the Detailed Study of Antibody-Antigen Interactions," *Vaccines*, 88:9.

79 Williams, W., D. Moss, T. Kieber-Emmons, J. Cohen, J. Myers, D. Weiner and M. Greene. 1989. "Development of Biologically Active Peptides Based on Antibody Structure," *Proc. Natl. Acad. Sci. USA*, 86:5537.

80 Saul, F. A., L. M. Amzel and R. J. Poljak. 1978. "Preliminary Refinement and Structural Analysis of the Fab' Fragment from Human Immunoglobulin NEW at 2.0 Å Resolution," *J. Biol. Chem.*, 25:585.

81 Gentsch, J. and A. Pacitti. 1985. "Effect of Neuraminidase Treatment of Cells and Effect of Soluble Glycoproteins on Type 3 Reovirus Attachment to Murine L Cells," *J. Virol.*, 56:356.

82 Pacitti, A. and J. Gentsch. 1987. "Inhibition of Reovirus Type 3 Binding to Host Cells by Sialylated Glycoproteins in Mediated through the Viral Attachment Protein," *J. Virol.*, 61:1407.

83 Burstin, S., D. Spriggs and B. Fields. 1982. "Evidence for Functional Domains on the Reovirus Type 3 Hemagglutinin," *Virology*, 117:146.

CHAPTER 4

NMR Spectroscopy of Peptides and Proteins in Membrane Environments

KI-JOON SHON[1]
STANLEY J. OPELLA[1]

INTRODUCTION

MANY important biological functions are expressed by peptides and proteins that are associated with membranes. Therefore, there is considerable interest in determining the structures and describing the dynamics of membrane bound peptides and proteins. Unfortunately, membrane environments present significant impediments for the use of the most powerful methods of structural biology—x-ray crystallography and multidimensional solution NMR spectroscopy. Detergent micelles in solution and hydrated lipid bilayers provide two model membranes that can be used for structural studies. X-ray diffraction studies are particularly difficult because so few membrane bound peptides or proteins have been crystallized from either detergent or lipid environments. Multidimensional solution NMR spectroscopy is problematic for peptide and proteins in micelles because they reorient rather slowly in solution and are inapplicable to peptides and proteins in bilayers because they do not reorient at all on the relevant timescales. Therefore, there exists strong motivation for developing NMR experiments capable of dealing with peptides and proteins in the membrane environments of micelles and bilayers.

Recently, substantial progress has been made in applying NMR spectroscopy to peptides and proteins in micelles and bilayers and, with additional improvements in instrumentation, it should become feasible to describe their structures and dynamics fully. As methods for crystallizing membrane bound peptides and proteins are developed, it may be possible in the future

[1]Department of Chemistry, University of Pennsylvania, Philadelphia, PA 19104, U.S.A.

to use NMR spectroscopy and x-ray crystallography to provide complementary information, just as is the case of globular proteins at the present time. The ability of NMR spectroscopy to determine the structures of proteins is a direct consequence of the development of one- and two-dimensional Fourier transform NMR methods, as recognized with the 1991 Nobel Prize in chemistry. Since multi-dimensional NMR methods can be used in both solution and solid-state NMR experiments, it is possible, in principle, to study peptides and proteins in both micelles and bilayers.

It must be emphasized that all peptides and proteins that exist in molecular complexes present substantial difficulties for solution NMR studies. If the proteins are immobile ($\tau_c > 10^{-3}$ s) in supramolecular structures or in solid samples, then the methods of solid-state NMR spectroscopy can be utilized to describe their structure and dynamics [1,2]. However, if the proteins are in solution and have moderate molecular weights (20–100 $\times$ 10^3 daltons) or are part of complexes, e.g., membrane-bound proteins in micelles, with effective rotational correlation times ($\tau_c > 20 \times 10^{-9}$ s), then solution NMR methods must be utilized even though in these cases the efficient transverse relaxation among the protons results in ^{1}H resonances with short T_2 values and correspondingly broad lines. The broad linewidths not only limit resolution and sensitivity in one-dimensional spectra but also have unfortunate consequences for two-dimensional experiments; in particular, they cause cancellation of cross-peak components in homonuclear correlated spectra [3]. In addition, the relatively long molecular correlation times enhance spin diffusion, making homonuclear ^{1}H Nuclear Overhauser Effect (NOE) measurements difficult to interpret.

The problems associated with solution NMR studies of relatively slowly reorienting proteins can be reduced by preparing protein samples labeled with stable isotopes. Uniform ^{15}N labeling greatly enhances the feasibility of many NMR experiments on proteins. Selective ^{15}N labeling offers obvious possibilities for improved resolution, resonance assignments, and obtaining structural information about specific residues with both one- and two-dimensional isotope-directed NOE measurements [4]. Uniform replacement of the ^{1}H nuclei bonded to carbons with ^{2}H nuclei effectively separates the amide protons from other protons and influences two important aspects of ^{1}H relaxation [5–8]. It lengthens T_2, narrowing the resonance linewidths and improving resolution and sensitivity, and it removes longitudinal relaxation pathways from amide protons to carbon-bound protons, attenuating spin-diffusion processes.

NMR SPECTROSCOPY OF MEMBRANE PROTEINS IN MICELLES

The multi-dimensional solution NMR methods that are so successful in determining the structures of globular proteins in solution can be adapted for peptides and proteins in micelles by taking advantage of both isotopic labeling and multi-dimensional NMR experiments. NMR spectroscopy of proteins in micelles benefits most dramatically from two- and higher-dimensional NMR experiments for several reasons. The extension of NMR spectroscopy to additional frequency dimensions greatly improves the effective spectral resolution. Many experiments yield a complete separation of resonances and spectral parameters because different nuclear spin interactions dominate the spectral features in different dimensions. This is accomplished by acquiring the experimental data in the form of intensities as a function of time and subsequently transforming the data, by Fourier transformation or other mathematical methods, into frequency domains. All multi-dimensional NMR experiments involve the application of radio-frequency pulses in timed sequences (pulse sequences) which can be described in terms of four separate time periods—preparation, evolution, mixing, and detection—as shown schematically in Figure 4.1. Representative examples of actual pulse sequences are shown in Figure 4.2. During the preparation period, the initial pulse (or set of pulses) tips the nuclear spin magnetization, originally developed along the longitudinal z axis, into the x,y plane, creating a coherent state of spins. The nuclear spins then precess at their Larmor frequencies, reflecting their individual chemical shifts, and become "labeled" with respect to frequency since the precession frequency and the length of the evolution period, t_1, determine the position of a particular spin in the x,y plane. At the end of the t_1 interval, additional pulses are applied to transfer the magnetization to other spins. The transfer occurs during the mixing period, which consists of a single pulse or a series of pulses and delays. During the detection period, the free induction decay (FID), which is the sum of all signal intensities as a function of time, is recorded as a function of t_2. The amplitude and/or phase of the signals that constitute the free induction decay depend upon the length of the time period t_1, the mixing process, and the precession frequency. Data sets are collected systematically by incrementing the value of t_1 by a fixed amount and averaging the signal collected during t_2 to improve the signal-to-noise ratio. Each stored FID results from a single t_1 value. As many as 500 t_1 increments are made in order to create a two-dimensional data matrix, s (t_1,t_2). The signal from each t_1 increment is Fourier transformed with respect to t_2, and then the signal corresponding to each

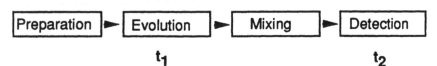

Figure 4.1 Distinction of four time periods in two-dimensional pulse sequences. t_1 and t_2 represent time dimensions that become frequency dimensions after the Fourier transformations.

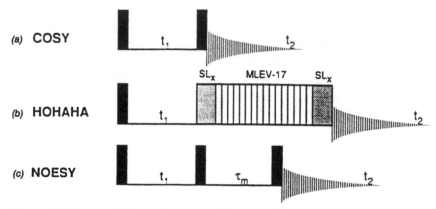

Figure 4.2 Most commonly used proton two-dimensional homonuclear pulse sequences: (a) COSY, correlation spectroscopy; (b) HOHAHA, homonuclear Hartmann-Hahn; (c) NOESY, nuclear Overhauser effect spectroscopy.

digitized t_2 point is again Fourier transformed as a function of t_1. The resulting two-dimensional spectrum, s (ω_1,ω_2), contains peaks with positions corresponding to precession frequencies ω_1 and ω_2.

Several different mixing methods are used in two-dimensional NMR experiments. These are broadly defined as coherent transfer, which is based on the existence of spin-spin coupling through-bond, and incoherent transfer, which is based on mutual relaxation from through-space dipolar interactions or chemical exchange of spins in spatial proximity. One of the many variations of two-dimensional homonuclear correlated spectroscopy (COSY) [9–12] is generally the first two-dimensional experiment to be used since it identifies scalar connectivities between protons separated by only a few chemical bonds. In a two-dimensional COSY spectrum the one-dimensional NMR spectrum lies along the diagonal and the off-diagonal cross-peaks are observed at the intersection of two spins that are coupled. The basic COSY pulse sequence is shown in Figure 4.2(a). In this experiment, two radio frequency pulses are applied with an evolution time, t_1. The second pulse is the mixing pulse that transfers coherence between coupled spins. Groups of different amino acids have distinctive coupling patterns, reflecting their spin systems, and the identification of these spin systems becomes an important tool for assigning resonances by amino acid residue type. Methods known as homonuclear Hartmann-Hahn (HOHAHA) [13] and total correlation spectroscopy (TOCSY) [14] are available for elucidating the connectivities in spin systems over a relatively large number of bonds. There are also conventional relay experiments capable of extending the correlations one bond at a time. These experiments allow the correlation of all spin coupled protons within a given spin coupling network, generally a single amino acid residue. The pulse sequence used in the HOHAHA experiment is quite complex, as depicted in Figure 4.2(b), in order to create Hartmann-Hahn mixing conditions. The integral number of repetitions of 49 pulses removes the effect of chemical shifts so that magnetization may transfer freely among protons. These experiments provide relatively high sensitivity and resolution because the coherence transfer during the mixing time is efficient.

Once spin systems are identified based on the type of amino acid, it is necessary to assign the resonance to the position of the residue in the peptide sequence by measuring short range inter-residue distances derived from nuclear Overhauser effect spectroscopy (NOESY) [15–18]. The pulse sequence for the basic NOESY experiment is shown in Figure 4.2(c). In this experiment the evolution period is followed by a 90° pulse, which converts transverse magnetization onto the longitudinal z axis. During the mixing time, τ_m, magnetization transfer between nearby protons occurs through cross relaxation. By varying the duration of the mixing time, the range of the effect can be controlled with the maximum observable distance being approximately 5 Å.

Coherence transfer can also be accomplished in heteronuclear experiments and this is extremely important in studies of peptides and proteins in micelles. The coupling constants between directly bonded hydrogens and other (X) nuclei, such as ^{13}C or ^{15}N, are relatively large and, therefore, the transfer of coherence between them is quite efficient. Figure 4.3(a) shows the pulse scheme of a proton detected heteronuclear multiple quantum chemical shift correlation (HMQC) [19,20] experiment. The first 90° pulse creates ^1H magnetization in the x,y plane where the two components resulting from spin-spin coupling to the ^{15}N or ^{13}C nucleus precess in opposite directions. The spin-spin coupling creates maximum antiphase magnetization at the end of the delay with the duration $1/2J$, where J is the magnitude of the heteronuclear spin-spin coupling constant. The 90° pulse near the ^{15}N or ^{13}C resonance frequency then creates multiple quantum coherence between a ^{15}N or ^{13}C spin and the directly coupled proton spin. During the evolution period t_1, the proton 180° pulse is given with the identical delays, $t_{1/2}$, before and after the pulse in order to decouple the ^1H-X scalar interaction in the t_1 dimension. The second 90° pulse at the X nucleus resonance frequency at the end of the evolution period converts the multiple quantum coherence into observable single quantum coherence. Another $1/2J$ delay allows the antiphase magnetization to refocus. During the acquisition period, a heteronuclear decoupling sequence is applied so that single line ^1H resonances can be observed.

^1H detected heteronuclear correlation spectroscopy is a powerful approach because it improves the spectral resolution by detecting only those protons directly bonded to X nuclei, eliminating intense diagonal

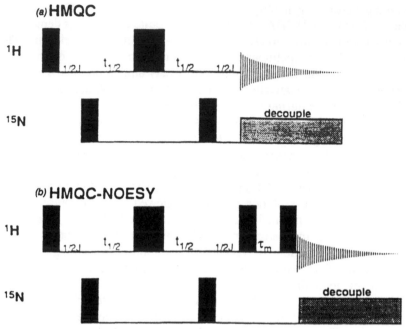

Figure 4.3 Pulse sequences of (a) two-dimensional heteronuclear multiple quantum correlation (HMQC) and (b) the combined two-dimensional HMQC with NOESY experiment.

resonances, which usually dominate homonuclear two-dimensional spectra, and adding an extra X nucleus frequency dimension. NMR experiments that combine ^{1}H heteronuclear correlation pulse sequences with other experiments, such as NOESY and COSY, were developed to obtain the greater spectral resolution possible with frequency dimensions with ^{15}N or ^{13}C nuclear spin parameters and the distance and coupling information needed for making assignments. There are several ways of combining two-dimensional experiments. Figure 4.3(b) shows one that we developed [5]. It combines the essential features of ^{1}H detected HMQC pulses in Figure 4.3(a) and those of ^{1}H homonuclear NOE pulses in Figure 4.2(c). During the first half of the pulse sequence, the resonances from protons directly bonded to ^{15}N nuclei are selectively filtered from those of the rest of the protons, and during the second half of the sequence, spin exchange through cross relaxation is allowed to take place between those protons. Systematic incrementation of the t_1 values generates a two-dimensional spectrum with ^{1}H resonance frequency along the first dimension and the corresponding ^{15}N resonance frequency along the second dimension. Figure 4.4 demonstrates the capability of the experiment for providing the secondary structural information of proteins. When the experiment is per-

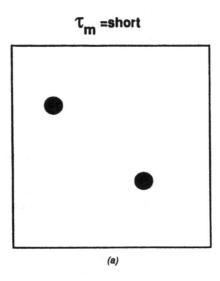

(a)

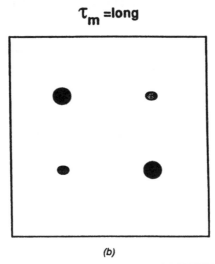

(b)

Figure 4.4 Schematic representation of the combined HMQC-NOESY spectra, (a) with short mixing time (correlation peaks only) and (b) with long mixing time (correlation peaks as well as NOE cross-peaks). Completely filled circles are N-H correlation peaks and half-filled circles are the NOE cross-peaks.

formed with a short mixing interval, each amide site gives rise to a single $^1H/^{15}N$ correlation resonance in the contour plot shown in Figure 4.4(a). When the experiment is performed with a long mixing interval, NOE cross-peaks are built up between neighboring amide protons separated by less than 5 Å, as illustrated in Figure 4.4(b). This experiment is particularly useful for proteins whose secondary structure is mostly helical, since the sequential NOE connectivities of amide protons can be easily mapped out [5].

The implementation of full three- (and higher-) dimensional NMR spectroscopy benefits from developments in both instrumentation and computers. Three-dimensional spectroscopy can be used to eliminate ambiguities present in two-dimensional spectra due to resonance overlaps or degeneracies (21–23). Figure 4.5 illustrates the power of the third dimension, by showing what appears to be a single resonance in a two-dimensional plot actually represents three separate resonances in a three-dimensional plot. This resolution enhancement contributes greatly to the determination of high resolution atomic level three-dimensional structures of proteins. Three-dimensional pulse sequences can be generated by combining two two-dimensional pulse sequences as illustrated in Figure 4.6 [24]. The two experiments are put together leaving out the detection

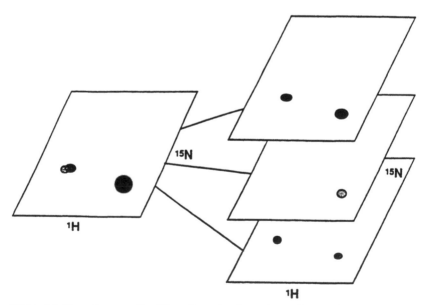

Figure 4.5 Shows the necessity of three-dimensional experiments for resolving resonance overlaps. The resonance overlaps shown in two-dimensional spectrum are completely resolved in three-dimensional spectrum even those overlaps that are not obvious.

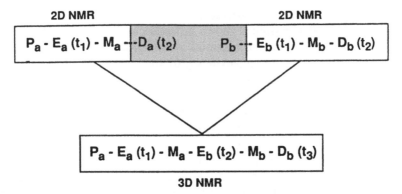

Figure 4.6 Demonstrates how three-dimensional pulse sequence is designed using two-dimensional pulse sequences: P, preparation; E, evolution; M, mixing; D, detection.

period of the first experiment and the preparation period of the second. In three-dimensional experiments, the FID is recorded as a function of t_3 with two additional time domains, t_1 and t_2, which are incremented independently. Three-dimensional data sets are collected as the matrix, s (t_1, t_2, t_3), that is subjected to triple Fourier transformation. A three-dimensional spectrum can be viewed as a stack of two-dimensional spectra. Each one-dimensional spectrum that contributes to the data matrix is obtained with two time variables kept constant while the FID representing the third time domain (t_3) is observed. For each two-dimensional spectrum, one of the two time variables, for example t_2, can be incremented as many times as required for the necessary spectral resolution. Once the data set for a two-dimensional spectrum is complete, t_1 is incremented by a fixed value and the next two-dimensional spectrum is obtained by incrementing t_2 repeatedly. Essentially any pair of pulse sequences for two-dimensional experiments can be combined to create a three-dimensional experiment, including the NOESY-HMQC [25] and HMQC-NOESY [22] experiments shown in Figure 4.7. The two major advantages to using heteronuclear instead of homonuclear experiments, are the efficient heteronuclear transfer step due to large spin-spin coupling constants and the requirement of only modest resolution in the heteronuclear dimension (i.e., ^{15}N or ^{13}C). As shown in Figure 4.6, the detection period of NOESY is replaced by the evolution period of HMQC in the design of the three-dimensional experiment and the rest of the pulses are kept the same as in two-dimensional experiments. The resulting pulse sequence contains t_1 and t_2 evolution periods, which represent the ^1H and ^{15}N dimensions, respectively, and the detection period, t_3. These three-dimensional experiments are designed to increase spectral resolution by inserting another proton dimension so that the amide proton as well as the alpha and other side chain protons can be resolved completely. A completely processed three-dimensional spectrum is shown schematically in Figure 4.8. Three-dimensional experiments are essential for assigning resonances of large proteins because of their complexities [26] and membrane proteins which are not only large in size but also have limited chemical shift dispersion due to their extensive helical secondary structure [6]. Another useful heteronuclear three-dimensional experiment is HOHAHA-HMQC, which is particularly effective in providing single as well as multiple bond correlations between scalar coupled ^{1}Hs for making resonance assignments.

Studies of peptides and proteins involve assignment of resonances and distance measurements. Complete ^{1}H resonance assignments are essential and Wuthrich and coworkers have established basic procedures for assigning ^{1}H resonances in proteins [24]. These assignment strategies utilizing the basic through-space and through-bond correlations observed in NOESY and COSY experiments, respectively, are based on the chemical properties of the covalently linked backbone structure of proteins. The COSY experiment observes direct through-bond connectivities between the NH and C_αH, C_αH and C_βH, and C_βH and C_γH protons, etc. Through-space correlation between closely spaced protons are essential for making sequential assignments. Short range NOEs are usually observed between backbone (C_αH, NH) protons, and between the backbone and C_βH on adjacent amino acids. Those NOEs also provide crucial information about the protein secondary structure. Long range NOEs are also observed and these are valuable for describing tertiary structure. Since short range sequential distances strongly depend on the type of secondary structure, they provide important constraints for identifying a variety of secondary structures in proteins. For example, the NH-NH distance, $d_{NN}(i, i + 1)$, is about 2.8 Å in an α helix and 4.2 Å in β sheets as tabulated in Table 4.1. The distance between C_αH of the residue i and the NH proton of the residue $i + 1$, $d_{\alpha N}(i, i + 1)$, is about 3.5 Å in an α helix and 2.2 Å in β sheets. Figure 4.9 shows those short and medium range NOE observable distances in secondary structures [28].

NMR SPECTROSCOPY OF MEMBRANE PEPTIDES IN BILAYERS

Solid-state NMR spectroscopy is capable of determining the complete structures of immobile proteins, such as those embedded in lipid bilayers, as long as the sample is oriented in one direction. Structure determination is possible when several spectral parameters are measured to characterize the angles between each of the peptide planes and the direction of sample orientation [1,2,29]. Once the secondary structure of a membrane-bound form of a protein in micelles in solution is established through the short

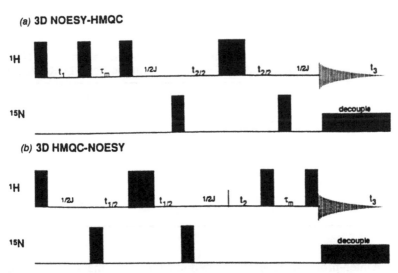

(a) **3D NOESY-HMQC**

¹H

t_1 τ_m $1/2J$ $t_2/2$ $t_2/2$ $1/2J$ t_3

¹⁵N

decouple

(b) **3D HMQC-NOESY**

¹H

$1/2J$ $t_1/2$ $t_1/2$ $1/2J$ t_2 τ_m t_3

¹⁵N

decouple

Figure 4.7 Three-dimensional pulse sequences of (a) NOESY-HMQC (t_1, the first time domain representing ¹H dimension; τ_m, the mixing time for NOE to build up between ¹Hs that are close in space; $1/2J$, scalar coupling constant arising from directly bonded ¹⁵N-¹H; $t_2/2$, the second time domain representing ¹⁵N dimension; t_3, the third time domain representing another ¹H dimension which is directly observed) and (b) HMQC-NOESY ($t_1/2$, the first time domain representing ¹⁵N dimension; t_2, the second time domain representing ¹H dimension; t_3, the third time domain representing another ¹H dimension).

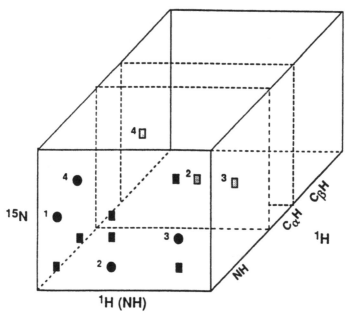

Figure 4.8 Schematic representation of three-dimensional NOESY-HMQC spectrum showing all three dimensions with NH correlation resonances (circles) as well as NOE cross-peaks (squares) arising from protons that are close in space.

TABLE 4.1. Short and Medium Range NOE Observable Distances (Å) in Polypeptide Chains (from *NMR of Proteins and Nucleic Acids* by K. Wuthrich).

Distance	α-helix	3_{10}-helix	βap	βp
$d_{\alpha N}$	3.5	3.4	2.2	2.2
$d_{\alpha N}(i, i + 2)$	4.4	3.8		
$d_{\alpha N}(i, i + 3)$	3.4	3.3		
$d_{\alpha N}(i, i + 4)$	4.2			
d_{NN}	2.8	2.6	4.3	4.2
$d_{NN}(i, i + 2)$	4.2	4.1		
$d_{\beta N}$	2.5–4.1	2.9–4.4	3.2–4.5	3.7–4.7
$d_{\alpha\beta}(i, i + 3)$	2.5–4.4	3.1–5.1		

range inter-proton distances measured in NOE experiments, a single spectral parameter, in this case the ^{15}N chemical shift, is sufficient to establish the orientations of the helices relative to the direction of sample orientation and the plane of the bilayer. Solid-state ^{15}N NMR spectra of oriented peptides and protein in lipid bilayers can be interpreted quantitatively through the use of graphical restriction plots. However, in many cases qualitative interpretations are quite informative and can be made by using the nearly axially symmetric ^{15}N amide chemical shift tensor as a guide to the orientation of the peptide groups in the helices. The calculated spectra of a powder pattern and those ^{15}N chemical shifts oriented parallel and perpendicular to the magnetic field are shown in Figure 4.10. The determination of helix orientations with respect to the lipid bilayer normal pro-

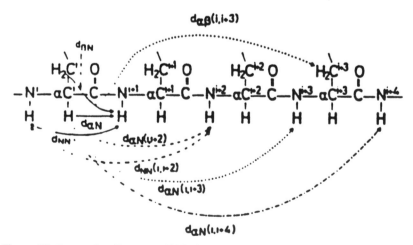

Figure 4.9 Short and medium range NOE observable distances in polypeptide chains displayed with dotted lines (from *NMR of Proteins and Nucleic Acids* by K. Wuthrich).

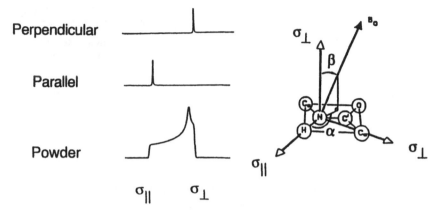

Figure 4.10 Calculated solid-state NMR spectra showing different ^{15}N chemical shift values depending on the orientation of amide bond with respect to magnetic field.

vides the tertiary structural information and this is essential for understanding the structure and function relationships of membrane proteins.

Magainins are a family of 20–25 residue peptides first found in the skin of frogs [30] that exhibit a broad range of antibacterial and other biological activities, possibly resulting from the formation of oligomeric peptide ion channels across membranes or some other mechanism for disrupting the electrochemical ionic gradient across cell membranes [31]. There is substantial evidence for strong interactions of magainins with bacterial membranes. However, these peptides do not lyse red blood cells, which suggests that they may interact quite differently with vertebrate membranes than with bacterial membranes. Two-dimensional solution NMR experiments indicate that these peptides are predominantly helical in detergent micelles [32] and trifluoroethanol/water mixtures [33] and unfolded in aqueous solution. The 23 residue Magainin2 peptide, GIGKFLHSAKKF-GKAFVGEIMNSamide, was synthesized with Ala$_{15}$ labeled with ^{15}N for NMR studies.

The major superfamilies of ion channels in biological membranes, such as the nicotinic acetylcholine receptor and voltage gated cation channels, are large and complex proteins. A promising approach to their analysis is to synthesize and study peptide sequences corresponding to segments of the protein [34,35]. The peptide M2 was selected from the δ subunit of the *torpedo* acetylcholine receptor, because homology and model studies suggest that this sequence specific motif is responsible for specific functions in the channel activity of the receptor [36]. M2δ differs substantially from Magainin2 in that it does lyse red blood cells [37] and closely mimics the ion channel properties of the receptor in model membranes. M2δ and similar peptides have been shown to be helical by solution NMR spectroscopy [6,38–42]. The 23 residue M2δ peptide, EKMSTAISVLL<u>A</u>QAVFLLLT-SQR, was synthesized with Ala$_{12}$ labeled with ^{15}N for these studies.

Figure 4.11 compares experimental solid-state ^{15}N NMR spectra of the specifically labeled Magainin2 and M2δ peptides in oriented phospholipid bilayers to a simulated ^{15}N amide chemical shift powder pattern. Each oriented peptide has a relatively narrow single line resonance from its one ^{15}N labeled amide site. The resonance frequencies observed in these two samples are quite different, varying by nearly the full breadth of the powder pattern, indicating that the planes containing the labeled peptide groups have very different orientations relative to the direction of the applied magnetic field. In order to fully determine the orientation of a labeled peptide plane, it would be necessary to measure at least one other spectral parameter associated with that site [1,2]. However, since the ^{15}N labeled residues in both Magainin2 [32,33] and M2δ [43] are known to adopt helical secondary structures in membrane environments from solution NMR experiments, the ^{15}N chemical shifts provide sufficient information to define the orientations of the helices.

The experimental spectra in Figures 4.11(a) and 11(b) can be readily interpreted qualitatively. The ^{15}N NMR spectrum in Figure 4.11(a) of ^{15}N-Ala$_{15}$ labeled Magainin2 consists of a single line with a resonance frequency near $\sigma_\perp$, therefore the N−H bond of Ala$_{15}$, as well as those of the other residues in the helical peptide, are approximately perpendicular to the direction of the magnetic field and parallel to the plane of the bilayer. The ^{15}N NMR spectrum in Figure 4.11(b) of ^{15}N-Ala$_{12}$ labeled M2δ has its resonance intensity near $\sigma_\parallel$, therefore the N−H bond of Ala$_{12}$, as well as those of the other residues in the helical peptide, are approximately parallel to the direction of the magnetic field and perpendicular to the plane of the bilayer.

Magainin2 is oriented approximately parallel to the plane of the bilayer. The drawing in Figure 4.12 places it at the interfacial region of the bilayer based on the expectation that an amphipathic peptide interacts with both the polar headgroups and the hydrocarbon chains of the lipids. M2δ is clearly a trans-membrane peptide, as shown in Figure 4.12, oriented perpendicular to the plane of the bilayer. Both of the peptides are visualized as monomers in Figure 4.12, however they are most likely associated as oligomers in the membranes, with each peptide having the same orientation relative to the plane of the membrane. These findings are consistent with the functional models of the M2δ peptide forming trans-membrane molecular channels. However, they suggest that the magainins, at least at equilibrium in this lipid system, do not cross the membrane, but rather reside in the interfacial regions.

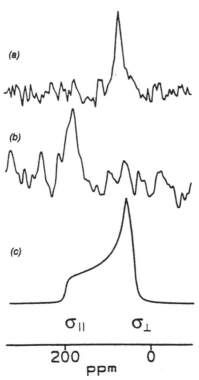

(a)

(b)

(c)

$\sigma_{\parallel}$ $\sigma_{\perp}$

200   0
ppm

Figure 4.11 ¹⁵N NMR spectra of peptides: (a) experimental spectrum of ¹⁵N-Ala₁₅-Magainin2 (3 mole %) in POPC/POPG (3:1) (1-palmitoyl-2-oleoly-sn glycero-3-phosphocholine/1-palmitoyl-2oleoyl-sn-glycero-3-phospholgycerol) bilayers oriented between glass plates at 40°C; (b) experimental spectrum of ¹⁵N-Ala₁₂-M2δ peptide (5 mole %) in DMPC/DMPG (4:1) (1,2-di-myristol-sn-glycero-3-phosphocholine/1,2-dimyristoyl-sn-glycero-3-phosphoglycerol) bilayers oriented between glass plates at 30°C.

M2δ   Magainin2

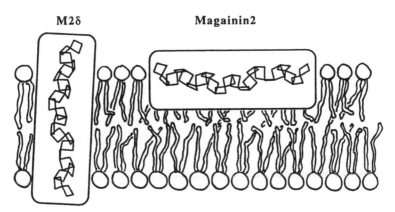

Figure 4.12 Schematic drawing of in-plane (Magainin2) and trans-membrane (M2δ) orientations of 23 residue amphipathic helical peptides in lipid bilayers. The helical backbones are represented by their 22 peptide bond planes whereas the white boxes indicate the extending side chains.

APPLICATION OF COMBINED NMR METHODS TO A MEMBRANE PROTEIN

The secondary structure of a protein is determined on the basis of distance measurements in micelles, while the arrangement of the major elements of secondary structure is derived from measurements of angular parameters in oriented bilayers in the combined approach using both multidimensional solution NMR spectroscopy and high-resolution solid-state NMR spectroscopy. The approach has shown the membrane-bound form of the 46-residue Pf1 coat protein to be surprisingly complex with five distinct regions; a long hydrophobic helix (residues 19 to 42) that spans the bilayer, a short amphipathic helix (residues 6 to 13) parallel to the plane of the bilayer, a mobile loop (residues 14 to 18) connecting the two helices, and mobile NH$_2$- and COOH-termini.

The resonance assignments and structure determination strategy of the heteronuclear alternative approach is outlined in Figure 4.13. As described earlier, isotope labeling of proteins becomes essential for improving spectral resolution as well as sensitivity in multi-dimensional experiments. The benefits of uniform deuteration for controlling spin-diffusion are demonstrated in Figure 4.14. One-dimensional slices out of a section of the two-dimensional spectra obtained from the coat protein isotopically labeled with ^{15}N only (top) and the coat protein labeled with both ^{15}N and ^{2}H (bottom) are presented in Figure 4.14. These two-dimensional experiments were run under identical spectrometer settings and sample conditions. As expected, there is a significant resonance line narrowing due to the increase in transverse relaxation time, T_2. The sensitivity enhancement and strong NOE cross-peaks, resulting from the line narrowing effect and the partial elimination of spin diffusion by the presence of deuterons, are obvious in the comparison. Uniform and selective ^{15}N labeling is very effective for improving spectral resolution. The HMQC spectrum contains resonances only from those protons directly coupled to ^{15}N nuclei. Further resolution enhancement is achieved with selective ^{15}N labeling, as demonstrated in Figure 4.15. There are only two Tyrosine residues in Pf1 coat protein and these are easily recognized by comparing the HMQC spectra of uniformly ^{15}N labeled and selectively ^{15}N-Tyr labeled protein samples. Once the identification of amide protons are completed based on their amino acid residue type, specific assignments can be made using sequential NOE connectivities between neighboring amide protons. The HMQC-NOESY spectrum in Figure 4.16 contains not only those correlation resonances from each amide proton of Pf1 coat protein in micelles, but also NOE cross-peaks arising from two closely spaced neighboring amide protons. The specific assignment of Tyrosine residue at position 40 can be easily made by comparing HMQC spectrum of selectively ^{15}N Tyrosine

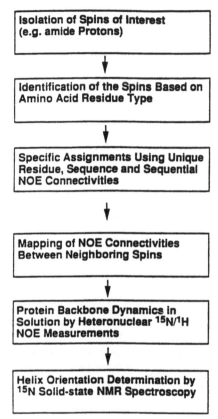

Figure 4.13 The outline of the alternative approach used to assign amide proton and nitrogen resonances and to determine the secondary as well as the tertiary structures of membrane-bound proteins.

labeled sample shown in Figure 4.15(a) with the HMQC spectrum of a single site ^{15}N-Tyr labeled sample shown in Figure 4.15(b). Then NOE connectivities can be used for making assignments of neighboring residues. For example, the neighboring residues of Tyr-40 are Serine-41 and Isoleuceine-39, and therefore one should be able to distinguish the resonance of the Ser-41 from those of the rest of the serine residues because of the presence of NOE cross-peaks between the resonances of Tyr-40 and one of the serine residues and, at the same time, select the Ile-39 resonance from the rest of the Isoleueine residues. Distance information on the protein in solution is obtained from ^{1}H-^{1}H homonuclear NOE measurements. Figure 4.16 is the result of the combined two-dimensional ^{1}H-^{15}N correlation and ^{1}H-^{1}H NOE spectrum of uniformly ^{2}H (80%) and ^{15}N (98%) labeled coat protein in dodecylphosphocholine (DPC) micelles.

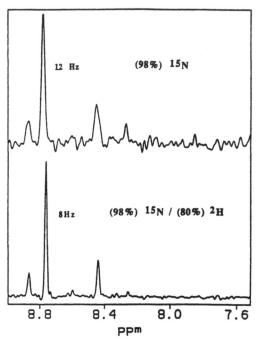

Figure 4.14 Demonstrates the resonance linewidth narrowing effect of protein deuteration. The one-dimensional slices are taken from two different spectra obtained under identical conditions. The frequency corresponding to ^{15}N dimension for these slices is the same.

The spectrum contains NOE cross-peaks between all amide correlation peaks from adjacent residues within α helices. The tracing of two continuous pathways of NOEs among the various amide ^{1}H atoms directly maps out the two stretches of α helix in the protein. The existence of these two α helices is strongly supported by the observation of many of the appropriate cross-peaks between amide ^{1}H and $C_\alpha{}^1$H resonances.

The measurements of heteronuclear NOEs from Pf1 coat protein in DPC micelles have not only identified the mobile residues on both terminal regions but also detected other mobile residues within the mid-section of the coat protein. The interesting result is that the region extending from residue 14 to 18 shows local backbone mobility that is slower than the terminal motions but faster than the overall tumbling motion of the complex. The implication derived from the observation is that the secondary structures involved within the mid-section of the coat protein is separated by a loosely structured mobile loop.

Solid-state NMR spectra of uniformly ^{15}N and selectively ^{15}N-Glu and ^{15}N-Tyr labeled coat proteins in oriented phospholipid bilayers are shown in Figure 4.17. The spectrum of uniformly ^{15}N labeled protein has two

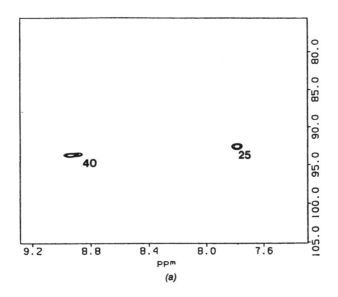

(a)

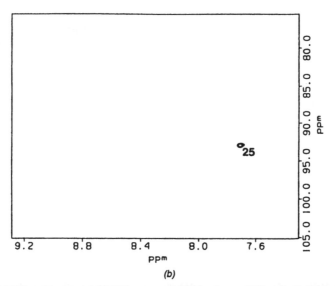

(b)

Figure 4.15 Two-dimensional HMQC spectrum showing its capability of selectively observing amide protons directly bonded to ^{15}N isotope: (a) HMQC spectrum of selectively ^{15}N-Tyr labeled protein showing two tyrosine residues 40 and 25; (b) HMQC spectrum of single site ^{15}N Tyr-25 labeled protein.

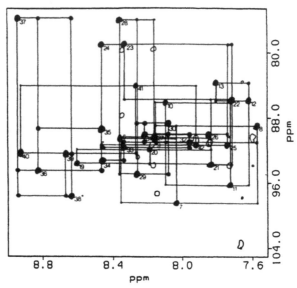

Figure 4.16 Two-dimensional HMQC-NOESY spectrum of uniformly ²H and ¹⁵N labeled Pf1 coat protein in DPC micelles at 50°C and pH 5.0. Each amide site gives rise to a single correlation peak in the contour plot. The lines connect the cross-peaks between correlation peaks from adjacent residues. Two α helices, hydrophobic and amphipathic, are mapped out by connecting NOE cross-peaks between adjacent amide protons. Those correlation peaks which are not connected are from mobile amide sites, the internal loop, and NH₂- and COOH-termini.

bands of signal intensity near the resonance frequencies associated with $\sigma_{\parallel}$ and $\sigma_{\perp}$ of the amide chemical shift tensor. Spectral resolution is greatly improved by using selectively ¹⁵N labeled protein samples. Since there is only one glutamic acid residue in Pf1 coat protein, the spectrum of ¹⁵N-Glu labeled Pf1 coat protein can be obtained with better resolution. It has a single line with a resonance frequency near $\sigma_{\perp}$, and therefore the N−H bond of Glu-9, representing the amphipathic helix orientation is approximately perpendicular to the direction of the magnetic field and parallel to the plane of the bilayer. The two tyrosine residues in Pf1 coat protein are in the hydrophobic helix, and therefore the spectrum of ¹⁵N-Tyr labeled Pf1 coat protein has overlapping resonance intensity near $\sigma_{\parallel}$. This result demonstrates that the N−H bonds of Tyr-25 and Tyr-40 (the hydrophobic helix) are approximately parallel to the direction of the magnetic field and perpendicular to the plane of the bilayer.

The results of the NMR experiments are summarized with the model of the protein in Figure 4.18. The protein has two α helices, as defined by the observation of the appropriate homonuclear ¹H-¹H NOEs in micelles in Figure 4.16. The data in Figure 4.17 demonstrate that the amphipathic

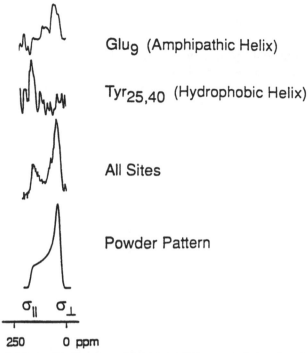

Glu$_9$ (Amphipathic Helix)

Tyr$_{25,40}$ (Hydrophobic Helix)

All Sites

Powder Pattern

$\sigma_\parallel$ $\sigma_\perp$

250   0 ppm

Figure 4.17 Solid-state NMR spectra of ^{15}N labeled Pf1 coat protein in oriented phospholipid bilayers. The experimental spectra are compared to a calculated ^{15}N amide chemical shift powder pattern with the positions of the principal components marked. The spectra were obtained on a home-built 8.5 T spectrometer.

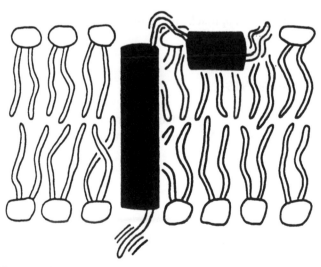

Figure 4.18 Model of Pf1 coat protein in lipid bilayers. The amphipathic helix parallel to the plane of the bilayer and the hydrophobic membrane spanning helix are represented as filled cylinders. The mobile terminal and loop regions are represented as ribbons.

helix is parallel to the plane of the bilayer and the hydrophobic helix is perpendicular to the plane of the bilayer. Negative heteronuclear NOE measurements indicate that the two rigid helices are connected by a mobile loop and that there are mobile residues at both the NH$_2$- and COOH-termini.

The structures of both photosynthetic reaction centers and bacteriorhodopsin are dominated by long hydrophobic membrane spanning helices connected by loops, some of which contain relatively short amphipathic bridging helices. Bacteriorhodopsin has been shown to have mobile amino and carboxyl terminal regions as well as mobile internal loops. It is quite surprising to find that the small Pf1 coat protein is remarkably rich with secondary structures consisting of five distinct regions that are identical with those found in much larger proteins like bacteriorhodopsin and the photosynthetic reaction center.

SUMMARY

Determination of the structure and dynamics of the filamentous bacteriophage Pf1 coat protein in its membrane-bound form by NMR spectroscopy, as described in this chapter, shows the way for studies of other membrane-bound systems which do not crystallize. The difficult problems associated with NMR studies of peptides in membrane environments can be overcome by using both multidimensional solution NMR and solid-state NMR. This same approach can be used with larger proteins in membrane environments.

ACKNOWLEDGEMENTS

This research is being supported by grants RO1 AI20770-08, RO1 GM29754-11, and RO1 GM24266-14 from the National Institutes of Health.

REFERENCES

1 Opella, S. J. and P. L. Stewart. 1989. *Methods in Enzymology, Vol. 176*, N. J. Oppenheimer and T. L. James, eds., San Diego, California: Academic Press, p. 242.

2 Opella, S. J., P. L. Stewart and K. G. Valentine. 1987. *Q. Rev. Biophys.*, 19:7, 1/2.

3 Neuhaus, D., G. Wagner, M. Vasak, J. H. R. Kagi and K. Wuthrich. 1985. *Eur. J. Biochem.*, 151:257.

4 Griffey, R. H. and A. G. Redfield. 1987. *Q. Rev. Biophys.*, 19:51, 1/2.

5 Shon, K. and S. J. Opella. 1989. *J. Magn. Reson.*, 82:193.

6 Shon, K., Y. Kim, L. A. Colnago and S. J. Opella. 1991. *Science*, 252:1303.

7 LeMaster, D. M. and F. M. Richards. 1988. *Biochemistry*, 27:142.

8 LeMaster, D. M. 1989. *Methods in Enzymology, Vol. 177*, N. J. Oppenheimer and T. L. James, eds., San Diego, California: Academic Press, p. 23.

9 Aue, W. P., E. Bartholdi and R. R. Ernst. 1976. *J. Chem. Phys.*, 64:2229.

10 Nagayama, K., A. Kumar, K. Wuthrich and R. R. Ernst. 1980. *J. Magn. Reson.*, 40:321.

11 Bax, A. and R. J. Freeman. 1981. *J. Magn. Reson.*, 44:542.

12 Wider, G., S. Macura, A. Kumar, R. R. Ernst and K. Wuthrich. 1984. *J. Magn. Reson.*, 56:207.

13 Davis, D. G. and A. Bax. 1985. *J. Am. Chem. Soc.*, 107:2820.

14 Braunschweiler, L. and R. R. Ernst. 1983. *J. Magn. Reson.*, 53:521.

15 Jeener, J., B. H. Meyer, P. Bachmann and R. R. Ernst. 1979. *J. Chem. Phys.*, 71:4546.

16 Macura, S. and R. R. Ernst. 1980. *Mol. Phys.*, 41:95.

17 Macura, S., Y. Huang, D. Suter and R. R. Ernst. 1981. *J. Magn. Reson.*, 43:259.

18 Kumar, A., R. R. Ernst and K. Wuthrich. *Biochem. Biophys. Res. Commun.*, 95:1.

19 Bax, A., R. H. Griffey and B. L. Hawkins. 1983. *J. Magn. Reson.*, 55:301.

20 Rance, M., O. W. Sorensen, G. Bodenhausen, G. Wagner, R. R. Ernst and K. Wuthrich. 1983. *Biochem. Biophys. Res. Commun.*, 117:479.

21 Griesinger, C., O. W. Sorensen and R. R. Ernst. 1987. *J. Magn. Reson.*, 73:574.

22 Fesik, S. W. and E. P. R. Zuiderweg. 1988. *J. Magn. Reson.*, 78:588; Vuister, G. W., R. Boelens and R. Kaptein. 1988. *J. Magn. Reson.*, 80:176.

23 Marion, D., L. E. Kay, S. W. Sparks, D. A. Torchia and A. Bax. 1989. *J. Am. Chem. Soc.*, 111:1515.

24 Oschkinat, H., C. Griesinger, P. J. Kraulis, O. W. Sorensen, R. R. Ernst, A. M. Gronenborn and G. M. Core. 1988. *Nature* (London), 332:374.

25 Kay, L. E., D. Marion and A. Bax. 1989. *J. Magn. Reson.*, 84:72.

26 Driscoll, P. C., G. M. Clore, D. Marion, P. T. Singfield and A. M. Gronenborn. 1990. *Biochemistry*, 29:3542.

27 Wuthrich, K. 1986. *NMR of Proteins and Nucleic Acids*, New York: Wiley-Interscience.

28 Wuthrich, K., M. Billeter and W. Braun. 1984. *J. Mol. Biol.*, 180:715.

29 Chirlian, L. E. and S. J. Opella. 1990. *S. J. Adv. Magn. Reson.*, 14:183.

30 Zasloff, M. 1987. *Proc. Natl. Acad. Sci. USA*, 84:5449–5453.

31 Urrutia, R., R. A. Cruciani, J. L. Barker and B. Kuchar. 1989. *FEBS Lett.*, 247:17–21.

32 Unpublished results.

33 Marion, D., M. Zasloff and A. Bax. 1988. *FEBS Lett.*, 227:21–26.

34 Montal, M. 1990. *Ion Channels Vol. 2* (Plenum) pp. 1–31.

35 Montal, M. 1990. *FASEB J.*, 9:2623–2635.

36 Oiki, S., W. Danho, V. Madison and M. Montal. 1988. *Proc. Natl. Acad. Sci. USA*, 85:8703–8707.

37 Kersh, J., J. Tomich and M. Montal. 1989. *Biochem. Biophys. Res. Commun.*, 162:352–356.
38 Brown, L. R., W. Braun, A. Kumar and K. Wuthrich. 1982. *Biophys. J.*, 37:319–328.
39 Braun, W., G. Wider, K. H. Lee and K. Wuthrich. 1983. *J. Mol. Biol.*, 169:921–948.
40 Lee, K. H., J. E. Fitton and K. Wuthrich. 1987. *Biochim. Biophys. Acta.*, 911:144–153.
41 Mulvery, D., G. F. King, R. M. Cooke, D. G. Doak, T. S. Harvey and I. D. Campbell. 1989. *FEBS Lett.*, 257:113–117.
42 Wennerberg, A. B. A., R. M. Cooke, M. Caarlquist, R. Rigler and I. D. Campbell. 1990. *Biochem. Biophys. Res. Commun.*, 166:1102–1109.
43 Unpublished results.

CHEMICAL SYNTHETIC ASPECTS OF PEPTIDE PRODUCTION

CHAPTER 5

Large Scale Peptide Production

MARIA-LUISA MACCECCHINI[1]

SUMMARY

SYNTHESIS of biologically active peptides and proteins can be achieved using several chemical, biochemical as well as recombinant strategies.

This chapter reviews several strategies and discusses their relevance to process scale up. We conclude that each peptide has its own dynamics and requires different scale up approaches. However, we can suggest guidelines for scale up in accordance with the size of the peptide and the amount of product needed. In general the best approach for production of large quantities of a short peptide, up to 15 amino acids in length, is solution synthesis; for a peptide of 20 to 45 amino acids in length is fragment condensation; and for a protein larger than 50 amino acids is recombinant technology. Smaller amounts of peptides in the 10 to 50 amino acid range are best synthesized by solid phase synthesis.

Advances most relevant to large scale peptide synthesis include enhanced versatility of solution synthesis, development of resins for synthesis of protected fragments, improvement of fragment condensations in solution or on the resin, and application of high pressure liquid chromatography together with ion exchange, and gel chromatography to peptide purification.

INTRODUCTION

Over the past 10 years, advances in peptide chemistry, genetic engineering, and other biotech-related techniques have resulted in a sharp rise in

[1]Symphony Pharmaceuticals, Inc., Philadelphia, PA 19104, U.S.A.

new peptide applications. Table 5.1 lists selected, existing and potential applications for peptides.

Insulin, isolated from the pancreas of cows, was one of the first peptides to be commercialized. Today, peptides and peptide analogs comprise a variety of well-known human health products such as captopril and enalapril for the treatment of hypertension; human growth hormone for pituitary dwarfism; cyclosporine as an immunosuppressant; interferons and interleukins as immunostimulants; and calcitonin for osteoporosis. Other common peptides include aspartame used as an artificial sweetener, glyphosate as an herbicide, and bacitracin as an antibiotic and growth promoter for animals. Many other peptides are currently in clinical trials or under investigation for such varied applications as AIDS, cancer, wound healing, flavor enhancers, pesticides, and specialty adhesives.

Worldwide consumption of peptides was $6.5 billion in 1990, up from $4.5 billion in 1987. U.S. consumption is estimated at $20 billion in 1995, versus $2.7 billion in 1988 and $2.1 billion in 1987. It accounts for almost 50% of worldwide consumption. Western Europe is responsible for about one-third of worldwide consumption, while Japanese consumption accounts for the other 20% (Table 5.2).

As new products and applications develop, worldwide consumption of peptides is forecast to increase at a compounded annual rate of 13% reaching $20 billion by 1995. Human health care is and will continue to be the largest market segment as many new products, including interleukins, colony stimulating factors, and growth factors, move through the regulatory process and are approved. Anticipated approval of bovine and porcine growth hormones will support rapid growth in the animal health sector. In Japan, such products as tuna and salmon growth promoters are expected to be more significant.

TABLE 5.1. **Peptide Applications.**

Human Health
AIDS, birth control, cancer, diabetes, growth, hypertension, immunostimulation, immunosuppression, infertility, pain control, wound healing

Agriculture
Herbicides, insecticides, plant metabolism

Food
Antioxidants, flavor enhancers, sweeteners

Animal Health
Growth promoters, hormones, veterinary drugs, vaccines

Industrial
Adhesives, high-performance fibers, research

Source: Strategic Analysis Inc.

TABLE 5.2 U.S. Consumption of Peptides by End-Use Market.

| | $ Million* | | |
	1987	1988	1989
Human Health	$1100	$1600	$2700
Food	700	750	900
Agriculture	250	300	350
Other**	50	50	50
Total	$2100	$2700	$4000

*Valued at manufacturer's levels.
**Includes animal health and industrial.
Source: Strategic Analysis Inc.

The development of pharmaceutically useful products has always been an important consideration in modern peptide research. However, in the past few years the explosive progress in peptide research, sparked by such discoveries as the hypothalamic releasing factors and endogeneous opioids, and the advent of molecular genetics and computer graphics have accelerated the pace for peptide drug development. Indeed, the opportunities for the commercial production of peptides, peptide mimetics, and proteins for use in medicine have never seemed to be better than at present.

PEPTIDE SYNTHESIS

SOLUTION PHASE SYNTHESIS

Experimental research on synthetic peptides had its inception in the early 1870s and was based on the assumption that the amino acids constituting the protein molecule are linked together via amide bonds. Such studies, initiated by Schaal in 1871 and extended by Grimaux some 10 years later, [1,2] involved the condensation of aspartic acid and asparagine to a mixture of polymeric products. Among early investigations, Leuchs [3] showed in 1906 that amino acids could be induced to polymerize, but despite the superficial resemblance of the polymeric substances to the protein molecule, the individual polymeric units were of different chain lengths, and the substances were amorphous and not conducive to characterization.

The 30-year search for a satisfactory acyl blocking group finally bore fruit in 1932, with the ingenious development of the "carbobenzoxy method" of Bergmann and Zervas [4]. Since its inception, the original

Bergmann-Zervas procedure, together with later modifications thereof, has been employed in the synthesis of some several hundred different peptides. Between 1906 and 1947 only a few significant studies were published [5] including the mechanism by which carboxyanhydrides of amino acids undergo polymer formation. In 1947, however, there was a resurgence of interest in macromolecular polypeptides as protein models, influenced by the brief announcement of Woodward and Schramm [6] that more complex linear peptides could be made through a refinement of the Leuchs' [3] procedure, as well as by the introduction of new analytical methods.

Today our understanding of solution peptide synthesis is as follows: a peptide linkage occurs through the direct condensation of the α-amino group of one amino acid with the α-carboxyl group of the other amino acid under elimination of a water molecule [7]. Peptide bond synthesis by direct condensation, as formulated above, requires suppression of the reactive character of the amino group of the first and of the carboxyl group of the second amino acid. The masking substituents must permit their ready removal, without inducing breakdown of the labile peptide molecule.

The major advantages of synthesis in solution are; availability of a multitude of coupling methods, a wide variety of protecting groups, opportunities for intermediate purification and linear scale up potential. In planning solution synthesis the strategy considerations include, (a) selection of main chain and side chain protective groups, (b) choice of activation method, (c) careful selection of segments in efforts to minimize racemization during segment condensation, and (d) solubility considerations. The problems faced during actual synthesis are unpredictable solubility and considerable racemization. Furthermore, solution peptide synthesis is a very labor intensive procedure.

SOLID PHASE PEPTIDE SYNTHESIS

Solid phase peptide synthesis (SPPS) was introduced by Bruce Merrifield in 1963 in an effort to overcome many of the problems encountered in solution synthesis [8,9]. SPPS uses an insoluble polymer for support of organic synthesis. Merrifield chose to attach the C-terminal residue of the peptide to a polymer and grow the peptide chain toward the amino end of the peptide [10,11]. After the desired sequence has been assembled on the support, the chain is cleaved and the finished peptide is released into the supernatant.

The great advantage of using a polymer-supported peptide chain is elimination of laborious purifications at intermediate steps. They are substituted by simple washing and filtration of the peptide resin. Mechanical loss of material during transfers is eliminated, so are losses associated with purification of intermediates.

The critical requirements for synthesis of homogeneous peptides by SPPS are that the deprotection and coupling reactions go fully to completion and that the side-chain blocking groups and the peptide-resin bond be completely stable throughout.

The deprotection reagent must be vigorous to remove all side-chain protecting groups and to cleave the peptide from the polymer matrix. Furthermore, the coupling reaction must be driven to completion with excess activated amino acids to reduce side products lacking one or more residues due to incomplete deprotection or coupling.

The greatest advantage of SPPS is its speed. With the "classical" system of Merrifield SPPS, peptide chains are usually assembled at the rate of one residue per four hours. Manual SPPS allows convenient elongation of peptide chains at the rate of two or three residues per day, and automatic synthesizers currently available can carry out synthesis at the rate of 12 or more residues per 24 hours. This speed and simplicity of SPPS has made it practical for individual peptide chemists to embark upon programs of analog synthesis which would be impractical using solution methods.

Several sets of combinations of resin linkers, protecting groups, blocking groups, and deprotection and cleavage reagents are given in Table 5.3, along with the purpose for which they have been used. While the classical system yields satisfactory results for synthesis of most small peptides, for larger peptides and for special purposes the choice of the proper combination of these factors is essential.

Boc Strategy

The system now considered standard for SPPS of small or medium-sized peptides uses as resin a 1% cross-linked polystyrene. The standard protecting group for α-amino functions is the tert-butyloxycarbonyl (Boc) group [12–14]. This group is removed with rather dilute solutions of strong acids such as 25% trifluoroacetic acid (TFA). The next Boc-amino acid is coupled to the aminoacyl resin, usually by use of dicyclohexylcarbodiimide (DCC). Following completion of assembly, the peptide-resin is treated with anhydrous hydrofluoric acid (HF) to cleave the benzyl ester link in order to liberate the free peptide. Side-chain functional groups are usually blocked during synthesis by benzyl-derived blocking groups, which are also cleaved by HF. The free peptide is then extracted from the resin with a suitable solvent, purified, and characterized.

Since acidolysis is used both for removal of the Boc groups during each step of the synthesis as well as cleavage of the side-chain blocking groups

TABLE 5.3. The Strategy of Solid Phase Peptide Synthesis.

System	Use	Resin Link	Alpha Protection	Deprotection Reagent	Side Chain	Cleavage
Classic	Stable	ObzI-R	Boc	TFA, HCl	Bzl	HF, HBr
	Amides	Pam-R	Boc	TFA, HCl	Bzl	HF, HBr
	Alcohol	MBHA, BHA	Boc	TFA, HCl	Bzl	HF
	Segments	OBzI-R	Boc	TFA, HCl	Bzl	LiBH$_4$
		Oxime-R	Boc	TFA	Bzl	HF
		OBzI-R	Bpoc	Dil. TFA	Bzl	HF
	Labile	OBzI-R	Bpoc	Dil. TFA	tBu	HF
		Ether-R	Bpoc	Dil. TFA	tBu	TFA
Orthogonal	Segments	Ether-R	Fmoc	Piperidine	tBu	TFA
		tBu-R	Fmoc	Piperidine	Bzl	TFA
		Hydrazide-R	Fmoc	Piperidine	Bzl	TFA
	Segments	Sasrin-R	Fmoc	Piperidine	tBu	TFA
	Amides	Fmoc-Amide-R	Fmoc	Piperidine	tBu	TFA

Adapted and complemented from Stewart [10].

118

and cleavage of the peptide from the resin at the end of the synthesis, successful SPPS requires a large difference in reactivity of these groups. The ester link of the C-terminal amino acid to the resin is not absolutely stable to deprotection conditions; up to 1% of peptide is lost from the resin at each step of synthesis. This difficulty can be overcome by use of either a more labile α-blocking group for the amino acids or a more stable peptide-resin link. Both these approaches have been used. The classical peptide-resin link can be used with Bpoc-amino acids, that require more dilute TFA for deprotection. On the other hand, Boc-amino acids can be used with a more stable peptide-resin link, such as that provided by the Pam-resin introduced by Merrifield. Peptide amides are extremely important, since many naturally-occurring peptide hormones are present in the amide form. In the Boc strategy amidated peptides can be obtained by use of benzhydrylamine and methylbenzhydrylamine resins which yield peptide amides directly upon cleavage with anhydrous HF.

Fmoc Strategy

In the procedures discussed above, the selectivity of cleavage of the side-chain blocking groups and of the peptide-resin link depends upon differences in the rate of acidolytic cleavage. Orthogonal systems have been introduced, where the side-chain blocking groups, and the peptide-resin link are completely stable to the reagent used to remove the α-protecting group at each step of the synthesis. The earliest approach to orthogonal SPPS involved use of Nps-amino acids. Instability and lack of commercial availability of the Nps-amino acids have inhibited development of this system. More attention recently has been given to the use of Fmoc-amino acids [15–17].

In the 9-fluorenylmethyloxycarbonyl (Fmoc) approach the side-chain protecting groups and the peptide-resin link are completely stable to secondary amines used for cleaving the N-α-Fmoc group. The side-chain protection and the peptide-resin link are cleaved by mild acidolysis. The repeated contact with base makes the Merrifield resin not suitable for Fmoc chemistry. Instead, p-alkoxybenzylesters linked to the resin are used as proposed by Wang [18]. Deprotection and cleavage are done by TFA treatment. A new super acid sensitive resin, Sasrin [26], uses Fmoc strategy and permits selective cleavage of protected peptide fragments. These can be isolated, purified, and further used for condensation either in solution or on the resin. Low racemization and high loading are further advantages of this novel resin. A new polymeric support for Fmoc synthesis of peptide amides was also developed [19]. The Fmoc-amide resin consists of a 4-methoxy-benzhydrylamine anchor linked to an aminomethyl resin through a spacer unit. A high loading capacity makes this resin very attractive.

Many problems are associated with the use of asparagine (Asn) and glutamine (Gln) in peptide synthesis such as dehydration, cyclization, pyroglutamic acid formation, deamidation, poor solubility of most derivatives and side reactions in the cleavage of Asn and Gln side-chain protecting groups. Introduction of the Trityl protected derivatives has facilitated synthesis as well as deprotection of peptides containing Asn and Gln. The protected amino acids are soluble in most organic solvents. Coupling is performed by standard procedures, and the group is easily removed by 95% TFA or TFA/dichloromethane. Another breakthrough for Fmoc SPPS is introduction of the pentamethylchroman-sulfonyl (Pmc) protecting group for arginine (Arg) [20]. Pmc can be easily removed with TFA in contrast to the original Tosyl group. These new resins and new protecting groups make working with the Fmoc strategy easier and more versatile.

Mixed and Combination Strategies

Using more than one chemistry allows us to take advantage of each chemistry's different properties. Boc was the original protecting group used during the development of SPPS and is removed by strong acids. Fmoc is removed by organic bases. Because some assembled peptides degrade under rigorous acidic procedures, Fmoc provides a milder alternative. An interesting example of dual chemistries applied to a single peptide is found in Applied Biosystems' "Characterization and Synthesis of the San Diego Test Peptide-3." In the most recent case, the test peptide was synthesized starting with a Fmoc-Lys(Boc) with Boc used during the first 10 amino acid couplings of the synthesis and Fmoc for the last 17 couplings of the peptide, resulting in a branched peptide.

The synthesis of peptides can be achieved by solution or solid phase methods or by a combination of the two—convergent peptide synthesis [21,22]: protected peptide segments built up on solid-phase are cleaved, purified, analyzed, and further used for fragment coupling either in solution or onto a peptide chain attached to a resin support.

Standard SPPS results in a crude product containing deletion peptides. Normal peptide purification procedures cannot always be expected to remove such contaminants unequivocally. In combination synthesis suitably blocked peptides are synthesized separately and then incorporated into the desired sequence. The deletion sequences will, therefore, differ from the desired sequence by more than a single amino acid residue and their removal will be simpler.

Segment condensation is also used to overcome difficult coupling problems in synthesis of long peptides. For example, extensive termination of peptide chains has been seen in certain sequences at glutamine (Gln) and proline (Pro) residues. The problems may often be overcome by synthesis of the peptide fragment containing the difficult sequence and coupling it to the peptide resin.

Several resins have been described that yield upon cleavage blocked peptides. Kaiser et al. describe an oxime support, which can be used in Boc SPPS to yield blocked peptides [23,24].

Sheppard and Williams synthesized an acid-labile anchor and coupled it to polydimethylacrylamide resin [25]. Mergler et al. [26,27] developed a super acid sensitive resin, Sasrin, mentioned earlier. The final resin is of higher loading and easier handling than the Sheppard resin. Protected fragments are synthesized by the Fmoc method and can be cleaved from Sasrin in mild conditions (0.5–1% TFA) at high yields and excellent purity. They can be coupled back to the resin or to a resin-bound peptide if desired.

Conventional solution peptide synthesis is cumbersome and time consuming, but it allows purification of fully protected intermediary fragments. This is an advantage over SPPS, in which case the final product has to be singled out from a mixture of similar fragments. Condensation of protected fragments made by SPPS combines the ease and speed of solid phase with the purification advantage of solution phase. Racemization at the C-terminus of the head fragment is one of the main problems of fragment coupling. Therefore, fragments with C-terminal Gly or Pro are selected whenever possible.

ENZYMATIC SYNTHESIS

Carboxypeptidase Y (CPD-Y) is a catabolic enzyme that degrades a peptide or protein from the carboxy terminus one amino acid at a time. Under appropriate conditions CPD-Y can be forced to reverse its activity and take on a synthetic function. CPD-Y has been used as a catalyst for the stepwise synthesis of several peptides. In the synthesis of the pentapeptide, Leuenkephalin, each peptide bond was formed by enzymatic catalysis using microquantities of the precursors (amino acids or peptide esters as acylcomponents and amino acid esters or amides as nucleophiles). High condensation yields were obtained suggesting that CPD-Y can be a useful tool for preparation of hormone peptides [28]. CPD-Y was also found to catalyze the carboxyterminal amidation of acyl amino acids and peptides using a transpeptidation method. Amides of amino acids and peptides were formed with yields up to 90%. Other enzymes can be made to reverse their activity and be used for fragment coupling and peptide synthesis (see Figure 5.1).

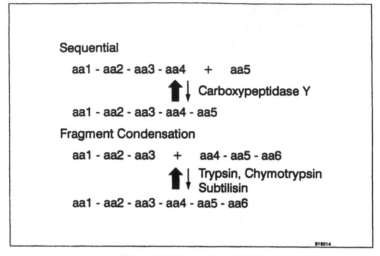

Figure 5.1 Enzymatic synthesis.

RECOMBINANT DNA BIOSYNTHESIS

Recombinant DNA—or gene-splicing—is rapidly becoming the most commercially exciting field in biological research. Recombinant DNA technology offers a method for programming living organisms to produce commercially important products. The major thrust of recombinant DNA technology so far has been in the area of pharmaceuticals. Already the new techniques have been used to produce such important drugs as human insulin, growth factors, lymphokines, vaccines, and human antibodies.

The gene coding for a desired protein is either synthesized or isolated and inserted into the bacterial cell via a vector—usually a plasmid. The bacterium into which the DNA piece is inserted is called a host. The recombinant bacterium is transformed so that it can now use its new genetic information to synthesize a commercially valuable protein product. In short, the steps necessary to engineer a recombinant bacterium are: identify and isolate the gene of interest, put the gene into a vector, infect a host, and induce the host to express the gene, thereby producing the corresponding protein.

The rapid growth of recombinant DNA technology and its applications are practically unparalleled. Production yields of bovine and porcine growth hormone are up to 20 g per liter of fermentation broth and the production costs are down to less than one U.S. dollar per gram. Systems in use today for expression of peptides and proteins of interest are: bacteria, yeast, insect cells, mammalian tissue culture cells, and whole transgenic animals.

SCALE UP

TECHNIQUES AND EXAMPLES

Efforts to utilize peptide hormones made by chemical synthesis in medicine date back to the middle 1950s when the Swiss pharmaceutical companies started their pioneering work. The first peptide drug was oxytocin developed by Sandoz. By 1977, 15 commercial drugs of nine different peptides had been introduced. The best known were corticotropin, thyrotropin releasing hormone and calcitonin.

The recent advances most relevant to large scale peptide synthesis include (a) enhanced versatility of synthesis in solution, (b) novel resins allowing synthesis of protected fragments, (c) considerable progress in solid phase peptide synthesis, (d) efficient solid phase peptide synthesizers, (e) high yield recombinant expression, and (f) application of reversed phase high performance liquid chromatography to peptide purification.

Examples of peptides synthesized in *solution* range in size from 2 to 70 amino acids long and in amounts from milligrams to tons. The largest synthetic production of any peptide at this time is that of aspartame (L-aspartyl-L-phenylalanine methyl ester) produced by Searle with an approximate annual output of 4000 tons. Merck Sharp and Dohme has developed scaled up synthesis of several thyrotropin-releasing hormone (TRH) analogs [29] in 10 to 100 gram quantities. Hoechst produces six peptide hormones in kilogram quantities, i.e., oxytocin, LHRH and its analog Buserelin, TRH, and ACTH. Hoffmann-La Roche scaled up grams of quality controlled material for clinical studies. Bachem Switzerland produces in solution kg of peptides ranging in size from 3 to 32 amino acids.

The advantages of large scale *solid phase* synthesis are: 2–4 cycles per working day, minimal racemization, few insolubility problems, convenient documentation of good manufacturing practices by computer printout. The synthetic disadvantages are: awkward monitoring, capping for incomplete reactions, strong HF acid cleavage required.

Representative of large scale solid phase synthesis is the production of gonadoliberin (LHRH) at Beckman Bioproducts and of two analogs of LHRH at Syntex [31,32]. Each was synthesized on benzhydrylamine resin, and yielded under optimized conditions about 50–55%. Merck, Sharp and Dohme has prepared a series of cyclic hexapeptides in 50 gram and up to 1 kilogram amounts. The Armour Company produces an estimated 250–300 grams/year of salmon calcitonin by solid phase synthesis with a Vega instrument containing a 5 liter capacity glass reactor vessel. After 32 cycles, the peptide is cleaved by liquid HF, is filtered and incubated in dilute aqueous solution at pH 7.5 to effect disulfide bond formation and is purified by chromatography.

Calcitonin is a peptide hormone of 32 amino acids that is used to treat Paget's disease and osteoporosis, conditions in which insufficient calcium is deposited in the bones. Calcitonin may at present be second to insulin as a peptide in terms of pharmaceutical sales. Using calcitonin as an example we can demonstrate how scale up and production approaches have shifted over the years. Originally, calcitonin was made by solution phase and still is at Sandoz, whereas the Armour Company produces it by SPPS. Bachem Switzerland produces calcitonin by solution phase synthesis, but is looking at *combination or convergent synthesis* (Table 5.4). Appropriate calcitonin fragments are selected according to their Gly and Pro distribution and synthesized by SPPS on Sasrin resin. They are cleaved with 1% TFA leaving all the protecting groups intact. Alternatively, one or several of the fragments can be made in solution. The first fragment containing the 2 cysteine residues is oxidized and purified by counter current distribution (CCD). The other two protected fragments are also purified on CCD and the three pieces are coupled in solution to each other. The final product is again purified on CCD deprotected with 50% TFA and extracted.

Recombinant processes for the production of calcitonin are being developed by a number of companies because they are cheaper than peptide synthesis. However, due to its small size calcitonin is degraded by bacterial proteases. The successful cloning strategy, therefore, involves expression of calcitonin as a fusion with another protein or with itself and subsequent cleavage and purification. Yeast and mammalian systems do express short sequences, but at lower yields than bacterial systems and are, as yet, uneconomical for production of kg quantities.

Recombinant processes are well suited for the production of large amounts of proteins, for after the initial investment in preparing the expression system, production output is very high and cost extremely low.

Scale up of *enzymatic* peptide synthesis was done with immobilized CPD-Y [33]. A packed-bed enzyme reactor with immobilized CPD-Y was used for the preparation of Bzl-Arg-Met-NH$_2$, from Bzl-Arg and Met-NH$_2$. The system was designed so that enzymatic peptide synthesis, separation by displacement chromatography, and column regeneration were carried out simultaneously. 460 mg of Bzl-Arg-Met-NH$_2$ with purity greater than 99% were obtained in 24 hours. Really long peptides have, so far, not been described as having been synthesized enzymatically.

RELEVANCE AND LIMITS OF VARIOUS TECHNIQUES

We discussed several technologies used for synthesis of peptides—from solution to solid phase synthesis, to recombinant expression in a host

TABLE 5.4. Calcitonin Synthesis, Oxidation and Purification.

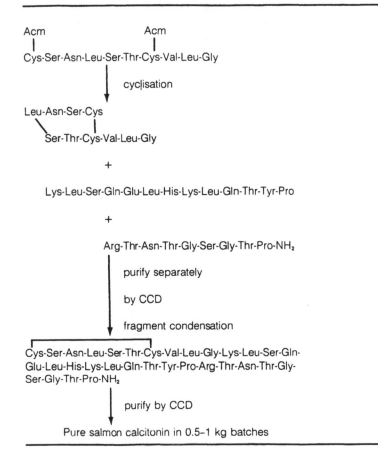

```
Acm                        Acm
 |                          |
Cys-Ser-Asn-Leu-Ser-Thr-Cys-Val-Leu-Gly
                    |
                    |  cyclisation
                    ↓

Leu-Asn-Ser-Cys
               \          |
                Ser-Thr-Cys-Val-Leu-Gly

                    +

       Lys-Leu-Ser-Gln-Glu-Leu-His-Lys-Leu-Gln-Thr-Tyr-Pro

                    +

       Arg-Thr-Asn-Thr-Gly-Ser-Gly-Thr-Pro-NH₂
                    |
                    |  purify separately
                    |
                    |  by CCD
                    |
                    ↓  fragment condensation

Cys-Ser-Asn-Leu-Ser-Thr-Cys-Val-Leu-Gly-Lys-Leu-Ser-Gln-
Glu-Leu-His-Lys-Leu-Gln-Thr-Tyr-Pro-Arg-Thr-Asn-Thr-Gly-
Ser-Gly-Thr-Pro-NH₂
                    |
                    |  purify by CCD
                    ↓
       Pure salmon calcitonin in 0.5–1 kg batches
```

system. What are the advantages and disadvantages of each technique, and how relevant are they for scale up of peptide synthesis? We can generalize by stating that solution phase synthesis is very useful for production of large amounts of short peptides. There is no question that 5 kg of a 5 amino acid peptide or 1 ton of aspartame will be prepared by solution phase.

Solid phase synthesis is extremely useful in the rapid synthesis of smaller amounts of longer peptides. Again 10 mg of a 20 to 70 amino acid long chain will be done by SPPS.

Recombinant techniques are best for large scale production of substantial quantities of long peptides and proteins. A ton of porcine growth hormone can only be made by expression in a host system.

So what is the best procedure for synthesizing 1 kg of calcitonin? Solution phase synthesis of calcitonin will lead to a very clean, well characterized product. The problem lies in the laborious intermediate purification steps and in the excessive amount of amino acid derivatives needed to fulfill the task.

SPPS will quickly yield the crude peptide with little manpower required, but the purification will be more difficult and will result in large losses due to the closely related nature of the impurities present in the crude preparation.

Expression of calcitonin as a recombinant protein in bacteria is burdened with degradation problems. The fusion protein approach will result in higher yields, a more cumbersome purification procedure, and a lower cost product.

As of 1990, the most advantageous way to make 1 kg of calcitonin is by combination of conventional and solid phase synthesis. Appropriate calcitonin fragments are synthesized, individually purified, and used for fragment condensation either on the resin or in solution, depending on their solubility. This combination approach takes advantage of the speed with which SPPS synthesizes fragments and of the ease with which solution phase allows for purification of the end product.

Technologies have been evolving quickly and new improvements in the synthetic and recombinant approach will change the considerations for choosing one technique versus another. However, I feel that for the moment we can represent the best technology to be used for a specific project as shown in Figure 5.2.

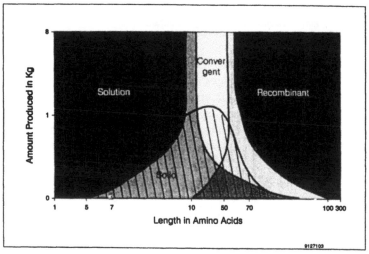

Figure 5.2 Choice of technique depending on peptide length and quantity needed.

PURIFICATION

COUNTER CURRENT DISTRIBUTION

Counter current distribution (CCD) has been used to purify many peptides synthesized by solution or solid phase [34,35]. Although long CCD runs are required for very high resolution, most moderate size peptides should be pure within 100 to 300 transfers.

A CCD solvent system must be used that provides a satisfactory partition coefficients k without causing degradation of the peptide or intractable emulsification. The principle relies on differential solubility between the peptide to be purified and its impurities. If the peptide has a purification coefficient $k = 1$, the most rapid purification will occur, because of

$$k = \frac{\text{concentration in upper phase}}{\text{concentration in lower phase}}$$

Practical limits are $0.2 < k > 5.0$. The real advantage of CCD is in the separation of protected peptides or peptide fragments obtained either by solution or solid phase peptide synthesis. These fragments can then be used for condensation in the production of large final peptide products.

ION EXCHANGE CHROMATOGRAPHY

Ion exchange column chromatography is a very widely used technique for separating and purifying peptides, because of its great versatility and extreme selectivity.

The basic principle of ion exchange is that separation is achieved on the basis of the charges carried by solute molecules. Ion exchange is capable of separating molecules differing by very small differences in charge, and is therefore a technique of very high resolving power.

The separation in ion exchange chromatography is obtained by reversible adsorption of substances having different affinities for the ion exchanger due to differences in their charge. In ion exchange chromatography one can choose whether to bind the substance of interest, or to adsorb out contaminants and allow the desired product to pass through the column. Generally it is more useful to adsorb the material to be purified, since this results in a greater degree of fractionation.

Ion exchange is a standard purification tool in biochemistry separating molecules on the basis of their charge differences. It is applicable in almost any purification protocol, and combines high resolution and concentration in a single method. When deciding on whether to use a cation or anion exchanger three factors have to be considered. The properties of your sample (charge, stability, size, etc.), the separation objectives you set, and the scale at which you are working. Ion exchange may be carried out in a column, by a batch procedure, or through derivatized membrane filtering. In all three cases definite stages are performed: equilibration of the ion exchanger, addition and binding of sample substances, change of conditions to produce selective desorption, and regeneration of the ion exchanger.

Chromatography on Dowex 1 [36,37] a strongly basic resin allows the entire range of peptides, from strongly basic to strongly acidic, to be chromatographed in a single run. Dowex 50 is a strongly acidic resin that elutes the entire range of peptides in the reverse order of a basic resin.

GEL CHROMATOGRAPHY

Gel chromatography is done with cross-linked dextran or polyacrylamide gels. It is a very useful technique for separating peptides from salt and other contaminants of low molecular weight, and for separating peptides on the basis of molecular weight. The size of column to be chosen should retain the entire quantity of the smaller molecules present in the sample, while still providing good separation from the desired peptide. For more refined separations such as removal of synthetic impurities from a desired peptide, a pore size should be chosen such that the desired peptide will be within the separation range, i.e., neither excluded nor totally included. Gel filtration is one of the most common techniques for separating biologically active molecules. It provides a relatively simple chromatographic pattern and immediate information on molecular size. It is an invaluable complement to other techniques, such as ion exchange, chromatofocusing, and reversed phase chromatography.

Gel filtration offers a variety of applications including molecular weight estimations, studies of conjugate formation and aggregation, group separation, protein purification, and screening of uncharacterized samples.

HIGH PERFORMANCE LIQUID CHROMATOGRAPHY

The application of high performance liquid chromatography (HPLC) to peptide research was first discussed 10 years ago [38,39]. Within a decade this technique has made major impacts on the isolation, purification, and analysis of natural and synthetic peptides. Major advances in SPPS were made, when it became apparent that reversed phase systems were capable of separating even the closest deletion peptides from the main product, and homogenous peptide samples were obtained. Development of HPLC has caused a revolution in peptide purification and analysis. It has greatly increased the resolving power and speed of operation of column chromatography. This improvement is primarily due to development of solid supports, which give high resolution and withstand high pressures of operation.

HPLC supports are generally small beads used alone or with attachment of surface functional groups. An organic functional layer may be covalently bonded to the surface, such as alkyl hydrocarbon chains reversedphase, rp; these may be 18 carbon chains C18, or shorter C8, C4, aromatic (phenyl), alkyl nitrile (CN), alcohol or ion exchange groups.

A primary rule in selection of HPLC conditions is that no solvents more basic than pH 8 be used. However, some dissolution takes place at any pH. A major problem with HPLC is the instability of the bonded phases; characteristics of the columns change continually during use due to loss of the organic layer. Columns have to be continuously monitored and restandardized.

AUTOMATION

In a modern laboratory, a new post doc needs a peptide in a hurry. The prepackaged chemicals are put into place, the sequence is programmed into the synthesizer's memory, a few adjustments are made, and the synthesis is started. Depending on the sequence, the peptide might be ready in a day [40].

Development of solid phase synthesis and automation took the chemical synthesis of peptides from the organic chemistry laboratory to the biochemist's benchtop, for production of vaccines, antibodies, and drugs. Essentially all automated synthesizers are designed for solid phase synthesis. There are four basic steps in SPPS: protection/deprotection, activation and coupling of the amino acid, cycling process to elongate the chain, and cleavage and deprotection. Expert systems take different factors into account and take a best guess at a synthetic strategy. These factors include the length of the peptide and the adjacent amino acids. Synthesizers can take care of the first two steps of SPPS. However, the steps from the completed peptide on the resin to the purification and verification of the peptide structure are the most problematic. The whole second part of the process of cleavage, deprotection and purification has so far not been automated and needs to be improved.

In contrast to peptide chemistry scale-up, fermentation technology has seen remarkable progress in automation [41]. Requirements for a pilot-plant system are quite different from those for a production plant, because in a pilot plant, the computer is used primarily as a research tool. It is necessary that the system be designed to be as flexible as possible. It should be particularly useful in obtaining kinetic data necessary for modeling the process, for developing control strategies aimed at process optimization, and for accommodating software development and software testing.

In a full-scale production plant the primary objective is to produce a product in an optimal manner. As a result, the computer is used for process control and optimization aimed at maintaining quality control and product uniformity.

In fermentation there are common calculations. These include computations for oxygen uptake rate, carbon dioxide evolution rate, respiratory quotient, overall mass transfer coefficient, heat balance, power requirements, cell mass, and cell growth rate. A computer system is a valuable tool for obtaining on-line information concerning the status of the fermentation process.

Computers have a variety of applications in the fermentation industry ranging from data logging and on-line analysis to process modeling, control, and optimization. So far a small fraction of the potential has been realized. Many groups are working on modeling, control, and optimization, for the real future lies in developing improved mathematical models and strategies for process control and optimization.

CONCLUSIONS

In concluding it is apparent that large scale peptide synthesis may be carried out either by solution, solid phase synthesis, combination synthesis, or recombinant technology. However, there are technical and operational differences. To obtain 1–10 kg of peptide by solution synthesis large amounts of protected amino acids (50 kg level), and protected fragments (10 kg level) have to be prepared and many manhours are required, but a pure product can be obtained. With solid phase synthesis that level of operation has not as yet been achieved. In general solid phase synthesis has not ventured beyond the kilogram level of operation, but this might be just a matter of time. The most attractive approach for scale up of peptide synthesis of a 30 amino acid peptide today, is the combination method: making fragments by solid phase and coupling them together by fragment condensation. For peptides longer than 40 amino acids the recombinant approach offers the best combination of parameters.

However, each peptide has its own dynamics and a different approach for scale up may have to be chosen. The future looks promising just considering three aspects: the cost of Fmoc amino acids have dropped substantially, which will make this method generally attractive; enzymatic synthesis offers the potential of producing large batches efficiently; and recombinant DNA synthesis unfolds exciting new opportunities with the development of new expression systems and host vectors.

ABBREVIATIONS

AA	amino acid
Ac	acetyl
Acm	acetamidomethyl
BHA	benzyhydrylamine (resin)
Boc	tert-butyloxycarbonyl
Bom	benzyloxy methyl
Bpoc	2-(4-biphenyl)propyl(2)oxycarbonyl
Bzl	benzyl
C-	carboxy-
Cbz	benzyloxycarbonyl
CCD	counter current distribution
DCC	dicyclohexylcarbodiimide
DMF	dimethylformamide
DMSO	dimethyl sulfoxide
Dnp	2,4-dinitrophenyl
DVB	1,4-divinylbenzene
Et	ethyl
EtOAc	ethyl acetate
EtOH	ethanol
Fmoc	9-fluorenylmethyloxycarbonyl
For	formyl
HF	hydrofluoric acid
HOAc	acetic acid
HOBt	1-hydroxybenzotriazole
HOSu	N-hydroxysuccinimide
HPLC	high performance liquid chromatography
IR	infrared (spectroscopy)
k	partition coefficient
MBHA	4-methylbenzhydrylamine (resin)
Mbs	4-methoxybenzenesulfonyl
Me	methyl
MeOH	methanol
MSA	methanesulfonic acid
NMR	nuclear magnetic resonance (spectroscopy)
OtBu	tert-butyl ester
OBzl	benzyl ester
OEt	ethyl ester
OMe	methyl ester
ONp	4-nitrophenyl ester
OSu	N-hydroxysuccinimide ester
-R	resin support

Pam	phenylacetamidomethyl
pc	partition chromatorgraphy
Ph	phenyl
Pmc	2,2,5,7,8-pentamethyl chroman-6-sulfonyl
rp	reversed phase (HPLC)
R.T.	room temperature
SPPS	solid phase peptide synthesis
tBu	tert-butyl
TEA	triethyl amine
TFA	trifluoroacetic acid
TFMSA	trifluoromethane sulfonic acid
TLC	thin layer chromatography
Tmob	2,4,6-trimethoxy benzyl
Tos	4-toluenesulfonyl (tosyl)
Trt	trityl
uv	ultraviolet (spectroscopy)
Z	benzyloxycarbonyl

ACKNOWLEDGEMENTS

To the Bachem Group for sharing its extensive knowledge on scale up of peptide synthesis and for its contribution in purification of peptides and proteins. Finally to Carla DuRant for working with me through all the revisions.

APPENDIX

Common Amino Acids

Alanine	Ala	A	Lysine	Lys	K
Arginine	Arg	R	Methionine	Met	M
Asparagine	Asn	N	Phenylalanine	Phe	F
Aspartic Acid	Asp	D	Proline	Pro	P
Cysteine	Cys	C	Pyroglutamyl	< Glu	< E
Glutamic Acid	Glu	E	Serine	Ser	S
Glutamine	Gln	Q	Threonine	Thr	T
Glycine	Gly	G	Tryptophan	Trp	W
Histidine	His	H	Tyrosine	Tyr	Y
Isoleucine	Ile	I	Valine	Val	V
Leucine	Leu	L			

Symbols for D-amino acids: DAla, DVal. Representation of blocking groups on amino acids: a symbol to the left and hyphenated is a blocking group on the alpha amino group: Boc-Gly = N-alpha-Boc-glycine; a symbol to the right and hyphenated is an ester on the alpha carboxyl: Gly-OHBT = hydroxybenzotriazole ester of glycine; a symbol in parentheses after the amino acid is a blocking group on the side chain: Tyr(Bzl) = O-benzyl tyrosine.

REFERENCES

1 Schaal, E. 1871. *Ann.*, 157:26.

2 Grimaux, E. 1882. *Bull. Soc. Chim.*, 38:64.

3 Leuchs, H. 1906. *Ber.*, 39:857.

4 Bergmann, M. and L. Zervas. 1932. *Ber.*, 65:1192.

5 Wessely, F. 1925. *Z. Physiol. Chem.*, 146:72.

6 Woodward, R. B. and C. H. Schramm. 1947. *J. Am. Chem. Soc.*, 69:1551.

7 Greenstein, J. P. and M. Winitz. 1986. *Chemistry of the Amino Acid, Vol. 2, 3rd Edition.* Krieger Publishing Company.

8 Merrifield, R. B. 1964. *Biochemistry*, 3:1385.

9 Merrifield, R. B. 1963. *J. Am. Chem. Soc.*, 86:304.

10 Stewart, J. M. and J. D. Young. 1984. *Solid Phase Peptide Synthesis, 2nd Edition.* Pierce Chemical Company.

11 Barany, G., N. Kneib-Cordonier and G. Mullen. 1987. "Solid Phase Peptide Synthesis: A Silver Anniversary Report," in *Int. J. Peptide Protein Res.*, 30:705.

12 Carpino, L. A. 1957. *J. Am. Chem. Soc.*, 79:4427.

13 McKay, F. C. and N. F. Albertson. 1957. *J. Am. Chem. Soc.*, 79:4686.

14 Anderson, G. W. and A. C. McGregor. 1957. *J. Am. Chem. Soc.*, 79:6180.

15 Carpino, L. A. and G. Y. Han. 1972. *J. Org. Chem.*, 37:3404.

16 Meienhofer, J., M. Waki, E. P. Heimer, T. J. Lambros, R. C. Makofske and C. D. Chang. 1979. *Int. J. Peptide Protein Res.*, 13:35.

17 Chang, C. D., M. Waki, M. Ahmad, J. Meienhofer, E. O. Lundell and J. D. Haug. 1980. *Int. J. Peptide Protein Res.*, 15:59.

18 Wang, S. S. 1973. *J. Am. Chem. Soc.*, 95:1328.

19 Breipohl, G., J. Knolle and W. Stuber. 1987. *Tetrahedron Letters*, 28:5651.

20 Ramage, R. and J. Green. 1987. *Tetrahedron Letters*, 28:2287.

21 Meienhofer, J., M. Waki, E. P. Heimer, T. J. Lambros, R. C. Makofske and C. D. Chang. 1979. *Int. J. Peptide Protein Res.*, 13:35.

22 Heimer, E. P., C. D. Chang, T. J. Lambros and J. Meienhofer. 1981. *Int. J. Peptide Protein Res.*, 18:237.

23 DeGrado, W. F. and E. T. Kaiser. 1980. *J. Org. Chem.*, 45:1295.

24 Kaiser, E. T., H. Mihara, G. A. LaForet, J. W. Kelly, L. Walters, M. A. Findeis and T. Sasaki. 1989. *Science*, 243:187.

25 Sheppard, R. C. and B. Williams. 1982. *Int. J. Peptide Protein Res.*, 20:451.

26 Mergler, M., R. Tanner, J. Gosteli and P. Grogg. 1988. *Tetrahedron Letters*, 29:4005.

27 Mergler, M., R. Nyfeler, R. Tanner, J. Gosteli and P. Grogg. 1988. *Tetrahedron Letters*, 29:4009.

28 Hellio, F., P. Gueguen and J. L. Morgat. 1988. *Biochimie*, 70(6):791.

29 Nutt, R. F., F. W. Holly, C. Homnick, R. Hirschmann, D. F. Verber and B. H. Arison. 1981. *J. Med. Chem.*, 24:692.

30 Felix, A. M., E. P. Heimer, C. T. Wang, T. J. Lambros, J. Swistok, M. Ahmad, M. Roszkowski, D. Confalone, J. Meienhofer, A. Trzeciak and D. Gillessen. 1983. *Peptides: Structure and Function*, V. Hruby and D. Rich, eds., Pierce Chemical Co., p. 889.

31 Nestor, J. J., Jr., T. L. Ho, R. A. Simpson, B. L. Horner, A. Jones, G. I. McRae and B. H. Vikery. 1982. *J. Med. Chem.*, 25:795.

32 Nestor, J. J. Jr., R. Tahilramany, T. L. Ho, G. I. McRae, B. H. Vickery and W. J. Brenmer. 1983. *Peptides: Structure and Function*, V. J. Hruby and D. H. Rich, eds., Pierce Chemical Co., p. 861.

33 Cramer, S. M., Z. Rassi and C. Horvath. 1987. *J. Chromatography*, 394(2):305.

34 Craig, L. C. and D. Craig. 1956. *Technique of Organic Chemistry, Vol. 3, Part 1, 2nd Edition*, A. Weissburg, ed., New York: Interscience, p. 149.

35 Craig, L. C., P. Alexander and R. J. Block, eds. 1960. *Analytical Methods of Protein Chemistry Vol. 1*. Oxford: Pergamon, p. 121.

36 Funatsu, G. 1964. *Biochemistry*, 3:1351.

37 Schroeder, W. A. 1967. In *Methods in Enzymology, Vol. 11*, C. H. W. Hirs, ed., Academic Press.

38 Burgus, R. and J. Rivier. 1976. In *Peptides 1976*, A. Loffet, ed., Brussels: Editions de 1 Universite de Bruxelles, p. 85.

39 Rivier, J. 1978. *J. Liquid Chrom.*, 1:343.

40 Gallagher, S. 1989. *Automation, Genetic Engineering News, Vol. 9*.

41 Arminger, W. B. and A. E. Humphrey. 1979. *Computer Application in Fermentation Technology, Vol. 2, 2nd Edition*. Academic Press.

CHAPTER 6

Advances in Peptide Synthesis

MOHMED K. ANWER[1]
SHABBIR A. KHAN[2]

D UE to the increasing number of applications of synthetic peptides in biological studies and as therapeutics, it is appropriate to briefly summarize the established as well as the emerging methods in the chemical synthesis of peptides. The advances in peptide synthesis have been comprehensively covered in numerous books and reviews [1–4], and specialized articles describing individual peptide hormones have been the subject of a monograph series [5]. The reader is encouraged to refer to the original literature for a flavor of the exciting developments in the realms of protecting groups, deprotection methods, and coupling procedures. Peptides synthesis, once considered a sophisticated task achievable only by synthetic organic chemists, has now extended to various biochemical laboratories due to the advent of automated solid-phase synthesis machines: this revolution was initiated with the introduction of the solid-phase method of peptide synthesis by Merrifield in 1963 [6]. Prior to this development, peptides were synthesized by the classical solution methods, which continue to be useful for synthesizing peptides containing unusual structural features [7–10]. Combining the advantageous features of solution methods, such as analytical control, with the ease and rapidity of automated solid-phase procedures has been the focus of recent endeavors in peptide chemistry. This chapter describes the prevailing art of peptide synthesis under the following categories: (1) protection of the reactive functional groups, (2) coupling methods, (3) deprotection methods, (4) solid-phase synthesis, and (5) peptide mimetics.

[1]Telios Pharmaceuticals, Inc., San Diego, CA 92121, U.S.A.
[2]The Wistar Institute, 3601 Spruce Street, Philadelphia, PA 19104, U.S.A.

PROTECTION OF THE REACTIVE FUNCTIONAL GROUPS

For the correct assembly of peptide sequence the N^{α}-amino protecting group should be specifically cleavable while leaving the side-chain protecting groups intact ("orthogonal" protection). Other reactive functional groups that require mandatory protection are side-chain amine (Lys), carboxylic acid (Asp, Glu), and the thiol (Cys) groups; protection of hydroxyl (Ser, Thr, Tyr), guanidino (Arg), imidazole (His), and the indole (Trp) groups while optional, is often preferred for minimizing the formation of side products. The overall selection of protecting groups is dictated by the synthetic strategy.

AMINO GROUP PROTECTION

Since the introduction of the benzyloxycarbonyl group by Bergmann and Zervas in 1932 [11], several variations of the alkoxycarbonyl type of amine protection have been developed [12–18]. Notable among these for the temporary protection of the N^{α}-amino group are tert-butyloxycarbonyl (Boc), tert-amyloxycarbonyl (Aoc), benzyloxycarbonyl (Z), 4-methoxybenzyloxycarbonyl (pMZ), 2-(3,5-dimethyloxyphenyl)propyl-2-oxycarbonyl (Ddz) and 9-fluorenylmethoxycarbonyl (Fmoc). Selection of the side-chain amino protecting group is based on the strategy of synthesis. The commonly used strategies encompass: (1) N^{α}-Boc, PMZ, Aoc, Ddz, or Fmoc and side-chain benzyl protection, (2) N^{α}-Z or Fmoc and side-chain tert-butyl based protection. Strategies that utilize other types of protecting groups, while novel, are not easily adoptable and have been sparingly used.

CARBOXYL GROUP PROTECTION

The carboxyl group is usually protected by conversion to an ester. The methyl, ethyl, benzyl, substituted benzyl, cyclohexyl, tert-butyl, or 9-fluorenylmethyl esters are widely used in peptide synthesis [19]. The unique properties of 4-picolyl, phenacyl, 4-methylphenacyl, 9-anthrylmethyl, 2-trimethysilylethyl, N-benzhydryl-glycolamide, and phthalimidomethyl esters have been shown to offer specific advantages in terms of selectivity [20–25]. The solid-phase approach also utilizes an ester group as a linker to the resin matrix [6,26,27] for the synthesis of peptides terminating in a carboxyl group.

THIOL GROUP PROTECTION

The highly nucleophilic thiol group requires protection. Thus, the Cys side chain is protected as thioether with 4-methylbenzyl (p-MeBzl) [28],

4-methoxybenzyl (p-MeOBzl) [29], trityl [30], S-tert-butyl [31], or acet-amidomethyl (Acm) [32] group. The use of S-tert-butylthio group has also been reported [33].

HYDROXYL GROUP PROTECTION

Though protection of the hydroxyl group is considered optional, a global protection strategy is generally adopted for minimizing side reactions. The hydroxyl group of Ser and Thr is often protected as its benzyl [34] or tert-butyl [35] ether. For the protection of the phenolic function of Tyr, 2-Bromobenzyloxycarbonyl (2-BrZ) [36,37] is preferred because the acidolytic removal of benzyl/2,6-dichlorobenzyl [38] results in the formation of significant amounts of Tyr-ring alkylated by-products. The O-tert-butyl group is used in the N^α-Fmoc strategy for hydroxyl group protection.

GUANIDINO GROUP PROTECTION

Mere protonation of the strongly basic guanidine side chain (Arg) offers sufficient protection during solution synthesis [39]. However, solubility considerations, possible acylation of the guanidine group during peptide coupling, and formation of lactam upon activation of the α-carboxyl group necessitate use of other types of protection for this functional group. Tosyl [40], methoxytrimethylphenylsulfonyl (Mtr) [41], mesitylenesulfonyl (Mts) [42], 2,2,5,7,8-pentamethylchroman-6-sulfonyl (Pmc) [43], ada-mantyloxycarbonyl (Adoc) [44], and nitro [45] groups have been successfully used.

IMIDAZOLE GROUP PROTECTION

The nucleophilic and weakly basic nature of the imidazole nucleus of His presents unique problems in synthesis if left unprotected. The N^τ-benzyloxymethyl (Bom) [46] appears to offer the most satisfactory protection. The tosyl [47] and trityl [48] groups, because of their location at the N^τ-position of His, are not entirely satisfactory in alleviating the racemization problem. The N^τ-tert-butyloxymethyl (Bum) [49] and trityl protection are compatible with Fmoc based synthetic strategies [50].

INDOLE GROUP PROTECTION

To prevent oxidation and alkylation of the indole nucleus during acidolytic treatment the indole nitrogen of Trp is protected by formyl [51] or mesitylenesulfonyl (Mts) [52] group. In the past, most syntheses used un-protected Trp because of the additional step required to remove the formyl group: concomitant removal of this group in the presence of a thiol reagent is an advantage of the "low-high" HF method [53].

COUPLING METHODS: FORMATION OF THE PEPTIDE BOND

The chemistry of the peptide-bond forming reactions was established by using the solution synthesis methods. Efficient formation of the peptide bond requires activation of the carboxyl group of the acylating component. To be suitable for synthesis, the coupling process should satisfy the following criteria: (1) free of racemization and side reactions, (2) facile, (3) safe to handle, and (4) economical. Of the numerous coupling reagents that meet these criteria, only a few have found general acceptance. N,N'-dicyclohexylcarbodiimide (DCC), DCC in presence of additives, and active esters are efficient coupling methods at ambient temperatures, and are convenient for both solution and solid-phase syntheses. Coupling methods that utilize an azide or mixed carbonic anhydrides are usually executed at < 0°C, and therefore are not easily amenable to solid-phase synthesis. However, these are an important part of the repertoire of solution synthesis and will be considered here.

AZIDE METHOD

The azide procedure has withstood the challenge of time, and is especially useful for segment condensations [54,55]. The azide intermediate is generated from an alkyl ester via a hydrazide. However, hydrazinolysis of the terminal ester necessitates the use of tert-butyl group for the protection of side-chain carboxyl functions in the acylating component. This limitation is overcome by using diphenylphosphoryl azide (DPPA), which furnishes an azide directly upon reaction with a carboxyl group [56,57]. While DPPA has been employed for cyclization [58] and stepwise assembly of peptides [56,57], its usefulness for segment condensation needs to be explored. However, the slow reactivity of azides and the formation of isocyanates by their disproportionation restrict the usefulness of this method.

ANHYDRIDE METHOD

The mixed carbonic anhydride method is widely used for the formation of peptide bond because of the facile removal of reaction by-products. The anhydride is formed upon reaction of the carboxylate anion with an alkyl chloroformate [59,60] or pivaloyl chloride [61]. The reason for this selection is to guide the attack of the amino component on to the carbonyl carbon of the acylating component. This is achieved in the former case due to the electron donating influence of the alkoxy group, and in the latter by the steric bulk of the tert-butyl group which obstructs attack on the wrong carbonyl group. Of the alkyl chloroformates, the most popular are isobutyl or isopropyl esters of chloroformic acid. Care should be exercised in using the proper stoichiometric equivalents of the reactants to minimize the formation of side products, particularly during the activation of β-branched amino acids. The mixed carbonic anhydride method requires the formation of the anhydride at low temperatures ($-10°C$), and hence not conducive to automated solid-phase synthesis. An obvious way of eliminating the wrong carbonyl attack is achieved by the formation of a symmetrical anhydride, albeit at the expense of an additional equivalent of the acylating amino acid. Alternatively, mixed anhydrides with phosphoric acid derivatives have also been successfully used. A special category of mixed anhydrides is represented by the N-carboxy (NCA) and N-thiocarboxy (NTA) anhydrides [62–64]. These conceptually simple and elegant procedures combine activation and protection in a single $-CO-O-$ or $-CS-O-$ group. However, to ensure product purity the reaction conditions need to be carefully optimized. The sensitivity of these reactive species of water, side reaction products formed by the attack on the wrong carbonyl, and double incorporation of the acylating amino acid due to premature decarboxylation have impeded their broad acceptance. The NCA/NTA method is well suited for polymerization of amino acids.

CARBODIIMIDE METHOD

Dicyclohexylcarbodiimide-mediated coupling introduced to peptide synthesis in 1955 [65] continues to be the method of choice in both solution and solid-phase strategies of peptide synthesis. Reaction of the carboxylic acid with DCC results in the formation of O-acylurea, which is similar to mixed anhydrides in its reactivity and general structure. The participation of symmetrical anhydride species in DCC-mediated coupling reactions has also been demonstrated [66]. Indeed, the popular method of preparing symmetrical anhydrides involves reaction of two equivalents of a suitably protected amino acid with one equivalent of DCC. The formation of inactive N-acylurea, resulting from O→N migration, is circumvented by converting the O-acylurea to active esters by reaction with N-hydroxy compounds. Among the N-hydroxy compounds, 1-hydroxybenzotriazole [67], 1-hydroxysuccinimide [68], 1-hydroxynorbornene carboxamide [69], and ethyl 2-hydroximino-2-cyanoacetate [70] have found general use. In addition to minimizing O→N migration, these additives also serve as catalysts during the coupling reaction [71] and assist in lowering racemization. Excess carbodiimide should be avoided to minimize the slow reaction of the reagent with the amine which results in guanidine derivatives. However, this is not a serious concern as the side reaction is too slow to compete with the rapid addition of the carboxyl group. The persistent trace amounts of DCU in products, while innocuous in terms of reactivity, is a practical nuisance. The two congeners of DCC namely diisopropylcarbodiimide (DIC) [72] and 1-(3-dimethylaminopropyl)-3-ethylcarbodiimide hydrochloride (water soluble carbodiimide) [73] have found special application. The solubility of diisopropylurea in dichloromethane makes DIC preferable to DCC in solid-phase synthesis. In the case of the water soluble carbodiimide, the solubility of the reagent and the ensuing urea make it attractive for coupling reactions which require the use of aqueous solvent media.

ACTIVE ESTER METHOD

Presence of electron withdrawing substituents on the alkoxy carbon of esters increases their susceptibility toward aminolysis. Thus, the cyanomethyl esters are highly reactive compared with the methyl esters. The high reactivity of esters of p-nitrophenol [74], polyhalogenated phenols [75,76], and N-hydroxy-compounds [67–70] has made these "active esters" useful in synthesis. Though the active esters, excepting pentafluorophenyl esters, do not stack up favorably with other coupling methods such as the DCC or the mixed anhydride in terms of reactivity, they are indeed the method of choice for coupling Asn or Gln. With DCC or mixed anhydride alone, the side-chain carboxamide group in these amino acids is transformed to the nitrile group because of dehydration [77]. While the *in situ* formed hydroxybenzotriazole esters of these amino acids are directly used, other active esters can be conveniently prepared using carbodiimide and are purified before use. The remarkable observation that 1-hydroxybenzotriazole can efficiently catalyze the aminolysis of active esters such as p-nitrophenyl, 2,4,5-trichlorophenyl, and pentachlorophenyl has enhanced the usefulness of these reagents [71,78,79]. The attractive features of active esters are ease of handling and reasonable shelf life. However, their sluggish reactivity and high cost have limited their application in solid-phase synthesis.

RECENT COUPLING REAGENTS

The last few years have witnessed development of benzotriazolyloxy-tris-(dimethylamino)phosphonium hexafluorophosphonate (BOP) [80] and its congeners [81] as advantageous coupling reagents. Their superior performance as compared to DCC-HOBt in difficult coupling reactions might be indicative of involvement of factors other than just the intermediacy of a benzotriazolyl ester [80]. Since the BOP coupling reaction is performed in a basic medium which has a beneficial influence on the active ester couplings, and certain chaotropic salts are also known to augment the coupling efficiencies [82], unequivocal conclusions are difficult to attain. Perhaps an evaluation of the DCC-HOBt reaction under the simulate BOP reaction conditions, namely in the presence of an added equivalent of a tert-amine hexafluorophosphonate salt and congruent basic conditions would provide an explanation for these claims. Advantages unique to the BOP and its congeners are the possibility of directly using Boc-amino acid dicyclohexylammonium salts and the omission of a separate neutralization step since the trifluoroacetate ion is not activated by these coupling reagents. Bromotris(dimethylamino)phosphonium hexafluorophosphate (BROP) [81] and bromotris(pyrrolidinyl)phosphonium hexafluorophosphate (PyBROP) [81] have been shown to be superior to Bop in difficult coupling reactions, such as those involving N-methylamino acid derivatives. This may be due in part to the participation of an acyl bromide intermediate. Both BROP and PyBROP compare favorably with the coupling efficiences obtained with bis(2-oxo-3-oxazolidinyl)-phosphinic chloride (Bop-Cl) [83,84] and diphenylphosphinyl chloride (Dpp-Cl) [85]. Other promising reagents are 2-(1H-benzotriazole-1-yl-1,1,3,3-tetramethyluronium tetrafluoroborate (TBTU) [86], 0-benzotriazolyl-N,N,N',N'-tetramethyluronium (HBTU) [87], and 1,1'-bis[6-(trifluoromethyl)benzotriazolyl] oxalate (BTBO) [88,89]. While BOP has found broader acceptance, its congeners and other novel reagents such as Dpp-Cl, Bop-Cl, and TBTU are beginning to receive attention.

DEPROTECTION METHODS

The deprotection method used during stepwise assembly of peptide chain and the final deblocking of all functional groups to yield the free peptide is determined by the synthetic strategy. Selective deprotection methods that can furnish peptides in a protected form suited for subsequent manipulations such as cyclization, selective modification, and segment condensation are complementary to the global deprotection procedures. On the basis of the nature of reagent used to effect the cleavage of protecting groups, the deprotection methods could be classified into three categories: (1) acidolysis, (2) base/nucleophile assisted methods, and (3) neutral cleavage methods. A successful synthetic strategy depends on a judicious selection of protecting groups susceptible to these conditions.

ACIDOLYTIC METHODS

Hydrogen chloride in organic solvents, trifluoroacetic acid (TFA), methanesulfonic acid (MSA), trifluoromethanesulfonic acid (TFMSA), and liquid hydrogen fluoride (HF) are typically employed for cleavage of acid labile protecting groups. While the first three reagents are generally employed for removal of the N^α-protecting group during synthesis, the latter two are routinely used for global deblocking. The various acidolytic methods will be discussed in context of the commonly employed synthetic strategies.

ACIDOLYTIC METHODS FOR USE WITH N^α-Boc, Pmz, Aoc, Ddz, AND SIDE-CHAIN BENZYL PROTECTION STRATEGY

The N^α-Boc/side-chain benzyl based strategy continues to be the most popular. Here, TFA in dichloromethane is used for removal of Boc, Aoc, Pmz, and Ddz protecting groups. Compatible side-chain protecting groups are benzyl based derivatives of carboxyl (Asp, Glu), hydroxyl (Ser, Thr, Tyr), amino (Lys, Orn), and imidazole (His). In addition, cyclohexyl esters of Asp and Glu are sometimes preferred to minimize side reactions [90]. The tosyl group (Arg, His) is compatible with this strategy. Suitable scavengers are included during sequential and final deprotections to minimize side reactions involving carbocations when dealing with sensitive amino acids (Tyr, Trp, Met, Cys). In solution synthesis, use of TFA for deblocking of N^α protecting group results in the formation of N-trifluoroacetyl derivative during the subsequent coupling reaction. Therefore, deprotection with HCl in organic solvents (dioxane, THF) is recommended. In some cases, deprotection with boron trifluoride-etherate [91], and MSA-formic acid [92] have been shown to be advantageous. This synthetic strategy utilizes HF [93–95] or TFMSA [96] for final deprotection. Recently, the "low-high" HF procedure has become popular because it minimizes side reactions and provides purer products [53].

ACIDOLYTIC METHODS FOR USE WITH N^α-Fmoc AND SIDE-CHAIN BENZYL TYPE PROTECTION

The intent of the introduction of Fmoc protection was to avoid exposure of the peptide chain to repetitive acid treatment. This objective is realized when the side-chain protecting groups are quantitatively cleaved under the final nonacidolytic conditions, such as hydrogenation; further, they should be stable to the secondary amine treatment used to cleave the N^α-Fmoc group. The restrictions imposed by hydrogenation such as exclusion of divalent sulfur functionalities or other soft bases which are potent poisons of palladium catalysts have resulted in the sparse use of this approach. However, in such instances TFMSA or HF can be used for final deprotection.

ACIDOLYTIC METHODS FOR USE WITH N$^\alpha$-Z AND SIDE-CHAIN TERT-BUTYL BASED PROTECTION

The utilization of N$^\alpha$-Z and side-chain tert-butanol derived groups (and extendable to other TFA-cleavable protecting groups) was elegantly demonstrated in the classical synthesis of glucagon [97] and ACTH [98]. The attractive feature of this strategy is the clean and quantitative removal of Z group by catalytic hydrogenation in presence of tert-butanol derived protecting groups. An annoying limitation, however, surfaces when the peptide has divalent sulfur groups. The final deprotection is achieved with TFA. The pMZ group [99] is unique in that it combines the desired features of both the Boc group (cleaved by TFA) and the Z group (hydrogenolyzable) [99]. This group is destined for prominent usage.

ACIDOLYTIC METHODS FOR USE WITH N$^\alpha$-Fmoc AND SIDE-CHAIN ACID-LABILE PROTECTION

A renaissance for the development of moderately acid labile (TFA) side-chain protecting groups compatible with the N$^\alpha$-Fmoc group was started upon the recognition of deleterious effects of exposing peptides to strong acid conditions (HF, TFMSA). Simultaneous advances in the development of linkers [100,101] for solid-phase synthesis, that can furnish peptides with C-terminal acid or amide group upon treatment with TFA, have resulted in wide practice of this strategy. Though hydrogenation results in the cleavage of the N$^\alpha$-Fmoc group [102,103], it is rarely used as a deblocking method.

BASE/NUCLEOPHILE ASSISTED METHODS FOR DEPROTECTION

The N$^\alpha$-Fmoc, primary alkyl esters, 2-bromo-benzyloxycarbonyl (Tyr), and tosyl (His) groups are cleaved upon exposure to basic/nucleophilic conditions [104]. From a practical aspect, the removal of Fmoc group by using secondary amines (pyrrolidine and piperidine) in suitable organic solvents is important [50].

CLEAVAGE OF ESTERS

The primary alkyl esters are generally cleaved by treatment with dilute alkali, benzyl esters are traditionally cleaved by hydrogenation. Recently, cleavage of alkyl esters including benzyl esters has been accomplished with tetra-n-butylammonium fluoride [104] and tetra-n-butylammonium carbonate [105]. The cleavage of benzyl esters by hydrogenation [106–109] has additional significance in solid-phase synthesis where a substituted benzyl ester links the peptide chain with the resin matrix. 9-Fluorenylmethyl esters are cleaved with secondary amines [110], whereas the glycolamide esters are cleaved with aqueous carbonate [25].

DEPROTECTION UNDER NEUTRAL CONDITIONS

Conceptually, cleavage of protecting groups under neutral conditions is highly desired for the following reasons. Such procedures would be: (1) free from racemization, (2) leave intact acid sensitive amino acids, (3) useful particularly in the synthesis of acid/base sensitive biologically active peptides, and (4) free of side reactions that are commonly observed in acidolysis and base treatment. Two such methods, catalytic hydrogenation [106,111,112] and catalytic transfer hydrogenation (CTH) [107,108,113–115] have become popular for the cleavage of benzyl and other hydrogenolyzable moieties. The only limitation being the intolerance of palladium catalysts to the presence of divalent sulfur. While hydrogenation with gaseous hydrogen is typically performed under high pressure (Parr apparatus), transfer hydrogenation is achieved under ambient pressure. Transfer hydrogenation procedures utilize simple organic molecules (cyclohexene [116], cyclohexadiene [117], formic acid [114], ammonium formate [115]) or inorganic compounds (phosphinic acid and its salts [117], hydrazine [118]) as *in situ* source of hydrogen. Ammonium formate, formic acid, and cyclohexadiene function as excellent hydrogen donors at room temperature and are therefore used at ambient temperature and pressure. Hydrazine, while an excellent hydrogen donor at room temperature precludes the presence of other ester moieties on the peptide due to its high nucleophilic nature. The utility of ammonium formate CTH for the deprotection of protecting groups [115], cleavage of peptides from Merrifield type resins [108], and for isotopic labeling of peptides [119] has been demonstrated. Of all the transfer hydrogenation and the conventional hydrogenation methods, ammonium formate-CTH has been shown to be superior [120,121].

SOLID-PHASE SYNTHESIS OF PEPTIDES

For selective and specific amide bond formation between two amino acids, the amino group of one amino acid and the carboxyl group of the other must be protected. The carboxyl group is protected in organic and classical peptide synthesis as its ester. If the ester group is rendered insoluble in solvents by attachment to a polymer, then the peptide could be assembled anchored to a solid support. Therefore, excess reagents and by-products could be removed by mere washing and filtration. The recognition by Merrifield of this simple but novel idea [6] is the genesis of a revolution that has shaped the present state of peptide and organic synthesis on solid supports.

The solid-phase peptide synthesis entails the following operations: (1) attachment of the C-terminal amino acid to an insoluble resin matrix, (2) assembly of the peptide chain, and (3) release of peptide from the resin matrix.

ATTACHMENT OF THE C-TERMINAL AMINO ACID

For the synthesis of peptides terminating in a carboxyl function, esterification via the nucleophilic displacement of a halogen functionalized resin support by the carboxylate anion [122–125] or coupling of the acid to the hydroxyl derivative of resin [126] accomplishes the attachment of the C-terminal amino acid. The most commonly used resins are the Merrifield resin, phenylacetamidomethyl (PAM) resin [127], and the alkoxy-substituted benzyl resins [128,129]; the amino acid esters of these resins are commercially available. For the synthesis of long peptide sequences using the classical Merrifield N^α-Boc-/side-chain benzyl type protection strategy, the relatively more acid stable PAM resin is employed. With the N^α-Fmoc/side-chain acid labile protecting groups scheme, the alkoxybenzyl resins are used. For the synthesis of peptides with C-terminal amide group, 4-Methylbenzhydrylamine resin [130] and substituted benzylamine (two or more strongly electron donating groups on the aromatic ring) resins [131,132] are used in the N^α-Boc and Fmoc strategies, respectively.

ASSEMBLY OF THE PEPTIDE CHAIN

This involves the following sequence of operations: (1) removal of the N^α-amine protection from the amino acid resin, (2) coupling of the next appropriately protected amino acid, and (3) monitoring of the coupling reaction. This sequence of operations is repeated for the stepwise build up of the desired peptide chain. Automated peptide synthesizers exploit the repetitive nature of this order of operations.

REMOVAL OF THE N^α-PROTECTION

In the N^α-Boc/pMZ/Aoc/DdZ and side-chain benzyl protection strategy, the N^α-masking group is removed by treatment with a suitable acid, such as trifluoroacetic acid. In the N^α-Fmoc and side-chain tert-butyl/benzyl strategy, the Fmoc group is conveniently removed by treatment with piperidine or pyrrolidine.

COUPLING REACTIONS

After liberating the amino function, the next sequential amino acid residue could be added by any of the coupling procedures previously described. However, the carbodiimide (with and without additives), active esters, and pre-formed symmetrical anhydride techniques are commonly used. The search for the ideal coupling reagent, one that would give coupling efficiencies of 99.9% or better with conservation of chiral integrity, continues despite the numerous coupling reagents that have been introduced thus far.

MONITORING OF COUPLING REACTIONS

Statistical analysis of the coupling efficiences indicates that the coupling reaction be better than 99.6% at each step for obtaining moderate size peptides in an acceptable level of purity. Equally important is the use of starting reagents of the utmost purity available. For monitoring of coupling efficiency, both the qualitative [133] and quantitative [134] ninhydrin test are useful. The continuous flow machines that utilize the N^α-Fmoc protection strategy are equipped with on-line coupling monitoring devices.

CLEAVAGE OF PEPTIDE FROM RESIN

Merrifield, in his classic revelation of the solid-phase concept, reported the use of alkali to cleave the ester bond between the peptide and the resin [6]. It is interesting that the nucleophile-assisted cleavage in its more recent adaptations has again become an area of activity, particularly for the preparation of protected peptide acids [104,105,135–137]. Acidolysis with HF, first proposed by Sakakibara [93], is currently, the most popular method for cleaving peptides attached to Merrifield type resins; previous to this method, acidolysis with HBr in TFA [138] was preferred. Another strong acid that recently has found wide acceptance is trifluoromethanesulfonic acid (TFMSA). Detailed studies concerning the manipulation of the various carbocation scavengers and their amounts have made the "low-high" modifications of HF [53] and TFMSA [96] methods attractive for the release and concomitant deprotection of peptides from resins. In some instances, hydrogenation and catalytic transfer hydrogenation techniques utilizing cyclohexene, formic acid, or ammonium formate are desirable to release peptides in a protected or free form. Powerful nucleophilic species such as carbonate (in the form of tetra-n-butylammonium carbonate

[105]), fluoride (tetra-n-butylammonium fluoride [104]), and lithium mer-captoethanol [139] have been used to release peptides bound to Merrifield and PAM resins. These procedures complement the strong acidolytic methods. Structural variants susceptible to photolysis [137] and other nucleophiles [139,140] have been developed as "handles" linking the peptide with the solid support. More recent is the development of acid-sensitive resins that are used with the N^α-Fmoc protection scheme [128,129,131]. Here, treatment of resin-peptide with TFA in the presence of suitable carbocation scavengers is used to release the peptide with concomitant deprotection of side-chain protecting groups.

PEPTIDE MIMETICS

The instense activity in the development of peptide mimetics is fueled by their pharmaceutical potential. Excellent summaries describing the various modifications of the peptide bond and the three segments of the amino acid, namely the α-nitrogen, α-carbon, and the carbonyl group, have appeared. The success achieved in the area of metalloenzyme inhibitors [141], Captopril [142] using this approach is being followed by incorporations of amide bond surrogates in hormones, such as somatostatin [143,144], enkephalins [145–147], and LH-RH [148] (see Chapter 8).

The objectives of such pursuits are to confer upon the peptide resistance to proteolytic degradation [149], improvements in the potencies of the agonist/antagonist response [150,151], elucidation of the necessary region of the peptide chain for its biological activity [145], and as probes to determine the conformational critical regions [58,105,145–147,152].

It should be pointed out that the incorporation of a single amide bond surrogate imparts stability to the entire molecule toward proteolytic breakdown [149]. The important structural features possessed by the divergent class of amide bond surrogates can be harvested in the design of analogues with a wide spectrum of biological, conformational, and structural profiles. Thus, the psi[CH=CH], a relatively lipophilic substitution, bears close conformational topology to the amide bond while lacking the hydrogen bond donor/acceptor characteristics. The thiomethylene ether, psi[CH$_2$S], is a flexible, lipophilic, and a nonparticipant in hydrogen bonding, has been shown to result in interesting variations in biological activity [150,151] and conformational features [58]. The psi[CH$_2$S] upon careful oxidation furnishes the optically distinct sulfoxides thus affording chiral amide bond surrogates, which often possess divergent biological activities. The psi[CH$_2$NH] is a hydrophilic, flexible amide bond surrogate which retains the hydrogen bond donor ability. It is easily incorporated into the solid-phase peptide synthesis methodology by the sodium cyanoborohydride reduction of the *in situ* formed Schiff base obtained by reaction of a suitably protected amino aldehyde with the amino component tethered to the resin support [144]. The thioamide, psi[CSNH], is a subtle modification of the amide bond: the first thioamide analogue, using oxytocin as a host, was reported by du Vigneaud. The pioneering studies of Lawesson et al. [153,154] have yielded a facile entry into this otherwise difficult class of endothiopeptides. The conformational studies of this surrogate suggest that it may be a better hydrogen bond donor participant than the amide bond [152]. The retro-inverso amide bond, psi[NHCO], extensively studied by Goodman et al. and others [145–147], has the elements of the peptide bond in the reverse order and therefore differs profoundly from the parent in its hydrogen bonding pattern. The retro-inverso bond surrogates are readily synthesized using I-I-bis(trifluoroacetoxy)iodobenzene [155,156]. Other surrogates such as methyleneoxy, psi[CH$_2$O], ketomethylene, psi[CH$_2$CO], etc., have been utilized in the structure-function studies of several hormones [8]. Finally, one can consider cyclosporin as nature's version of a peptide mimetic. It is interesting to note that all the NHs in cyclosporin are involved in intramolecular hydrogen bonding while the exposed peptide bonds are N-methylated!

ACKNOWLEDGEMENTS

We thank Dr. Manoj K. Das, The Wistar Institute, for assistance in the organization of the references in the manuscript.

REFERENCES

1 Bodanszky, M. 1984. *Principals of Peptide Synthesis.* Berlin: Springer-Verlag.

2 Bodanszky, M. and A. Bodanszky. 1984. *The Practice of Peptide Synthesis.* New York: Springer-Verlag.

3 Wunsch, E. 1974. In *Houben-Weyl, Methoden der Organischen Chemie, Vol. 15/l.* Stuttgart: Thieme, p. 800.

4 Gross, E. and J. Meienhofer, eds. *The Peptides, Vol. 1–9.* New York: Academic Press.

5 Li, C. H., ed. *Hormonal Peptides and Proteins, Vol. 1–10.* New York: Academic Press.

6 Merrifield, R. B. 1963. *J. Am. Chem. Soc.,* 86:304.

7 Khan, S. A. and B. W. Erickson. 1982. *J. Am. Chem. Soc.,* 104:4283.

8 Spatola, A. F. 1983. In *Chemistry and Biochemistry of Amino Acids, Peptides, and Proteins,* 7:267.

9 Franklin, T. J. and G. A. Snow. 1981. *Biochemistry of Antimicrobial Action.* London: Chapman and Hall.

10 Sturgeon, C. M. 1982. *Carbohydr. Chem.*, 13:572.

11 Bergman, M. and L. Zervas. 1932. *Ber. Dtsch. Chem. Ges.*, 65:1192.

12 Mckay, F. C. and N. F. Albertson. 1957. *J. Am. Chem. Soc.*, 79:4686.

13 Carpino, L. A. 1957. *J. Am. Chem. Soc.*, 79:4427.

14 Sakakibara, S., M. Shin, M. Fujino, Y. Shimonishi, S. Inoue and N. Inukai. 1965. *Bull. Chem. Soc. Japan*, 38:1522.

15 Weygand, F. and K. Hunger. 1962. *Chem. Ber.*, 95:1.

16 Birr, C., W. Lochinger, G. Stahnke and P. Lang. 1972. *Liebigs Ann. Chem.*, 763:162.

17 Carpino, L. A. and C. Y. Han. 1970. *J. Am. Chem. Soc.*, 92:5748.

18 Geiger, R. and W. Konig. 1981. In *The Peptides Analysis, Synthesis, Biology, Vol. 3*, E. Gross and J. Meienhofer, eds., New York: Academic Press, p. 3.

19 Roeske, R. W. 1981. In *The Peptides Analysis, Synthesis, Biology, Vol. 3*, E. Gross and J. Meienhofer, eds., New York: Academic Press, p. 101.

20 Garner, R. and G. T. Young. 1971. *J. Chem. Soc. C.*, p. 50.

21 Kuramizo, K. and J. Meienhofer. 1974. *J. Am. Chem. Soc.*, 96:4978.

22 Tam, J. P., W. F. Cunningham-Rundles, B. W. Erickson and R. B. Merrifield. 1977. *Tetrahedron Lett.*, p. 4001.

23 Stewart, F. H. C. 1965. *Aust. J. Chem.*, 18:1699.

24 Sieber, P., R. Andreatta, K. Eisler, B. Kamber, B. Riniker and H. Rink. 1977. In *Peptides, Proc. Fifth Amer. Pept. Symp.*, M. Goodman and J. Meienhofer, eds., New York: Wiley, p. 543.

25 Amblard, M., M. Rodriguez and J. Martinez. 1988. *Tetrahedron*, 44:5101.

26 Barany, G. and R. B. Merrifield. 1980. In *The Peptides, Vol. 2*, E. Gross and J. Meienhofer, eds., New York: Academic Press, p. 1.

27 Fields, G. B. and R. L. Noble. 1990. *Int. J. Peptide Protein Res.*, 35:161.

28 Erickson, B. W. and R. B. Merrifield. 1973. *J. Am. Chem. Soc.*, 95:3750.

29 Yamashiro, D., R. L. Noble and C. H. Li. 1973. *J. Org. Chem.*, 38:3561.

30 Zervas, L., I. Photaki and I. Phocas. 1968. *Chem. Ber.*, 101:3332.

31 Beyerman, H. C. 1963. In *The Peptides 1962*, G. T. Young, ed., Oxford: Pergamon, p. 53.

32 Kamber, B. 1971. *Helv. Chim. Acta*, 54:927.

33 Hartter, P. and U. Weber. 1973. *Hoppe-Seyler's Z. Physiol. Chem.*, 354:365.

34 Hruby, V. J. and K. W. Ehler. 1970. *J. Org. Chem.*, 35:1690.

35 Wunsch, E. and G. Wendelberger. 1968. *Chem. Ber.*, 101:3659.

36 Yamashiro, D. and C. H. Li. 1973. *J. Org. Chem.*, 38:591.

37 Stewart, J. M. 1981. In *The Peptides Analysis, Synthesis, Biology, Vol. 3*, E. Gross and J. Meienhofer, eds., New York: Academic Press, pp. 170–201.

38 Erickson, B. W. and R. B. Merrifield. 1973. *J. Am. Chem. Soc.*, 95:3750.

39 Anderson, G. W. 1953. *J. Am. Chem. Soc.*, 75:6081.

40 Schwyzer, R. and C. H. Li. 1958. *Nature*, 182:1669.

41 Fujino, M., M. Wakimasu and C. Kitada. 1981. *Chem. Pharm. Bull.*, 29:2825.

42 Yajima, H., M. Takeyama, J. Kanaki and K. Mitani. 1978. *J. Chem. Soc. Chem. Commun.*, p. 482.

43 Ramage, R. and J. Green. 1987. *Tetrahedron Lett.*, p. 2287.

44 Jager, G. and R. Geiger. 1970. *Chem. Ber.*, 103:1727.

45 Bergmann, M., L. Zervas and H. Rinke. 1934. *Hoppe-Seyler's Z. Physiol. Chem.*, 224:40.

46 Brown, T., J. H. Jones and J. D. Wallis. 1982. *J. Chem. Soc. Perkin Trans. 1*, p. 3045.

47 Sakakibara, S. and T. Fujii. 1967. *Bull. Chem. Soc. Japan*, 42:1466.

48 Stelakatos, G. C., D. M. Theodoropoulos and L. Zervas. 1959. *J. Am. Chem. Soc.*, 81:2884.

49 Colombo, R., F. Colombo and J. H. Jones. 1984. *J. Chem. Soc. Chem. Commun.*, p. 292.

50 Atherton, E. and R. C. Sheppard. 1987. In *The Peptides Analysis, Synthesis, Biology, Vol. 9*, S. Udenfriend and J. Meienhofer, eds., New York: Academic Press, p. 1.

51 Ohno, M., S. Tsukamoto, S. Sato and N. Izumiya. 1973. *Bull. Chem. Soc. Japan*, 46:3280.

52 Fujii, N., S. Futaki, K. Yasumura and H. Yajima. 1984. *Chem. Pharm. Bull.*, 32:2660.

53 Tam, J. P., W. F. Heath and R. B. Merrifield. 1983. *J. Am. Chem. Soc.*, 105:6442.

54 Yajima, H. and N. Fujii. 1981. *J. Am. Chem. Soc.*, 103:5867.

55 Meienhofer, J. 1979. In *The Peptides Analysis, Synthesis, Biology, Vol. 1*, E. Gross and J. Meienhofer, eds., New York: Academic Press, p. 197.

56 Shioiri, T., K. Ninomiya and S. Yamada. 1972. *J. Am. Chem. Soc.*, 94:6203.

57 Yamada, S., Y. Yokoyama and T. Shioiri. 1974. *J. Org. Chem.*, 39:3302.

58 Spatola, A. F., M. K. Anwer, A. Rockwell and L. M. Geirasch. 1986. *J. Am. Chem. Soc.*, 108:825.

59 Vaughan, J. R., Jr. and R. L. Osato. 1952. *J. Am. Chem. Soc.*, 74:676.

60 Meienhofer, J. 1979. In *The Peptides, Vol. 1*, E. Gross and J. Meienhofer, eds., New York: Academic Press, pp. 263–314.

61 Zaoral, M. 1962. *Coll. Czech. Chem. Commun.*, 27:1273.

62 Leuchs, H. 1906. *Ber. Dtsch. Chim. Ges.*, 39:857.

63 Bailey, J. L. 1949. *Nature*, 164:889.

64 Blacklock, T. J., R. Hirschmann and D. F. Veber. 1987. In *The Peptides Analysis, Synthesis, Biology, Vol. 9*, S. Udenfriend and J. Meienhofer, eds., New York: Academic Press, p. 39.

65 Sheehan, J. C. and G. P. Hess. 1955. *J. Am. Chem. Soc.*, 77:1067.

66 Rich, D. H. and J. Singh. 1979. In *The Peptides, Vol. 1*, E. Gross and J. Meienhofer, eds., New York: Academic Press, p. 241.

67 Konig, W. and R. Geiger. 1970. *Chem. Ber.*, 103:788.

68 Zimmerman, J. E. and G. W. Anderson. 1967. *J. Am. Chem. Soc.*, 89:7151.

69 Fujino, M., S. Kobayashi, M. Obayashi, F. Tsunehiko, S. Shinagawa and O. Nishimura. 1974. *Chem. Pharm. Bull. Tokyo*, 22:1851.

70 Itoh, M. 1973. *Bull. Chem. Soc. Japan*, 46:2219.

71 Konig, W. and R. Geiger. 1973. *Chem. Ber.*, 106:3626.

72 Sheehan, J. C. and G. P. Hess. 1955. *J. Am. Chem. Soc.*, 77:1067.

73 Sheehan, J. C. and J. J. Hlavka. 1956. *J. Org. Chem.*, 21:439.

74 Bodanszky, M. and V. du Vigneand. 1959. *Nature*, 183:1324.

75 Pless, J. and R. A. Boissonas. 1963. *Helv. Chim. Acta*, 46:1609.

76 Kovacs, J., L. Kisfaludy and M. Q. Ceprini. 1967. *J. Am. Chem. Soc.*, 89:183.

77 Gish, D. T., P. G. Katsoyannis, G. P. Hess and R. J. Stedman. 1956. *J. Am. Chem. Soc.*, 78:5954.

78 Ressler, C. and H. Ratzkin. 1961. *J. Org. Chem.*, 26:3356.

79 Khan, S. A. and K. M. Sivanandaiah. 1978. *Int. J. Peptide Protein Res.*, 1212:164.

80 Castro, B., J. R. Dormoy, G. Evin and C. Selve. 1975. *Tetrahedron Lett.*, p. 1219.

81 Coste, J., M. N. Dufour, D. Le-Nguyen and B. Castro. 1990. In *Peptides Chemistry, Structure, Biology, Proc. of 11th Amer. Pept. Symp.*, J. E. Rivier and G. R. Marshall, eds., Leiden: Escom Science Publishers, p. 885.

82 Klis, W. A. and J. M. Stewart. 1990. In *Peptides Chemistry, Structure, Biology, Proc. of 11th Am. Pept. Symp.*, J. E. Rivier and G. R. Marshall, eds., Leiden: Escom Science Publishers, p. 904.

83 Diago-Messegner, J., A. L. Palomo-Coll, J. R. Fernandez-Lizarbe and A. Zugazo-Bilbao. 1980. *Synthesis*, p. 547.

84 Tung, R. D. and D. H. Rich. 1985. *J. Am. Chem. Soc.*, 107:4342.

85 Kenner, G. W., G. A. Moore and R. Ramage. 1976. *Tetrahedron Lett.*, p. 3623.

86 Knorr, R., A. Trzeciak, W. Bannworth and D. Gillessen. 1989. *Tetrahedron Lett.*, p. 1927.

87 Knorr, R., A. Trzeciak, W. Bannworth and D. Gillessen. 1989. *Tetrahedron Lett.*, p. 1929.

88 Dourtoglou, V., J.-C. Ziegler and B. Castro. 1978. *Tetrahedron Lett.*, p. 1269.

89 Dourtoglou, V., B. Gross, V. Lamproglou and C. Ziodrou. 1984. *Synthesis*, p. 527.

90 Tam, J. P., T. Wong, M. W. Riemen, F. Tjoeng and R. B. Merrifield. 1979. *Tetrahedron Lett.*, p. 4033.

91 Williard, P. G. and C. B. Fryhle. 1980. *Tetrahedron Lett.*, p. 3731.

92 Khan, S. A., G. J. Merkel, J. M. Becker and F. Naider. 1981. *Int. J. Pept. Prot. Res.*, 17:219.

93 Sakakibara, S. and Y. Shimonishi. 1965. *Bull. Chem. Soc. Japan*, 38:4921.

94 Sakakibara. S. 1971. In *Chemistry and Biochemistry of Amino Acids, Peptides and Proteins, Vol. 1*, B. Weinstein, ed., New York, Marcel Dekker, p. 51.

95 Tam, J. P., W. F. Heath and R. B. Merrifield. 1983. *J. Am. Chem. Soc.*, 105:6442.

96 Yajima, H., N. Fujii, H. Ogawa and H. Kawatani. 1974. *J. Chem. Soc. Chem. Commun.*, p. 107.

97 Wunsch, E. and S. Drees. 1966. *Chem. Ber.*, 99:110.

98 Schwyzer, R. and P. Seiber. 1963. *Nature*, 199:172.

99 Weygand, F. and K. Hunger. 1962. *Chem. Ber.*, 95:1.

100 Wang, S. S. 1973. *J. Am. Chem. Soc.*, 95:1328.

101 Colombo, R. 1982. *Int. J. Pept. Prot. Res.*, 19:71.

102 Atherton, E., R. C. Sheppard and B. J. Williams. 1979. In *Peptides 1978, Proc. 15th Eur. Pept. Symp.*, Wroclaw, Poland: Wroclaw Univ. Press, p. 207.

103 Martinez, J., J. C. Tolle and M. Bodanszky. 1979. *J. Org. Chem.*, 44:3596.

104 Ueki, M., K. Kafi and M. Amemiya, et al. 1988. *J. Chem. Soc. Chem. Commun.*, 414.

105 Anwer, M. K., D. B. Sherman and A. F. Spatola. 1990. *Int. J. Peptide Protein Res.*, 36:392.

106 Schlatter, J. M., R. H. Mazur and O. Goodmonson. 1977. *Tetrahedron Lett.*, p. 2851.

107 Khan, S. A. and K. M. Sivanandaiah. 1978. *Synthesis*, p. 750.

108 Anwer, M. K. and A. F. Spatola. 1981. *Tetrahedron Lett.*, p. 4369.

109 Anwer, M. K., A. F. Spatola and C. D. Bossinger. 1983. *J. Org. Chem.*, 38:3503.

110 Bednarek, M. A. and M. Bodanszky. 1983. *Int. J. Pept. Prot. Res.*, 21:196.

111 Rylander, R. 1974. *Catalytic Hydrogenation in Organic Synthesis.* New York: Academic Press.

112 Kieboom, A. P. and R. Van Rantwijk. 1977. *Hydrogenation and Hydrogenolysis in Synthetic Organic Chemistry.* Delft, Netherlands: Delft University Press.

113 Anantharamaiah, G. M. and K. M. Sivanandaiah. 1977. *J. Chem. Soc. Perkin Trans. 1*, 5:490.

114 ElAmin, B., G. M. Anantharamaiah, G. P. Royer and G. E. Means. 1979. *J. Org. Chem.*, 44:3442.

115 Anwer, M. K. and A. F. Spatola. 1980. *Synthesis*, p. 929.

116 Entwistle, I. D., R. A. Johnston and E. J. Povall. 1975. *J. Chem. Soc. Perkins 1*, p. 1300.

117 Felix, A. M., E. P. Heimer, T. J. Lambros, C. Tzongraki and J. Meienhofer. 1978. *J. Org. Chem.*, 43:4194.

118 Anwer, M. K., S. A. Khan and K. M. Sivanandaiah. 1978. *Synthesis*, p. 751.

119 Anwer, M. K., R. Porter and A. F. Spatola. 1987. *Int. J. Peptide Protein Res.*, 30:489.

120 Anwer, M. K., D. B. Sherman, J. G. Roney and A. F. Spatola. 1989. *J. Org. Chem.*, 554:1285.

121 Ram, S. and R. Ehrenkaufer. 1988. *Synthesis*, p. 91.

122 Merrifield, R. B. 1964. *Biochemistry*, 3:1385.

123 Marglin. A. 1971. *Tetrahedron Lett.*, p. 3145.

124 Gisin, B. F. 1973. *Helv. Chim. Acta*, 56:1476.

125 Roeske, R. W. and P. D. Gesselchen. 1976. *Tetrahedron Lett.*, p. 3369.

126 Wang, S. S. 1975. *J. Org. Chem.*, 40:1235.

127 Mitchell, A. R., S. B. H. Kent, M. Engelhard and R. B. Merrifield. 1978. *J. Org. Chem.*, 43:2845.

128 Wang, S. S. 1973. *J. Am. Chem. Soc.*, 95:1328.

129 Mergler, M., R. Tanner, J. Gosteli and P. Grogg. 1988. *Tetrahedron Lett.*, p. 4005.

130 Matsueda, G. R. and J. M. Stewart. 1981. *Peptides*, 2:45.

131 Bernatowicz, M. S., S. B. Daniels and H. Kaster. 1989. *Tetrahedron Lett.*, p. 4645.

132 Rink, H. 1987. *Tetrahedron Lett.*, p. 3787.

133 Kaiser, E., R. L. Colescott, C. D. Bossinger and P. I. Cook. 1970. *Anal. Biochem.*, 34:595.

134 Sarin, V. K., S. B. H. Kent, J. P. Tam and R. B. Merrifield. 1981. *Anal. Biochem.*, 117:147.

135 Degrado, W. F. and E. T. Kaiser. 1980. *J. Org. Chem.*, 45:1295.

136 Lobl, T. and L. L. Maggiora. 1988. *J. Org. Chem.*, 53:1979.

137 Wang, S. W. 1976. *J. Org. Chem.*, 41:3258.

138 Ben-Ishai, D. and A. Berger. 1952. *J. Org. Chem.*, 17:1564.

139 Shekhani, M. S., G. Grubler, H. Echler and W. Volter. 1990. *Tetrahedron Lett.*, p. 339.

140 Ceccato, M. L., J. Chenu and J. Mery, et al. 1990. *Tetrahedron Lett.*, p. 6189.

141 Condon, M. E., E. W. Petrillo, D. E. Riono, et al. 1982. *J. Med. Chem.*, 25:250.

142 Patchett, A. A., E. Harris, E. W. Tristram, et al. 1980. *Nature*, 288:279.

143 Sasaki, Y., W. A. Murphy and M. Heiman, et al. 1987. *J. Med. Chem.*, 30:1162.

144 Coy, D. H., S. J. Hocharts and Y. Sasaki. 1988. *Tetrahedron*, 34:835.

145 Spatola, A. F., H. Saneii and J. V. Edwards. 1986. *Life Sciences*, 38:1243.

146 Richman, S. J., M. Goodman, T. M. Nguiyen and P. Schiller. 1985. *Int. J. Peptide Protein Res.*, 25:648.

147 Berman, J. and M. Goodman. 1984. *Int. J. Peptide Protein Res.*, 23:610.

148 Spatola, A. F., A. L. Bettag and N. S. Agarwal. 1981. In *LH-RH Peptides as Female and Male Contraceptives*, G. I. Zatuchni, J. D. Shelton and J. Sciarra, eds., New York: Harper and Row, p. 24.

149 Benovitz, D. E. and A. F. Spatola. 1985. *Peptides*, 6:257.

150 Spatola, A. F., F. Formaggio and P. Shiller, et al. 1989. In *2nd Forum on Peptides*, A. Aubry, M. Marrand and B. Vitona, eds., Colloques Iserm, John Libbey, Eurotext Ltd., 174:45.

151 Sherman, D. B., A. F. Spatola and W. Wire. 1989. *Biophys. Biochem. Res. Commun.*, 162:1126.

152 Sherman, D. B. and A. F. Spatola. 1990. *J. Am. Chem. Soc.*, 112:433.

153 Scheibye, S., B. S. Pederson and S. O. Lowesson. 1978. *Bull. Soc. Chim. Belgium*, 87:229.

154 Klauson, K., M. Thorsen and S. O. Lowesson. 1981. *Tetrahedron*, 37:3635.

155 Parham, M. E. and G. M. Louden. 1978. *Biophys. Biochem. Res. Commun.*, 80:1.

156 Radhakrishna, A., M. E. Parham, R. N. Riggs and G. M. Louden. 1979. *J. Org. Chem.*, 44:1247.

CHAPTER 7

Development of Chemically Modified Peptides

LASZLO OTVOS, JR.[1]
MIKLOS HOLLOSI[1,2]

OVERVIEW

MANY proteins contain modified amino acids for which no codons exist in the genome. They are products of post-translational modifications of certain residues of the nascent protein. Important examples are pyroglutamic acid, 5-hydroxy-lysine, 4-hydroxyproline, the acetyl group at the N-termini of a number of protein chains, 6-N-mono- and dimethyl-lysines as well as phosphates and sulphates of tyrosine. However, the two most frequent forms of post-translational modifications are the phosphorylation and glycosylation of hydroxy amino acids and the glycosylation of the asparagine residue. Both the oligosaccharide antennae and the negatively charged phosphoryl groups are located on the surface of the molecule, and are known to play a crucial role in recognition processes, not only at macromolecular but also at cell levels. The structure and biological significance of glycosylated and phosphorylated proteins have been discussed in a great variety of review articles (for selected monographs see References [1–10]).

An important similarity of the two chemically different groups of modified proteins is that glycosylated and phosphorylated residues are frequently involved in reverse turns [11]. The sequence Asn-Xxx-Ser(Thr) was observed to occur at the site of N-glycosylation [12]. Phosphorylation seems to require both the presence of basic amino acid residues (i.e., Lys, Arg, or His) and a β-turn, within or adjacent to the sequence containing the Ser or Thr residue to be phosphorylated [13,14]. As shown by studies

[1]The Wistar Institute of Anatomy and Biology, Philadelphia, PA 19104, U.S.A.
[2]Department of Organic Chemistry, L. Eotvos University, Budapest, Hungary.

on β-turns [15–18], hydrophilic interactions between the peptide backbone and Ser, Thr, and Asn side-chain groups are of primary importance in supporting the β-turns and determining their type [19,20]. X-ray structural analysis of tripeptide models confirmed the hypothesis that H-bonds between the side chain carbonyl group of Asn and the hydroxyl of Ser or Thr facilitates the attachment of sugar to Asn by decreasing the dissociation constant of the amide group [21]. In real proteins, established phosphorylation and glycosylation sites appear to be on both class I (III) or class II predicted or spectroscopically determined β-turns [22–25]. All these findings raise the question of whether a special signal or *sequential* code is required for glycosylation of phosphorylation of a given residue. An answer to this question is expected from detailed statistical analysis of phosphoproteins and glycoproteins with well-established recognition sites.

The other, possibly more intriguing, question concerns the conformation of the polypeptide chain around the glycosylated or phosphorylated residue when post-translational modifications are complete. Oligosaccharide antennae have many interactive groups ($-NHCOCH_3$, $-OH$, $-O-$, $-COOH$), which through H-bondings or ionic interactions with the backbone and side-chain groups of the polypeptide, may alter the polypeptide conformation and support or orient the branched oligosaccharide chains. Physical-chemical or spectroscopic experiments [26–29] as well as electron microscopic studies [30] on glycoproteins indicate that the peptide chain stiffens around the sugar-binding residue and increases the apparent dimension of the protein [31]. Shortening the carbohydrate chain seems not to result in a dramatic conformational change, unlike the removal of the first one or two carbohydrate moieties [30,31]. This conformational change is more clearly expressed in O-glycoproteins than in N-glycosylated ones [31]. The altered and presumably fixed steric structure of both the polypeptide and the oligosaccharide may play a key role as recognition determinants in host pathogen and cell-cell interactions.

Both supporting and dissenting papers have been published about the possible influence of the incorporated phosphate group on the conformation of proteins [23,24,32–34]. The supporting studies indicate that intrapeptide salt bridges result from ionic forces between the negatively charged serine- or threonine-linked phosphoryl and the positive lysine, arginine or histidine side-chain groups. These local interactions may be strong enough to alter the conformation of the peptide chain and form the molecular basis of the biological function of phosphoproteins [35]. Actual changes of the membrane protein structure, due to abnormal phosphorylation, have been shown to be associated with various disease states [36–39].

Interest is growing in the chemical synthesis of glycosylated and phosphorylated peptides of biological importance. A glycosylated peptide is protected from proteolytic attack or has increased hydrophilicity in certain of its regions. Indeed, increasing levels of monosaccharide incorporation reduce the retention time on reversed-phase HPLC [40], and the main determinant of elution time is the total number of monosaccharide units. Moreover, glycosylation facilitates the transport of certain peptides or their mobilization to the cell surface [41]. In spite of the promising prospects of using oligosaccharide-linked peptides as antigens for synthetic vaccines [42–44], relatively little is known about the role glycopeptides may play in the immune response. Indications of both stimulatory [45] and inhibitory [46] effects on the immune recognition of glycosylated T-cell epitopic peptides have been reported. The presence of carbohydrate has been reported to influence the immune response of antisera to retrovirus and influenza virus glycoprotein antigens [47]. The removal of the carbohydrate from the epitope causes a shift in the conformation of the polypeptide backbone such that the epitope is no longer recognized. In another study, conformation of the glycoproteins, determined by 2D NMR studies [48] has been shown to have no effect on the biological activity [49]. Virulent and avirulent influenza viruses differ only in the degree of glycosylation; the virulent strain lacks an asparagine-linked carbohydrate on a hemagglutinin subunit [50].

An increasing amount of glycopeptide synthetic work, like ours [51] is accomplished to corroborate and extend work that elucidates the effect of glycosylation on immune response especially since T-cell epitopic regions often fall close or within proposed glycosylation sites [52]. Natural killer cell-mediated cytolysis is also affected by modification of N-linked oligosaccharides [53]. Although phosphorylation is recognized as a major regulatory process mediated by protein kinases [54] much less is known about the role of phosphorylation in immune recognition. Phosphorylated sequences are found in a highly hydrophilic environment, making these structures excellent antigens [55]. At the same time, T-cell activity of phosphopeptides has not been reported so far. We used synthetic phosphopeptides in "epitope analysis" to identify the multiphosphorylation repeats of mammalian neurofilaments [56,57]. We also demonstrated the existence of immunological similarities between these multiphosphorylation repeats and the neurofibrillary tangles of Alzheimer's disease [35]. Differential recognition after incorporation of the phosphate group could be correlated with secondary structural changes on the peptide [58].

Recently, the chemical synthesis of several small (< 10 residues) glycosylated and phosphorylated peptides of biological importance has been reported. However, an effective study of the function of post-translational modifications requires a large number of mid-size (> 10 residues) selectively phosphorylated and glycosylated peptides. Obviously, the method of choice to generate them would be by solid-phase peptide synthesis [59].

The synthesis of peptides corresponding to the third most often occurring post-translational modification, acetylation, seems to be resolved. Pentafluorophenyl acetate selectively acetylates amino groups in the absence of a tertiary base and acetylates hydroxyl groups in the presence of a base in solution [60]. Unlike pentafluorophenyl formate, used for formylation reactions [61], pentafluorophenyl acetate is a useful reagent for acetylation of both amino [62] and unprotected primary hydroxyl groups [51] on solid support as well.

While a simple synthetic protocol is desired for synthesis of phosphoserine- or phosphothreonine-containing peptides, the final and distant goal of glycopeptide synthesis is the preparation of long polypeptide chains bearing the natural complex (mostly branched) oligosaccharide antennae of glycoproteins. In this chapter we plan to outline the *state of the art* and give perspectives on the chemical synthesis of glycopeptides and phosphopeptides. We will not be covering backbone modifications, like peptide synthesis containing thioamides [63], or synthesis of peptides with various amide-linked N-terminal groups (like peptidoglycans of cell wall) or fatty acid coupled peptides used for preparation of liposomes [64].

CHEMICAL SYNTHESIS OF GLYCOPEPTIDES

SOLUTION TECHNIQUES

At the beginning of the 1970s the discovery of sugar-nucleotide compounds was followed by a revolution of glycoconjugate chemistry and biochemistry. The first step was to learn how to synthesize oligosaccharides larger than di- and trisaccharides. Until the late 1970s the preparation of trisaccharides with various monomers and types of linkages was only sporadically successful. Oligosaccharide synthesis entails the coupling of two or more polyfunctional reaction partners. The reactive areas of all components must be selectively blocked. In the *glycosyl component* the anomeric center must be selectively exposed and functionalized. In the *hydroxyl component* it is the acceptor OH group which must be selectively deblocked prior to the glycosylation step. The reactivities of the anomeric center and the acceptor OH strongly depend on the blocking pattern of the reaction partners. To avoid expensive anomer separation, the coupling step should result in only one of the possible anomers.

Large oligosaccharides were best obtained by using glycosyl halides. Their reactivity can be modified by blocking groups (neighboring group-assisted procedures) and by selecting suitable catalysts (heterogenous catalyst procedures) [65]. The fundamental reaction strategies which are most suitable for building up larger oligosaccharides are discussed by Paulsen [66]. Other glycoside linking techniques, such as the trifluoromethanesulfonic (triflic) anhydride method [67–70], application of glycosyl fluorides in the presence of metallocene-AgClO$_4$ catalyst [71,72], glycosylation with thioglycosides [73] or trichloroimidates [74], redox glycosylation [75], and unusual (e.g., photoremovable [76]) hydroxyl group protections have also been suggested. One of the triflic anhydride catalyzed methods can be applied even for direct glycosylation of an amide nitrogen [70]. So far these approaches have, however, been used only rarely for the preparation of larger oligosaccharides.

The chemical synthesis of glycopeptides is governed by the principles of carbohydrate and peptide chemistry. The coupling step between carbohydrate and peptide should proceed as stereoselectively as possible. Apart from the problem of compatibility of the blocking techniques used in the two different fields, the sensitivity of the O-glycosyl-, especially fucosyl- (found in tumor antigens) serine and threonine linkages requires the use of protecting groups which can be removed under almost neutral conditions [77–81]. In N-glycosides the 2-acetamido-2-deoxy-β-D-glucopyranosyl-amine is attached to aspartic acid through a secondary amine linkage which compares in stability with the peptide bond.

The first attempts to synthesize glycopeptides were made by sugar chemists, who, inspired by the idea that the specificity of many natural polymers is determined by the carbohydrate portion [82], concentrated on large oligosaccharides linked to one single amino acid residue. In terms of peptide chemistry these molecules are not true glycopeptides. The other extreme is one carbohydrate moiety linked to the peptide chain. This approach is based on the idea that such an oligosaccharide structure with limited carbohydrate residues will allow custom synthesis of glycopeptides, and the glycopeptides will bear the biological and conformational properties of glycoproteins. Sometimes conjugates consisting of one protected or nonprotected amino acid and sugar residue are also called glycopeptides. These molecules are cores of glycopeptides and in many cases they can be used for preparing true glycopeptides by elongating the peptide or carbohydrate chain. Early glycopeptide syntheses dealt solely with the synthesis of mono- and disaccharide-linked amino acids [83–86] but preparation of novel reagents (or/and building blocks) have been published recently [51, 87–89]. In the course of preparing the reagents chemists learn how to form selectively α or β O- and N-glycosidic linkages [90] and to synthesize glycopeptides with more complex oligosaccharide side-chains [91]. An excellent review was published in 1985 on synthetic glycopeptides by Garg and Jeanloz [92]. Another review-like article by Paulsen et al. [91], surveying the chemical synthesis of O-glycosylated peptides, appeared in 1988.

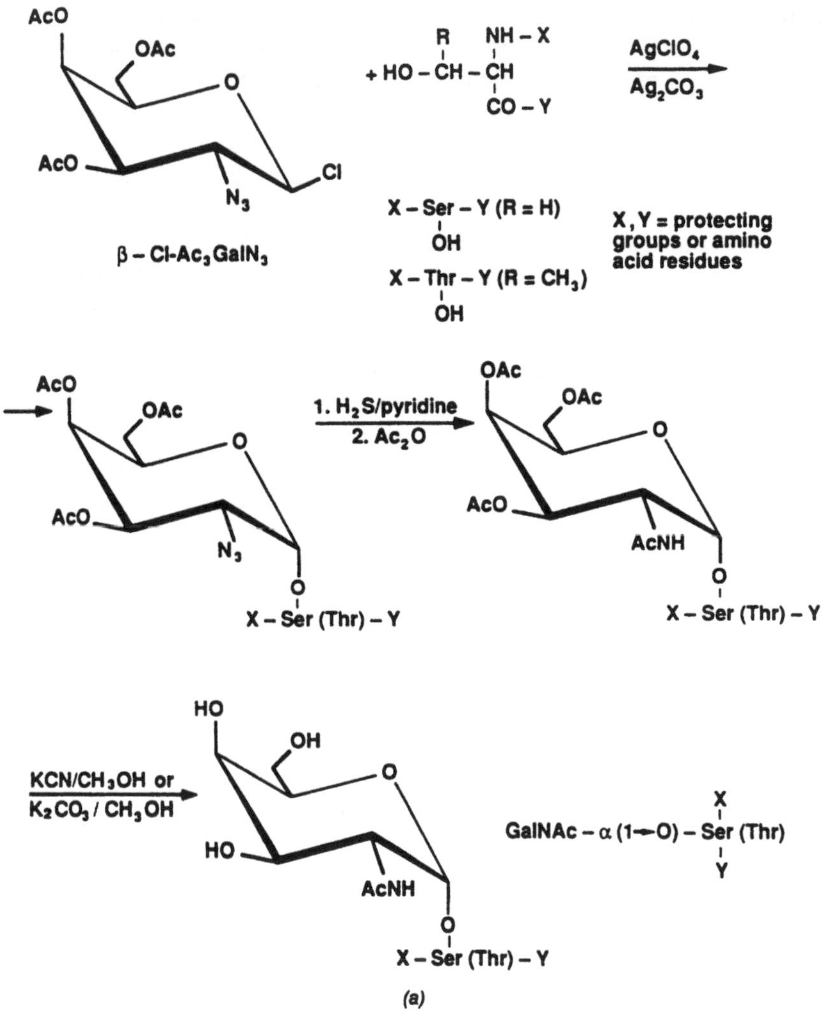

AgClO₄ → $\dfrac{AgClO_4}{Ag_2CO_3}$

R   NH – X
+ HO – CH – CH
            CO – Y

β – Cl-Ac₃ GalN₃

X – Ser – Y (R = H)
        |
        OH

X – Thr – Y (R = CH₃)
        |
        OH

X, Y = protecting
groups or amino
acid residues

1. H₂S/pyridine
2. Ac₂O

X – Ser (Thr) – Y

X – Ser (Thr) – Y

KCN/CH₃OH or
K₂CO₃ / CH₃OH

GalNAc – α (1→O) – Ser (Thr)

X – Ser (Thr) – Y

(a)

Scheme 7.1 (a) Typical stereoselective synthesis of O-glycosides with natural α-glycosidic linkage (Koenigs-Knorr method).

160

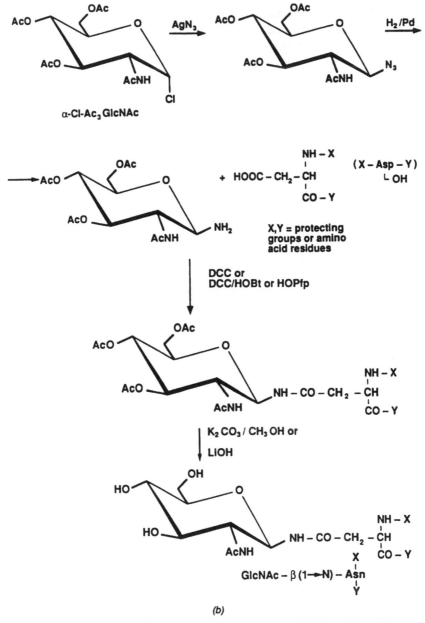

Scheme 7.1 (continued) (b) Typical stereoselective synthesis of N-glycosides with natural β-glycosidic linkage.

Table 7.1 gives a selection of glycopeptides synthesized after 1983 and serves to present the latest trends in glycopeptide synthesis. The largest group of conjugates comprises fragments of glycoproteins such as anti-freeze glycoprotein, glycophorin, interleukin, mucin, etc. An interesting example of more sophisticated glycopeptides is a hexapeptide of gly-cophorin A that bears two serine-linked disaccharide units [121]. Glyco-sylated peptide hormones and epitopes of immunologically active pro-teins, usually with one monosaccharide moiety, are used for evaluating the effect of glycosylation on the biological activity of the parent peptide.

To address pharmacological questions, such as the stabilization of po-tentially active peptides against enzymatic degradation, and in a relatively easier synthetic solution, amide-type connection of carbohydrate to pep-tides (found in muramyl-dipeptides [122]) was employed to attach sugar to tuftsin and rigin [118,119]. An early idea was the incorporation of 2-acetamido-1-N-(β-L-aspartyl)-2-deoxy-β-glucopyranosylamine into hydan-toin, thiohydantoin, dioxopiperazine and p-toluenesulfonamide derivatives of pharmacological importance [123]. A new approach couples glycopep-tides to proteins through a heterobifunctional coupling reagent [124]. Aldonate coupling [125] and reductive amination [126] were also used to prepare carbohydrate-protein conjugates.

Recently interest has grown in the synthesis of partially protected glyco-peptides which are suitable models for spectroscopic and conformational studies. High-field ^{1}H and ^{13}C NMR model studies date back to the early 1980s [127–129]. The first optical rotatory dispersion (ORD) and circular dichroism (CD) measurements on glycopeptides were performed to iden-tify synthetic glycosylated amino acids [130–132]. Conformational studies using CD spectroscopy have been reported on antifreeze glycopeptides [133] and galactofuranosyl-containing glycopeptides [134].

A series of glycosylated models of β-turns were prepared in our labora-tories to study the effect of glycosylation on the peptide backbone. We found that peracetylated glycosides of Pro-L-Ser and Val-L-Ser dipeptides have a tendency to form type I (III) β-turns, while the Pro-D-Ser and Val-D-Ser models will likely adopt type II or distorted type II β-turn confor-mations. Based on circular dichroism data [135,136], the configuration at C-2 of the carbohydrate residue [gluco (galacto) or manno] has no effect on the turn-forming ability of the peptide. The intensity ratios of the free and intra H-bonded NH bands in the infrared spectra, measured in CCl_4 and CH_2Cl_2, show that the glycosylated models are present as mixtures of single- and double-H-bonded conformers in dilute nonpolar solution and the gluco- and galactoconjugates (equatorial acetoxy group at C-2) have a higher tendency than do the mannoconjugates (axial acetoxy at C-2) to form double H-bonded conformers. In a hetero NOE experiment per-formed on Boc-Pro-Ser[β-(1→O)Ac$_4$Glc]-NHCH$_3$ in CDCl$_3$ at $-20°C$,

TABLE 7.1. A Selection of Glycopeptides Synthesized after 1983.

Peptide Component (the glycosylated amino acid is marked by *)	Carbohydrate Component and Type of Linkage	Glycosylation Method	Study Aimed at	References
Glycophorin etc., glycoprotein sequences				
Z-Val-Ser*-Glu(OBzl)-Ile-Ser*-Val-OBzl	Ac_4Glc-$\beta(1\to3)$-$Bzl_2GlcNAc$-$\alpha(1\to O)$	Coupling glycosylated Fmoc-Ser or Thr-OH	Synthesis	93
Triglycosylated pentapeptides of glycophorin A^N and A^{MC} (H-Leu-Ser*-Thr*-Thr*-Glu-OH and H-Ser-Ser*-Thr*-Thr*-Glu-OH)	$GalNAc$-$\alpha(1\to O)$	Tf_2O using $GalN_3$-OH	Synthesis, ^{13}C-NMR characterization	94
Ser*-Ser*-OH, H-Thr*-Ser*-Ser*-Ser*-OH	Gal-$\alpha(1\to3)$-$GalNAc$-$\alpha(1\to O)$	KK1, EEDQ coupling of Fmoc-derivatives	Synthesis	95
3 glycophorin A^M N-terminal pentapeptides (H-Ser-Ser-Thr-Thr-Gly) O-glycosylated at Ser^2, Thr^3, or Thr^4	$GalNac$-$\alpha(1\to O)$	coupling with Fmoc-Ser $(GalN_3)$-ONp or Fmoc-Thr$(GalN_3)$-OSu	Synthesis, ^{13}C NMR characterization	96
H-Ser-Ser*-Thr*-Thr*-Gly-OH	Bzl_3GalN_3-$\alpha(1\to O)$	Tf_2O	Synthesis	97
Glycopeptide models				
H-Ala-Thr*-Ala-OH	Bzl_4-Gal-$\beta(1\to3)$-Bzl_3Gal-$\alpha(1\to O)$	AgOTf	Synthesis	98
CF_3COOH·H-Asn*-Phe-Thr-OAll	$Ac_4GlcNAc$-β-$(1\to4)$-$Ac_2GlcNAc$-$\beta(1\to N)$	Coupling of glycosylated Boc-Asn-OH	Preparation of disaccharide containing Boc-Asn-OAll derivative, synthesis.	99

(continued)

163

TABLE 7.1. (continued).

Peptide Component (the glycosylated amino acid is marked by*)	Carbohydrate Component and Type of Linkage	Glycosylation Method	Study Aimed at	References
Z-Ala-Thr*-Ala-OMe	Ac_3GalN_3-$\alpha(1\rightarrow O)$	Tf_2O	Glycosylation of sterically hindered Thr	100
H-Ala-Ser*-Gly-Ile-OH	Ac_3Xyl-$\beta(1\rightarrow O)$ or Bzl_3Xyl-$\beta(1\rightarrow O)$	TMSOTf from 1-acetyl or DMTST from 1-ethylmercapto derivatives	Synthesis	101
Boc-Asn*-Gly-NHMe, Boc-Gly-Asn*-NHMe	$Ac_3GlcNAc$-$\beta(1\rightarrow N)$	EEDQ coupling of $Ac_3GlcNAc$-NH_2	Synthesis, ¹H-NMR, conformation	102
Z-Thr*-Ala-Ala-OMe, Ac-Ala-Ala-Thr*-OMe, Ac-Ala-Thr*-Ala-OMe, Ac-Thr*-Ala-Ala-OMe	$Ac_3GalNAc$-$\alpha(1\rightarrow O)$	KK2	¹H-NMR carbohydrate-peptide interaction	103
Z-Thr*-Ala-Ala-OMe, Ac-Thr*-Ala-Ala-OMe	$Ac_3GalNAc$-$\alpha(1\rightarrow O)$	KK2	¹H-NMR, carbohydrate-peptide interaction	104
Ac-Thr*-Ala-Ala-OMe	$GalNAc$-$\alpha(1\rightarrow O)$	TEA/MeOH deacetylation	¹H-NMR, carbohydrate-peptide interaction	105
H-*Ala-D-iGln-OH and H-*Ala-D-Gln-Buⁿ	MurNAc amide linkage	Peptide coupling	¹H-NMR, conformation	106,107

TABLE 7.1. (continued).

Peptide Component (the glycosylated amino acid is marked by*)	Carbohydrate Component and Type of Linkage	Glycosylation Method	Study Aimed at	References
Z-Thr*-Ala-OMe, Z-Ala-Thr*-OMe	Ac₃GalNAc-α(1→O)	KK2	¹H-NMR, peptide sugar interaction	108
9 Tripeptides (e.g., Z-Pro-Thr*-Ala-OBzl) and Boc-Gly-Phe-Leu-Ser*-Gly-OMe	Ac₃Glc, GalAc₃Man, Tal; α(1→O)	I-Su procedure	Synthesis	109
Aloc-Ala-Leu-Asn*-Leu-Thr-Asn-O¹Bu	Ac₃FucGlcNAc-α(1→6)-AcGlcNAc-β(1→4)-Ac₃GlcNAc-β(1→N)	EEDQ to Aloc-Asp-O¹Bu	Synthesis	110
H-Asn*-Val-Phe-OBu	Ac₃GlcNAc-β(1→N)	Incorporation of Noc-Asn(Ac₃GlcNAc)-OH	Synthesis, Noc protection	77
H-Asn*-Glu-Thr-Ile-Val-OH	Ac₃GlcNAc-β(1→N)	Incorporation of Boc-Asn(Ac₃GlcNAc)-OH	Synthesis, allyl protection	111
Glycosylated peptide hormones Protected opioid peptides (Boc-Tyr(Bzl)-Gly-Gly-Phe*-Oh and Boc-Tyr(Bzl)-Gly-Phe-Leu*-OH	α- and β-anomeric esters of Glc-OH (α, β10 type)	DCC/CuCl coupling	Synthesis, ¹H- and ¹³C-NMR characterization	112
[Leu⁵] enkephalin (H-Tyr-Gly-Gly-Phe-Leu*-OH)	β10 and 60 esters of Glc-OH	DTC/CuCl; OPcp/Im	Synthesis, opioid activity	113
[D-Met², Pro⁵] enkephalin amide, H-Tyr-D-Met-Gly-Phe-Pro-NH₂*	Glc-β(1→N)	DCC coupling of β-Ac₄Glc-NH₂ NH₃/MeOH deacetylation	synthesis, opioid activity 2D-NMR, conformation	114

(continued)

165

TABLE 7.1. (continued).

Peptide Component (the glycosylated amino acid is marked by *)	Carbohydrate Component and Type of Linkage	Glycosylation Method	Study Aimed at	References
[D-Met², Hyp⁵] enkephalin amide, H-Tyr-D-Met-Gly-Phe-Hyp*-NH₂	Gal-β(1→O)	KK2	Synthesis 2D-NMR, conformation	115
Opioid peptides (H-Tyr*-Gly-Gly-Phe-Oh and H-Tyr*-Gly-Gly-Phe-Leu-OH)	Glc-β(1→O)	DCC/CuCl coupling with Bzl₄Glc-OH	Synthesis and opioid activity	116
Protected tetrapeptide of vespulakinin 1 [Z-Thr (OBuᵗ)-Ala-Thr*-Thr(OBuᵗ)-NH-NH-Boc]	Bzl₄ Gal-α(1→O)	Incorporation of Fmoc-Thr(Bzl₄Gal)-OSu	Synthesis, ¹H-NMR characterization	117
Immunogenic peptides				
Tuftsin derivatives, H-Thr*-Lys-Pro-Arg-OH; H-Thr-Lys-Pro-Arg*-NH₂	Nα-gluconyl-(Thr) (Arg)-NHGlc; α,β(1→O)Thr	lacton acylation; mixed anhydride; Tf₂O	Synthesis	118
Rigin derivatives, H-Gly-Glu*-Pro-Arg-OH; H-Gly-Gln-Pro-Arg*-OH; H-Gly*-Gln-Pro-Arg-OH; H-Gly*-Glu-Pro-Arg-OH	γ-glutamyl-D-glucosamine; arginyl-D-glucosamine; Nᵃ¹ gluconyl-Gly	Azide coupling	Synthesis, binding and phagocytosis assay	119
Interleukin 2 (H-Ala-Pro-Thr*-Ser-Ser-Ser-Thr-Lys-Lys-THr-OH)	GalNAc-α(1→O) or GalNAc-β(1→3)-Bzl₂GalNAc-α(1→O)	Fmoc- Thr(Ac₄Gal)-OBu prepared by KK1 method	Synthesis	120

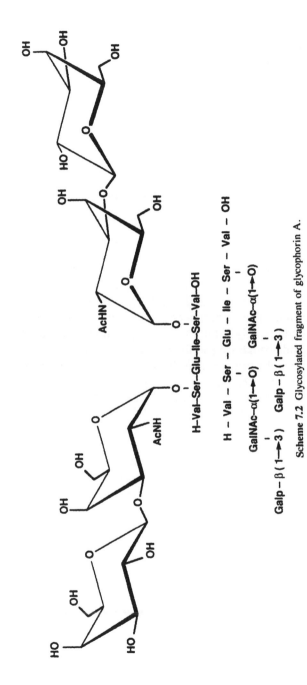

H–Val–Ser–Glu–Ile–Ser–Val–OH

H – Val – Ser – Glu – Ile – Ser – Val – OH
　　　　　　 |　　　　　 |
　　GalNAc–α(1→O)　　GalNAc–α(1→O)
　　　　　　 |　　　　　 |
　　Galp – β (1→3)　　Galp – β (1→3)
　　　　　　 |
Galp – β (1→3)

Scheme 7.2 Glycosylated fragment of glycophorin A.

167

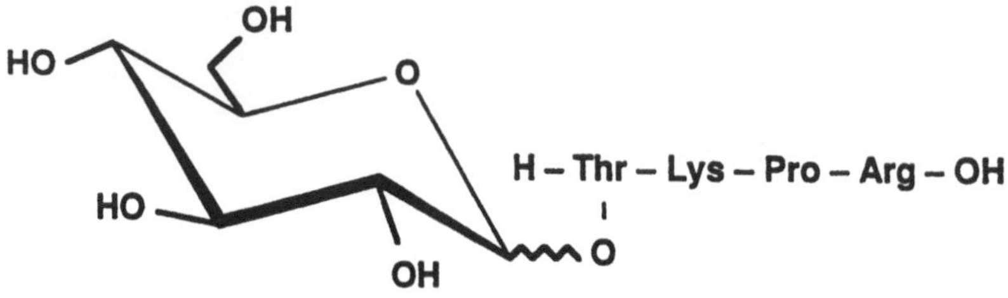

(α + β) **anomeric mixture of**

O – glucosyl – tuftsin

(Glc – α, β (1 → O) tuftsin)

Scheme 7.3 Anomeric mixture of O-glycosyl-tuftsin.

selective irradiation of the NH(CH$_3$) proton at 400 MHz caused a definite enhancement of the intensity of the carbonyl resonance of C-2 acetoxy in the ^{13}C spectrum. This experiment gives direct support to the idea that turn-like structures (glyco-turns), fixed by intramolecular H-bonds between the peptide backbone and the first sugar residue may play an important role in fixing the oligosaccharide antennae of glycoproteins. A similar glyco-turn was found recently in Ac-Thr[α(1 → O)GalNAc]-Ala-Ala-OMe [105]. In this case the peptide-carbohydrate intramolecular H-bond is formed between the amide proton of GalNAc and the carbonyl oxygen of the Thr residue. Most recently, we found that incorporation of GlcNAc residue in mid-chain position of a dodekapeptide broke the α-helical conformation of the parent peptide. Chitobiose and cellobiose acted similarly to GlcNAc [137]. Obviously, detailed spectroscopic studies on well-selected models are required to learn the possible types of glyco-turns and their conformational effect on the peptide backbone.

Until recently there were only a few examples of synthetic glycopeptides which contained both long peptide and long oligosaccharide chains, or more than one oligosaccharide. One of the most notable chemical efforts is the synthesis of a tetrapeptide sequence, H-Thr-Ser-Ser-Ser-OH, with four disaccharide chains [95]. Apparently, classical (in solution) chemical synthesis of glycopeptides has its limits and further synthetic studies are required to generate more sophisticated glycopeptide models.

SOLID-PHASE METHODS

Solid-phase peptide synthesis is the method of choice to prepare medium-size or longer unmodified peptides today. This method provides

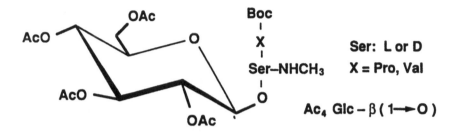

Ser: L or D   X = Pro, Val

Ac$_4$ Glc – β (1 → O)

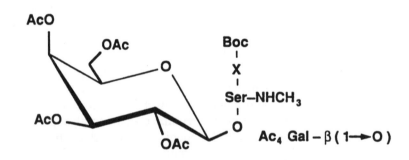

Ac$_4$ Gal – β (1 → O)

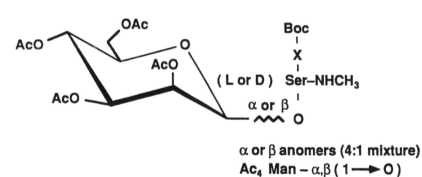

α or β anomers (4:1 mixture)

Ac$_4$ Man – α,β (1 → O)

Scheme 7.4 Glycosylated models of β-turns.

synthesis without isolation of the intermediate products. The attachment of the C-terminal residue to the solid support must be strong enough to withstand the repetitive cleavage of the N-terminal protecting groups and the steps of washing and sometimes neutralization. This strong attachment is traditionally achieved by an acid-cleavable connection. The acid lability of the peptide-resin bond varies from 1% trifluoroacetic acid (TFA), used for selective cleavage of side-chain protected peptides, to liquid HF used in conventional Merrifield synthesis. N-terminal deprotection is accomplished with a base or an acid which leaves the peptide attached to the resin. These strategies are compatible with the synthesis of N-monoglycosylated peptides, where the asparagine-sugar connection is similar to the peptide bond.

On the other hand the O-glycosidic linkage (whether it is between a hydroxy-amino acid and a carbohydrate or between two sugar moieties) is extremely acid sensitive. This acid sensitivity is not independent from the other parts of the molecule. TFA was found to cleave the intersaccharide fucosidic bonds if the carbohydrate side-chain was not protected by acetylation [110]. The fucosidic bond is markedly more acid-labile than the corresponding galactosidic bond [138]. Acetyl side-chain protection was used for solid-phase synthesis of threonine-containing glycopeptides corresponding to bovine submaxially mucin, porcine glycophorin [91,139] and fibronectin [140]. The acetyl groups were removed from the sugar moieties with methanol/methoxide ion. The other favorite sugar-protecting group is the benzyl ether, which is removed with catalytic hydrogenolysis. Side reactions such as incomplete removal, isomerization of isoglutamine residues [122], racemization, and β-elimination may occur and unsuccessful attempts to obtain fully deblocked synthetic glycopeptides have been reported [141]. Kunz and Dombo [142] suggested the use of a polymeric support with allylic anchor groups for synthesis of a fully protected glycosylated tripeptide. The peptide-resin connection is cleaved selectively and quantitatively by $[(C_6H_5)_3P_4]Pd$ and morpholine in tetrahydrofuran [111]. The commercial unavailability of C-terminal amino acids attached to this Pd^0 cleavable "Hycram" resin restricts widespread application of the method in the biotechnology sector.

The second problem is related to the size of the acylating agent. It is well known that coupling efficiency is a crucial point in successful solid-phase synthesis [143]. Coupling efficiencies less than 98–99% (depending upon the size of the peptide being synthesized) lead to heterogeneous final products. Amino acids with bulky side-chains like isoleucine, valine, and protected threonine residues are known to couple slowly. Apparently solid-phase peptide synthesis incorporates glycosylated amino acids rather than glycosylates unprotected amino acids. Steric hindrance leads to low coupling efficiencies when bulky glycosylated amino acids are incorporated

[111,122] in the same way that steric hindrance prevents direct glycosylation of N-terminally substituted threonine residue [100].

We examined the coupling efficiencies of variously protected glycosylated asparagine residue to a dodekapeptide and to glycine attached to 4-methoxy-4'-alkoxy-benzhydrylamine resin [51]. We found that coupling rates decreased as the size of the acylating agent increased. When the sugar-hydroxyls were acetylated only 50–60% glycoamino acid addition was detected with double couplings. This value prohibited the use of protected glycoamino acids on automated synthesizers. We introduced the synthesis and application of a new reagent, O-unprotected Fmoc-Asn (GlcNAc)-OH. This glycoamino acid can be prepared easily from commercially available components. Our coupling rates rose to >90%. Couplings were performed with preformed pentafluorophenol esters (-OPfp), followed by symmetrical anhydrides for subsequent amino acids. Based on successful experiments with minimal side-chain protection [144] we have shown [145] that symmetrical anhydrides do not acylate unprotected hydroxyl groups on solid support. The glycosylated asparagine residue already on the resin did not decrease the coupling efficiency of the next amino acid. A simple preparation of 1-amino-GlcNAc [used for synthesis of Fmoc-Asn(GlcNAc)-OH] and the corresponding 1-amino-disaccharide (chitobiose) is reported [146]. Later we extended this synthetic strategy to Fmoc-Asn(chitobiose)-OH [147], Fmoc-Asn(cellobiose)-OH [137], Fmoc-Asn(chitotriose)-OH, Fmoc-Asn(Glc)-OH, and Fmoc-Asn(maltose)-OH [148]. Coupling efficiencies varied between 70 and 100%. No cleavage of the O-glycosidic bond was found for either of the oligosaccharides during standard TFA treatment.

Similarly, sugar-unprotected Fmoc-Thr(β-Gal)-OPfp has been used to synthesize tuftsin peptides by the continuous flow variant of the Fmoc-polyamide method [141]. Ninety-five percent TFA was used for detachment of the peptide from the resin, and no carbohydrate-cleavage was reported. The otherwise fully protected, N-acetylated, serine-unprotected peptide-resin [145] was utilized for O-linked glycopeptide synthesis. Glycosylation was made with 3,4,6-O-triacetyl-glycose and galactose-oxazolines [149]. Gluco- and galactoserine-containing peptides were obtained after cleavage and deacetylation. Once again, no cleavage of the O-glycosidic bond was detected during standard TFA cleavages from the resin. If the activation step of the unprotected sugar is long, the sugar can lactonize [122]. The shorter the activation is, the higher the coupling rates are. Another side-reaction is an intramolecular O-acylation of urethane-type N-protected hydroxyamino-acids during C-terminal saponification [150]. Glycopeptides are purified on reversed-phase HPLC [151,152] and their structure can be verified by fast-atom bombardment mass spectrometry and peptide sequencing [151].

CHEMICAL SYNTHESIS OF PHOSPHOPEPTIDES

SOLUTION TECHNIQUES

The simplest way to prepare phosphorylated peptides and proteins is to use enzymatic methods. However, due to the high specificity of enzyme reactions, this approach is limited to well-selected substrate sequences. The other generally applicable method is chemical phosphorylation. Although the synthesis of a true phosphoric acid monoester derivative of a protein, by using phosphorous oxychloride, was accomplished in 1901, the first phosphoserine-containing peptides were prepared after 1955 [153–155]. The literature on the synthesis and properties of N-, O-, and S-phospho derivatives of amino acids, peptides and proteins is covered by an excellent review published in 1984 [1].

Polyphosphoric acid, made *in situ* from H_3PO_4 and P_2O_5 was used to phosphorylate proteins [156]. We used this procedure for synthesis of per-phosphorylated human neurofilament fragments [24]. The sequence Lys-Ser-Pro-Val-Pro-Lys-Ser-Pro-Val-Glu-Glu-Lys-Gly is repeated six times in the natural protein. We prepared the tridekapeptide and three repeats thereof and determined their conformation. Phosphorylation for three days resulted in complete phosphorylation of all serine residues. When the reaction was stopped after 12 hours, equal amounts of all three possible phosphate forms of a single repeat unit (and the nonphosphorylated tridekapeptide) was found. Separation of these differentially phosphorylated forms was achieved by reversed-phase HPLC [145]. The possibility of separating the monophosphorylated isomers suggests a conformational orientation on the surface of the bonded phase [157]. Ion exchange chromatography was used to separate phosphonodipeptide diastereomers [158]. Conformational analysis of phosphoserines by ^{1}H- and ^{13}C-NMR revealed a planar W-type arrangement of the H_α-C_α-C_β-O-P atoms [159]. NMR is very useful for verifying the structure of synthetic phosphopeptides, because the application of fast atom bombardment mass spectrometry, suggested by Johns et al. [160], is restricted to phosphopeptides without strong ionic character [157].

Polyphosphoric acid uniformly modifies all serine residues, but it is often difficult to establish whether or not each serine indeed corresponds to authentic *in vivo* phosphorylation sites. Moreover, the extended dialysis required to remove all inorganic salts (introduced by aqueous acidic hydrolysis of the formed N-phosphates and following neutralization) leads to tremendous synthetic loss, especially of the smaller peptides.

There are two basic approaches to the synthesis of phosphorylated peptides. The first introduces the phosphate after synthesis is complete. This procedure requires orthogonal protection or incorporation of unprotected serines or threonines. Awkward stereochemistry may hinder the phosphorylation of larger peptides [161]. The alternative approach uses properly protected phospho amino acids or small phosphopeptides as synthons [161,162]. Synthesis of some phosphorylated hydroxy-amino acid derivatives was outlined by Riley et al. [163] using diphenyl-phosphochloridate. Cleavage of the protecting phenyl groups was accomplished by hydrogenolysis. Alewood, Perich, and Johns reported on several aspects of the latter synthetic strategy [165-167,170,171]. First dibenzyl phosphochloridate [164] was used to prepare phosphorylated serine residue and the resulting protected phosphoserine was incorporated in a tripeptide [165,166]. Ninety-eight percent formic acid was used to remove the Boc group that protected the N-terminal, since usual acidolytic reagents (4 M HCl/dioxan, TFA) caused considerable debenzylation. Later the above-mentioned group used diphenyl phosphochloridate to circumvent the problem. Boc-Ser(diPhP)-OH was used for the preparation of H-Glu-Ser(P)-Leu-OH [167]. After the synthesis was completed, the phenyl groups were removed by catalytic hydrogenation using PtO_2 in 40% TFA/AcOH. Similar conditions were applied to the hydrogenolytic cleavage of the phenyl-O bond during the synthesis of a peptide containing two adjacent phosphoserine residues [168,169]. Phenyl protection was used in synthesis of an octapeptide-amide containing four phosphoserine residues [170]. Perich, Alewood, and Johns [171] reported an efficient one-pot synthesis of phenyl protected Z- and Boc-phosphoserine, phosphothreonine and phosphotyrosine by oxidative (I_2) aqueous workup.

The newest method to introduce the phosphate moiety to the hydroxyl function of serine, threonine, or tyrosine residues uses N,N-diethylamino-dibenzyl-phosphoramidite followed by oxidation of the phosphite with excess ′butyl hydroperoxide [172]. This strategy was used for synthesis of a relatively difficult pentapeptide, H-Lys-Arg-Thr(P)-Leu-Arg-OH [173]. Phosphorylation was done after the third cycle, on Boc-Thr-Leu-Arg (MBS)-OMe.

A series of phosphoserine-containing protected model peptides was synthesized in our laboratory. Freshly prepared dibenzyl phosphochloridate in dry pyridine was used to introduce the dibenzyl-phosphoryl group following peptide synthesis. The benzyl groups were removed by catalytic hydrogenation using 10% Pd/C catalyst. The low (40-60%) yields and the difficulties in purifying the products were due to side reactions [166] during the crucial phosphorylation step. After characterization, the phosphorylated peptides were used for conformational and metal ion binding studies.

Forty percent TFA in dichloromethane was reported to remove the benzyl groups from O-phosphotyrosine during synthesis of H-Tyr(P)-Leu-Gly-OH [174]. It was also found that liquid HF effects complete dephosphorylation of the O-phosphotyrosyl residue.

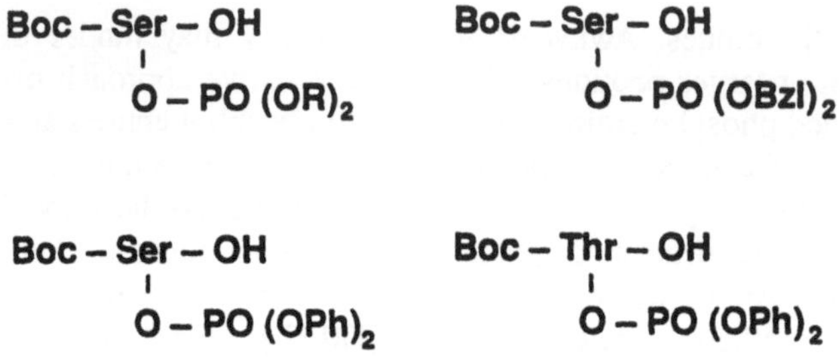

Boc – Ser – OH   Boc – Ser – OH
    | |
    O – PO (OR)$_2$ O – PO (OBzl)$_2$

Boc – Ser – OH   Boc – Thr – OH
    | |
    O – PO (OPh)$_2$ O – PO (OPh)$_2$

R = CH$_3$ or C$_2$H$_5$; Bzl = C$_6$H$_5$CH$_2$; Ph = C$_6$H$_5$

Scheme 7.5 Synthons for solution synthesis of phosphopeptides.

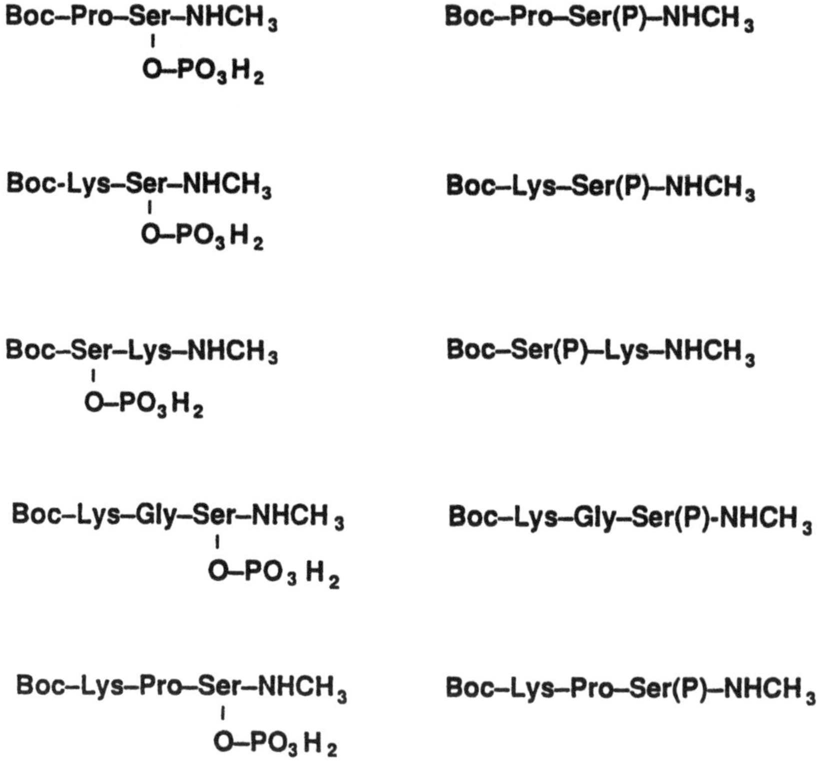

Boc–Pro–Ser–NHCH$_3$ Boc–Pro–Ser(P)–NHCH$_3$
         |
         O–PO$_3$H$_2$

Boc-Lys–Ser–NHCH$_3$ Boc–Lys–Ser(P)–NHCH$_3$
         |
         O–PO$_3$H$_2$

Boc–Ser–Lys–NHCH$_3$ Boc–Ser(P)–Lys–NHCH$_3$
       |
       O–PO$_3$H$_2$

Boc–Lys–Gly–Ser–NHCH$_3$ Boc–Lys–Gly–Ser(P)-NHCH$_3$
             |
             O–PO$_3$H$_2$

Boc–Lys–Pro–Ser–NHCH$_3$ Boc–Lys–Pro–Ser(P)–NHCH$_3$
             |
             O–PO$_3$H$_2$

Scheme 7.6 Phosphorylated models of β-turns.

SOLID-PHASE METHODS

The acid stability of the amino acid phosphate esters is in the center of many discussions today. The opposite of N-phosphates, O-phosphates are known to be acid stable and base labile [1]. Indeed, 2N HCl, used for N-phosphate cleavage does not hydrolyze the phosphoserines during the post-synthetic phosphorylation protocol [156]. Considering the different strategies for solid-phase synthesis of phosphopeptides, we found that liquid HF cleaves off the phosphate from phosphoserine, and although the phospho-serine is more stable in trifluormethanesulfonic acid (TFMSA) in TFA, decomposition is still observed during the workshop [175]. This finding suggests that Merrifield-type resins cannot be used in solid-phase synthesis of phosphopeptides, and is in accordance with earlier studies [168]. In spite of this, Arendt et al. [176] reported solid-phase phosphopeptide synthesis on Pam-resin. H-Leu-Arg-Arg-Ala-Ser(P)-Leu-Gly-OH and H-Leu-Arg-Arg-Ala-Thr(P)-Leu-Gly-OH was synthesized, when Boc-diphenyl-phosphoserine and threonine was incorporated into the growing peptide chain. After cleavage with HF (and TFMSA) removal of phenyl groups was achieved with catalytic hydrogenolysis in 40% TFA/AcOH. In another case the phenyl protecting groups were cleaved with concomitant release of a phosphotripeptide from the solid support [177]. Boc-dimethylphos-phono-tyrosine was used to synthesize a phosphotyrosine containing heptapeptide [178].

Based on our experiences with the limited acid stability of phospho-serine, we decided to follow the Fmoc-N-terminal protecting strategy with TFA to cleave the ready phosphopeptides from the solid support. We did not find the other part of the above outlined [176,177] strategy suitable for custom solid-phase synthesis of phosphopeptides, since in our hands the activation and coupling of N-Fmoc-O-dibenzyl- (or diphenyl) phospho-serine with acceptable yield was unsuccessful (similar to our glycopeptide synthesis). To introduce the protected phosphate and to continue coupling further amino acids was also less advantageous due to the base-lability of the phosphate, since piperidine was used for repetitive N-terminal de-blocking. Since neither the activated esters, nor the symmetrical anhy-drides [145,175] acylate unprotected serine hydroxyls in solid-phase, in our strategy Fmoc-Ser-OPfp (made *in situ*) was incorporated in the peptide, and phosphorylation was accomplished after assembly of the peptide chain. Our synthetic strategy initiated further reports [179]. In determining the optimal phosphoric acid chloride, we observed that the benzyl group could be removed from the dibenzyl phosphate, while the diphenyl phosphate remained intact under the conditions used to cleave the peptides from the p-alkoxy-benzylalcohol resin, an observation similar to a previous report [161]. A model heptapeptide, H-(and Ac)-Gly-Lys-Ser(P)-Pro-Val-

Glu-Lys-OH and three selectively phosphorylated peptides corresponding the human neurofilament protein middle-sized subunit H-Lys-Ser(P or nP)-Pro-Val-Pro-Lys-Ser(P or nP)-Pro-Val-Glu-Glu-Lys-Gly-OH (nP = nonphosphorylated) were synthesized [175]. Figure 7.1 shows the strategy for synthesis of Ser^2 nonphosphorylated, Ser^7 phosphorylated peptide. These peptides can be used to characterize anti-neurofilament antibodies through their selective recognition of the location of the phosphate group. Selectively phosphorylated peptides corresponding to several neuronal proteins can be utilized to identify regions of abnormal phosphorylation that can play a role in deposition of neurofibrillary tangles of Alzheimer's disease.

SUMMARY AND FUTURE TRENDS

In the past, the synthesis of chemically modified peptides was a "self-entertainment" for peptide chemists. In recent years, however, new phosphorylating and glycosylating agents have been developed at an exponentially increasing rate. Phosphopeptide (and mostly) glycopeptide synthesis have become separate sections at the American and European peptide Symposia and even at the Solid-Phase Synthesis Conference and have become integrated parts of the biotechnology sector. The conformational change made by glycosylation can be purposefully designed [180] to make small changes in the conformation (caused by the numerous slightly different sugar moieties) of hypervariable regions (e.g., the envelope glycoprotein of human immunodeficiency virus) that may break tolerance *in vivo* [181]. Since the carbohydrate chain is assembled entirely before it is attached to the growing protein chain, glycosylation is expected to take place on engineered positions by synthesizing glycopeptides, where the first sugar is incorporated at nonnatural positions of the peptide chain, and afterward appropriate enzymes are added. While glycosylation is considered highly effective at certain asparagine residues, phosphorylation is random. Our preliminary results show that accidental phosphorylation of serine residues of epitopes can result in diminished T-cell response, allowing viruses to escape immune surveillance [182]. We also expect breakthrough discoveries in phosphopeptide immunology in the foreseeable future. Today, a reviewer in this field can probably peruse 80% of the literature. The field is growing at such a rate, however, that within five years a scientist will be hard pressed to cover 20% of the reports.

ABBREVIATIONS

Ac	acetyl
Ac$_3$D	3,4,6-tri-O-acetyl-2-deoxy

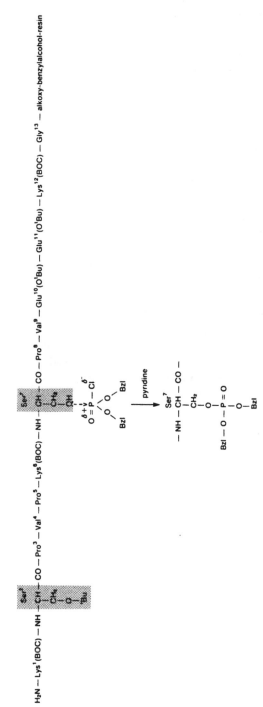

Figure 7.1 Strategy for solid-phase synthesis of selectively phosphorylated neurofilament peptide.

Ac$_3$	DI,3,4,6-tri-O-acetyl-2-deoxy-2-iodo
Ac$_3$GlcNAc	3,4,6-tri-O-acetyl-2-acetamido-2-deoxy-D-glycopyranosyl
All	allyl
Aloc	allyloxy-carbonyl
Boc	tert-butyloxy-carbonyl
Bu^n	n-butyl
Bu^t	tert-butyl
Bzl	benzyl
Bzl$_4$Glcp	2,3,4,6-tetra-O-benzyl-D-glucopyranosyl
DCC	dicyclohexyl-carbodiimide
DMTST	Dimethyl(methylmercapto)sulfonium-trifluoromethylsulfon-ate
DTC	di-p-tolyl-carbodiimide
EEDQ	2-ethoxy-1-ethoxycarbonyl-1,2-dihydroquinoline
Fmoc	9-fluorenylmethoxy carbonyl
Fuc	1-D-fucosyl
Gal N$_3$	2-azido-2-deoxy-D-galactopyranosyl
Gal	1-D-galactopyranosyl
GalNAc	2-acetamido-2-deoxy-D-galactopyranosyl
GlcNAc	2-acetamido-2-deoxy-D-glycopyranosyl
GlcN$_3$	2-azido-2-deoxy-D-glucopyranosyl
Glc	1-D-glucopyranosyl
I-Su	N-iodosuccinimide
iGln	isoglutamine
Im	imidazol
KK1	Koenigs-Knorr glycosylation of hydroxy-amino acids with O-protected 2-azido-2-deoxy-α-D-gluco(galacto)parano-syl-halogenide derivatives in the presence of AgClO$_4$ catalyst
KK2	Koenigs-Knorr glycosylation of hydroxy-amino acids with O-protected 2-azido-2-deoxy-α-D-gluco(galacto)pyrano-syl-halogenide derivatives in the presence of Hg(CN)$_2$/HgCl$_2$ catalyst
Mbs	4-Methoxy-benzene sulfonyl
MeOH	methanol
MurNAc	N-acetyl-muramyl
Noc	p-nitrocinnamyloxy-carbonyl
nP	nonphosphorylated
ONp	p-nitrophenyl ester
OPcp	pentachlorophenyl ester
OPfp	pentafluorophenyl ester
OSu	N-hydroxy-succinimide ester
P	phosphorylated or phosphoryl

Pam	phenyl acetamidomethyl
Ph	phenyl
Tal	D-talopyranosyl
TEA	triethylamine
TFA	trifluoroacetic acid
Tf$_2$O	trifluoromethanesulfonic anhydride
TMS	trimethylsilyl
TMSOTf	trimethylsilyl-triflate
Xyl	1-D-xylopyranosyl
Z	benzyloxy-carbonyl

ACKNOWLEDGEMENTS

The authors wish to thank Shirley Peterson for editing the manuscript and Cathy Taylor for production of molecule diagrams. This work was supported by NIH grant #GM 45011 and funds have been provided by Alzheimer's Disease Research, a program of the American Health Assistance Foundation, Rockville, Maryland (to Laszlo Otvos).

REFERENCES

1 Frank, A. W. 1984. "Synthesis and Properties of N-, O-, and S-phospho Derivatives of Amino Acids, Peptides, and Proteins," *CRC Crit. Rev. Biochem.*, 16:51–101.

2 Thomas, G., E. J. Podesta and J. Gordon, eds. 1980. *Protein Phosphosphorylation and Bio-Regulation*. Basel, Switzerland: S. Karger.

3 Hemmings, H. C., Jr., A. C. Nairn, T. L. Guiness, R. L. Huganir and P. Greengard. 1989. *FASEB J.*, 3:1583–1592.

4 Bourret, R. B., J. F. Hess, K. A. Borkowich, A. A. Pakula and M. I. Simon. 1989. *J. Biol. Chem.*, 264:7085–7088.

5 Shenolikar, S. 1986–1987. "Control of Cell Function by Reversible Protein Phosphorylation," *J. Cyclic Nucleotide Protein Phosphor. Res.*, 11:531–541.

6 Gottschalk, A., ed. 1972. *Glycoproteins: Their Composition, Structure and Function, Vol. 5A*. New York, NY: Elsevier.

7 Kornfeld, R. and S. Kornfeld. 1976. *Annu. Rev. Biochem.*, 45:217–237.

8 Kornfeld, R. and S. Kornfeld. 1985. *Annu. Rev. Biochem.*, 54:631–664.

9 Montreuil, J. 1980. *Adv. Carbohydr. Chem. Biochem.*, 37:157–223.

10 Horowitz, M. I. and W. Pigman, eds. 1977. *The Glycoconjugates*. New York, NY: Academic Press.

11 Smith, F. A. and L. A. Pease. 1980. *CRC Crit. Rev. Biochem.*, 8:315–399.

12 Mononen, I. and E. Karjalainen. 1984. *Biochim. Biophys. Acta*, 788:364–367.

13 Williams, R. E. 1976. "Phosphorylated Sites in Substrates of Intracellular Protein Kinases: A Common Feature in Amino Acid Sequences," *Science*, 192:473–474.

14 Small, D., P. Y. Chou and G. D. Fasman. 1977. *Biochem. Biophys. Res. Commun.*, 79:341–346.

15 Marraud, M. and A. Aubry. 1984. *Int. J. Pept. Protein Res.*, 23:123–133.

16 Aubry, A., N. Ghermany and M. Marraud. 1984. *Int. J. Pept. Protein Res.*, 23:113–122.

17 Carbone, F. R. and S. J. Leach. 1985. *Int. J. Pept. Protein Res.*, 26:498–508.

18 Hollosi, M., K. E. Kover, S. Holly, L. Radics and G. D. Fasman. 1987. *Biopolymers*, 26:1555–1572.

19 Venkatachalam, C. M. 1968. "Stereochemical Criteria for Polypeptides and Proteins. V. Conformation of a System of Three Linked Peptide Units," *Biopolymers*, 6:1425–1436.

20 Lewis, P. N., F. A. Momany and H. A. Scheraga. 1973. *Biochim. Biophys. Acta*, 303:211–229.

21 Pichon-Pesme, V., A. Aubry, A. Abbadi, G. Boussard and M. Marraud. 1988. *Int. J. Pept. Protein Res.*, 32:175–182.

22 Welphy, J. K., P. Shenbagamurth, W. J. Lennarz and F. Naider. 1983. *J. Biol. Chem.*, 258:11856–11863.

23 Hider, R. C., U. Ragnarson and O. Zetterqvist. 1985. *Biochem. J.*, 229:485–489.

24 Otvos, L., Jr., M. Hollosi, A. Perczel, B. Dietzschold and G. D. Fasman. 1988. *J. Protein Chem.*, 7:365–376.

25 Chessa, G., G. Borin, F. Marchiori, F. Meggio, A. M. Brunati and L. A. Pinna. 1983. *Eur. J. Biochem.*, 135:609–614.

26 Sheehan, J. K. and I. Carlstedt. 1984. *Biochem. J.*, 217:93–101.

27 Shogren, R. L., A. M. Jamieson, J. Blackwell and W. Fentoff. 1986. *Biopolymers*, 25:1505–1517.

28 Bush, C. A., S. Ralapati, G. M. Matson, R. B. Yamashaki, D. T. Osuga, Y. Yeh and R. E. Feeney. 1984. *Arch. Biochem. Biophys.*, 232:624–631.

29 Lamblin, G., M. Lhermitte, P. Degand, P. Roussel and H. S. Slayter. 1979. *Biochimie*, 61:23–43.

30 Rose, M. C., W. A. Voter, H. Saage, C. F. Brown and B. Kauftmann. 1984. *J. Biol. Chem.*, 259:3167–3172.

31 Gerken, T., K. J. Butenhof and R. Shogren. 1989. *Biochemistry*, 28:5536–5543.

32 Chaplin, L. C., D. C. Clark and L. J. Smith. 1988. *Biochim. Biophys. Acta*, 956:162–172.

33 Kaplan, L. J., R. Bauer, E. Morrison, T. A. Langan and G. D. Fasman. 1984. *J. Biol. Chem.*, 259:8777–8785.

34 Ratanabanangkoon, K., H. T. Keutmann, K. Kitzmann and R. J. Ryan. 1983. *J. Biol. Chem.*, 258:14527–14531.

35 Lee, V. M.-Y., L. Otvos, Jr., M. L. Schmidt and J. Q. Trojanowski. 1989. *Proc. Natl. Acad. Sci. USA*, 85:7384–7388.

36 Roses, A. D. and S. H. Appel. 1975. *J. Membrane Biol.*, 20:51–58.

37 Beutler, E., E. Guinto and C. Johnson. 1976. *Blood*, 48:887–898.

38 Greenquist, A. C. and S. B. Shohet. 1976. *Blood*, 48:877–886.

39 Bancher, C., C. Brunner, H. Lassmann, H. Budka, K. Jellinger, G. Wiche, F. Seitelberger, I. Grundke-Iqbal and H. M. Wisniewski. 1989. *Brain Res.*, 477:90–99.

40 Morehead, H., P. McKay and R. Wetzel. 1982. *Anal. Biochem.*, 126:29–36.

41 Neurath, N. and R. L. Hill, eds. 1982. *The Proteins, Vol. 5*. New York, NY: Academic Press.

42 Ivanov, V. T., T. M. Andronova, M. V. Bezrukov, V. A. Rar, E. A. Makarov, S. A. Kozmin, M. V. Astapova, T. A. Barkova and V. A. Nesmeyanov. 1987. *Pure Appl. Chem.*, 59:317–324.

43 Arnon, R., M. Sela, M. Parant and L. Chedid. 1980. *Proc. Natl. Acad. Sci. USA*, 77:6769–6772.

44 Audibert, F., M. Jolivet, L. Chedid, R. Arnon and M. Sela. 1982. *Proc. Natl. Acad. Sci. USA*, 79:5042–5046.

45 Macfarlan, R. I., B. Dietzschold, T. J. Wiktor, M. Kiel, R. Houghten, R. A. Lerner, J. R. Sutcliffe and H. Koprowski. 1984. *J. Immunol.*, 133:2748–2752.

46 Brown, L. E., R. A. Ffrench, J. M. Gawler, D. C. Jackson, M. L. Dyall-Smith, E. M. Anders, G. W. Tregear, L. Duncan, P. A. Underwood and D. O. White. 1988. *J. Virol.*, 62:305–312.

47 Alexander, S. and J. H. Elder. 1984. *Science*, 226:1328–1330.

48 Bechtel, B., J. A. Wand, K. Wroblewski, H. Koprowski and J. Thurin. 1990. *J. Biol. Chem.*, 265:2028–2037.

49 Torres, J. L., H. Pepermans, G. Valencia, F. Reig, J. M. Garcia-Anton and G. Van Binst. 1990. "Conformational Analysis of Galactosyl Enkephalin Analogues Showing High Analgesic Activity," in *Peptides*, J. E. Rivier and G. R. Marshall, eds., Leiden, Holland: ESCOM, pp. 339–340.

50 Deshpande, K. L., V. A. Fried, M. Ando and R. G. Webster. 1987. *Proc. Natl. Acad. Sci. USA*, 84:36–40.

51 Otvos, L., Jr., K. Wroblewski, E. Kollat, A. Perczel, M. Hollosi, G. D. Fasman, H. C. J. Ertl and J. Thurin. 1989. *Pept. Res.*, 2:362–366.

52 Cease, K. B., H. Margalit, J. L. Cornette, S. D. Putney, W. G. Robey, C. Quyang, H. Z. Streicher, P. J. Fishinger, R. C. Gallo, C. DeLisi and J. A. Berzofski. 1987. *Proc. Natl. Acad. Sci. USA*, 84:4249–4253.

53 Ahrens, P. B. and H. Ankel. 1987. *J. Biol. Chem.*, 262:7575–7579.

54 Krebs, E. G. and J. A. Beavo. 1979. *Annu. Rev. Biochem.*, 48:923–959.

55 Lee, V. M.-Y., M. J. Carden, W. W. Schlaepfer and J. Q. Trojanowski. 1987. *Neurosci.*, 7:3474–3488.

56 Lee, V. M.-Y., L. Otvos, Jr., M. J. Carden, M. Hollosi, B. Dietzschold and R. A. Lazzarini. 1988. *Proc. Natl. Acad. Sci. USA*, 85:1988–2002.

57 Trojanowski, J. Q., M. L. Schmidt, L. Otvos, Jr., H. Arai, W. D. Hill and V. M.-Y. Lee. 1991. *Ann. Rev. Gerontol. Geriatr.*, 10:167–182.

58 Otvos, L., Jr., V. M.-Y. Lee, M. Hollosi, A. Perczel and B. Dietzschold. 1988. "Phosphorylation of Synthetic Mid-Sized Neurofilament Protein Fragment Changes the Secondary Structure and Antibody Recognition of This Peptide," in *Peptide Chemistry 1987*, T. Shiba and S. Sakakibara, eds., Osaka, Japan: Protein Research Foundation, pp. 799–802.

59 Barany, G., N. Kneib-Cordonier and D. G. Mullen. 1987. *Int. J. Pept. Protein Res.*, 30:705–739.

60 Kisfaludy, L., T. Mohacsi, M. Low and F. Drexler. 1979. *J. Org. Chem.*, 44: 325–327.

61 Kisfaludy, L. and L. Otvos, Jr. 1987. *Synthesis*, p. 510.

62 Otvos, L., Jr., B. Dietzschold and L. Kisfaludy. 1987. *Int J. Pept. Protein Res.*, 30:511–514.

63 Lankiewicz, L., D. B. Sherman and A. F. Spatola. 1990. "Subtle Amide Bond Surrogates: The Effect of Backbone Thioamides on the Physical Properties Conformation, and Biological Activities of Peptides," in *Peptides*, J. E. Rivier and G. R. Marshall, eds., Leiden, Holland: ESCOM, pp. 976–977.

64 Jung, G., K.-H. Weismuller, G. Becker, H.-J. Buhring and W. G. Bessler. 1985. *Angew. Chem.*, 24:872–873.

65 Schmidt, R. R. 1986. "New Methods for the Synthesis of Glycosides and Oligosaccharides—Are There Alternatives to the Koenigs-Knorr Method?" *Angew. Chem. Int. Ed. Engl.*, 25:212–235.

66 Paulsen, H. 1985. In "Strategies in Oligosaccharide Synthesis," in *Organic Syntheses: Interdisciplinary Challenge*, J. Streich, H. Prinzbach and G. Schill, eds., Oxford, UK: Blackwell, pp. 317–335.

67 Leroux, J. and A. S. Perlin. 1976. *Carbohydr. Res.*, 47:c8–c10.

68 Leroux, J. and A. S. Perlin. 1978. *Carbohydr. Res.*, 67:163–178.

69 Pavia, A. A., J.-M. Rocheville and S. N. Ung. 1980. *Carbohydr. Res.*, 79:79–89.

70 Kahne, D., S. Walker, Y. Cheng and D. Van Engen. 1989. *J. Am. Chem. Soc.*, 111:6881–6882.

71 Matsumoto, T., H. Maeta, K. Suzuki and G. Tsuchihashi. 1988. *Tetrahedron Lett.*, 29:3567–3570.

72 Suzuki, K., H. Maeta, T. Matsumoto and G. Tsuchihashi. 1988. *Tetrahedron Lett.*, 29:3571–3574.

73 Paulsen, H., W. Rauwald and U. Weichert. 1988. *Liebigs Ann. Chem.*, pp. 75–86.

74 Rathore, H., T. Hashimoto, Q. Igarashi, H. Nukaya and D. S. Fullerton. 1985. *Tetrahedron*, 41:5427–5438.

75 Barrett, A. G. M., B. C. B. Bezuidenhoudt, A. F. Gasiecki, A. R. Howell and M. A. Russel. 1989. *J. Am. Chem. Soc.*, 111:1392–1396.

76 Binkley, R. W. and D. J. Koholic. 1989. *J. Org. Chem.*, 54:3577–3581.

77 Kunz, H. and J. Marz. 1988. *Angew. Chem. Int. Ed. Engl.*, 27:1375–1377.

78 Bergmann, M. and L. Zervas. 1932. *Chem. Ber.*, 65:1201–1205.

79 Kunz, H. and S. Birnbach. 1986. *Angew. Chem. Int. Ed. Engl.*, 25:360–362.

80 Kunz, H. and H. Waldmann. 1984. *Angew. Chem. Int. Ed. Engl.*, 23:71–72.

81 Kunz, H. and C. Unverzagt. 1984. *Angew. Chem. Int. Ed. Engl.*, 23:436–437.

82 Sharon, N. 1975. *Complex Carbohydrates. Their Chemistry, Biosynthesis and Functions*. Reading, MA: Addison Wesley.

83 Bolton, C. H. and R. W. Jeanloz. 1963. *J. Org. Chem.*, 28:3228–3230.

84 Spinola, M. and R. W. Jeanloz. 1970. *J. Biol. Chem.*, 245:4158–4162.

85 Paulsen, H. and M. Paal. 1984. *Carbohydr. Res.*, 135:71–84.

86 Shaban, M. A. E.-M. and R. W. Jeanloz. 1981. *Bull. Chem. Soc. Jpn.*, 54:3570–3576.

87 Chadwick, R. J., J. C. Heesom, J. S. Thompson and G. Tomalin. "Strategy for the Solid-Phase Synthesis of Glycopeptides," in *Innovations and Perspectives in Solid-Phase Synthesis*, R. Epton, ed., Birmingham, UK: Solid-Phase Conference Coordination, pp. 379–388.

88 Kinzy, W. and R. R. Schmidt. 1987. *Carbohydr. Res*, 166:265–276.

89 Nakabayashi, S., C. D. Warren and R. W. Jeanloz. 1988. *Carbohydr. Res.*, 174:279–289.

90 Iijima, H. and T. Ogawa. 1988. *Carbohydr. Res.*, 172:183–193.

91 Paulsen, H., K. Adermann, G. Merz, M. Schultz and U. Weichert. 1988. *Stärke*, 40:465–472.
92 Garg, H. G. and R. W. Jeanloz. 1985. *Adv. Carbohydr. Chem. Biochem.*, 43: 135–201.
93 Paulsen, H. and M. Schultz. 1987. *Carbohydr. Res.*, 159:37–52.
94 Ferrari, B. and A. A. Pavia. 1985. *Tetrahedron*, 41:1939–1944.
95 Paulsen, H. and M. Schultz. 1986. *Liebigs Ann. Chem.*, pp. 1435–1447.
96 Dill, K. and D. Carter. 1986. *Carbohydr. Res.*, 152:217–228.
97 Ferrari, B. and A. A. Pavia. 1983. *Int. J. Pept. Protein Res.*, 22:549–559.
98 Anisuzzaman, A. K. M., L. Anderson and J. N. Navia. 1988. *Carbohydr. Res.*, 174:265–278.
99 Kunz, H., H. Waldmann and J. Marz. 1989. *Liebigs Ann. Chem.*, pp. 45–49.
100 Maeji, N. J., Y. Inoue and R. Chujo. 1986. *Carbohydr. Res.*, 146:174–176.
101 Paulsen, H. and M. Brenken. 1988. *Liebigs Ann. Chem.*, pp. 649–654.
102 Ishii, H., Y. Inoue and R. Chujo. 1984. *J. Pept. Protein Res.*, 24:421–429.
103 Maeji, N. J., Y. Inoue and R. Chujo. 1987. *Carbohydr. Res.*, 162:c4–c8.
104 Maeji, N. J., Y. Inoue and R. Chujo. 1987. *Biopolymers*, 26:1753–1767.
105 Mimura, Y., Y. Inoue, N. J. Maeji and R. Chujo. 1989. *Int. J. Pept. Protein Res.*, 34:363–368.
106 Fermandjian, S., B. Perly, M. Level and P. Lefrancier. 1987. *Carbohydr. Res.*, 162:23–32.
107 Sizun, P., B. Perly, M. Level, P. Lefrancier and S. Fermandjian. 1988. *Tetrahedron*, 44:991–997.
108 Maeji, N. J., Y. Inoue and R. Chujo. 1987. *Int. J. Pept. Protein Res.*, 29:699–707.
109 Kessler, H., M. Kottenhahn, A. Kling and C. Kolar. 1987. *Angew. Chem. Int. Ed. Engl.*, 26:888–890.
110 Kunz, H. and C. Unverzagt. 1988. *Angew. Chem. Int. Ed. Engl.*, 27:1697–1699.
111 Kunz, H. and H. Waldmann. 1985. *Helvetica Chim. Acta*, 68:618–622.
112 Horvat, S., L. Varga and J. Horvat. 1986. *Synthesis*, pp. 209–211.
113 Horvat, J., S. Horvat, C. Lemieux and P. W. Schiller. 1988. *Int. J. Pept. Protein Res.*, 31:499–507.
114 Torres, J. L., F. Reig, G. Valencia, R. E. Rodriguez and J. M. Garcia-Anton. 1988. *Int. J. Pept. Protein Res.*, 31:474–480.
115 Torres, J. L., I. Haro, G. Valencia, F. Reig and J. M. Garcia-Anton. 1989. *Experientia*, 45:574–576.
116 Varga, L., S. Horvat, C. Lemieux and P. W. Schiller. 1987. *Int. J. Pept. Protein Res.*, 30:371–378.
117 Gobbo, M., L. Biondi, F. Filira, R. Rocchi and V. Lucchini. 1988. *Tetrahedron*, 44:887–893.
118 Rocchi, R., L. Biondi, F. Filira, M. Gobbo, S. Dagan and M. Fridkin. 1987. *Int. J. Pept. Protein Res.*, 29:250–261.
119 Rocchi, R., L. Biondi, F. Cavaggion, F. Filira, M. Gobbo, S. Dagan and M. Fridkin. 1987. *Int. J. Pept. Protein Res.*, 29:262–275.
120 Paulsen, H. and K. Adermann. 1989. *Liebigs Ann. Chem.*, pp. 751–769.
121 Paulsen, H. and M. Schultz. 1987. *M Carbohydr. Res.*, 159:37–52.
122 Keglevich, D. 1989. "Synthesis and Reactions of O-acetylated Benzyl α-gly-

cosides of 6-O-(2-acetamido-2-deoxy-β-D-glucopyranosyl)-N-acetyl-muramoyl-L-alanyl-D-isoglutamine Esters: The Base-Catalised Isoglutamine-Glutamine Rearrangement in Peptidoglycan-Related Structures," *Carbohydr. Res.*, 186: 63–75.

123 Shen, T. Y., J. P. Li, C. P. Dorn, D. Ebel, R. Bugianesi and R. Fecher. 1972. *Carbohydr. Res.*, 23:87–102.

124 Lee, R. T., T.-C. Wong, R. Lee, L. Yue and Y. C. Lee. 1989. *Biochemistry*, 28: 856–1861.

125 Lonngren, J., I. J. Goldstein and J. E. Niederhuber. 1976. *Arch. Biochem. Biophys.*, 175:661–669.

126 Gray, G. R. 1978. "Antibodies to Carbohydrates: Preparation of Antigens by Coupling Carbohydrates to Proteins by Reductive Amination with Cyanoborohydride," *Meth. Enzymol.*, 50:155–160.

127 Williamson, M. P., M. J. Hall and B. K. Handa. 1986. *Eur. J. Biochem.*, 158:527–536.

128 Wilson, I., J. J. Skehal and D. C. Wiley. 1981. *Nature*, 289:366–373.

129 Brisson, J.-R. and J. P. Carver. 1983. *Biochemistry*, 22:1362–1368.

130 Pace, N., C. Tanford and E. A. Davidson. 1964. *J. Am. Chem. Soc.*, 86: 3160–3162.

131 Beychok, S. and E. A. Kabat. 1965. *Biochemistry*, 4:2565–2574.

132 Austin, B. M. and R. D. Marshall. 1970. *Biochim. Biophys. Acta*, 215:559–561.

133 Bush, C. A., R. E. Feeney, D. T. Oscegai, S. Ralapati and Y. Yeh. 1981. *Int. J. Pept. Protein Res.*, 17:125–129.

134 Herschlag, D., E. S. Stevens and J. E. Gander. 1983. *Int. J. Pept. Protein Res.*, 22:16–20.

135 Hollosi, M., A. Perczel and G. D. Fasman. 1990. *Biopolymers*, 29:1549–1564.

136 Hollosi, M., A. Perczel, G. Szokan, P. Sandor and G. D. Fasman. 1990. "Glyco-β-Turns Anchor the Antennae Systems in Glycoproteins," in *Peptides*, J. E. Rivier and G. R. Marshall, eds., Leiden, Holland: ESCOM, pp. 800–801.

137 Otvos, L., Jr., J. Thurin, E. Kollat, L. Urge, H. H. Mantsch and M. Hollosi. 1991. *Int. J. Pept. Protein Res.*, 38:476–482.

138 Overend, W. G., C. W. Rees and J. S. Sequiera. 1962. *J. Chem. Soc.*, pp. 3429–3440.

139 Paulsen, H., G. Merz and U. Weichert. 1988. *Angew. Chem. Int. Ed. Engl.*, 27: 1365–1367.

140 Luning, B., T. Norberg and J. Tejbrant. 1989. *J. Chem. Soc. Chem. Commun.*, pp. 1267–1268.

141 Filira, F., L. Biondi, F. Cavaggion, B. Scolaro and R. Rocchi. 1990. "Unprotected O-Glycosylated Fmoc-Threonine Derivatives in the Synthesis of Glycopeptides," in *Peptides*, J. E. Rivier and G. R. Marshall, eds., Leiden, Holland: ESCOM, pp. 804–805.

142 Kunz, H. and B. Dombo. 1988. *Angew. Chem. Int. Ed. Engl.*, 27:711–713.

143 Kaiser, E., R. L. Colescott, C. D. Bossinger and P. I. Cook. 1970. *Anal. Biochem.*, 34:595–598.

144 Storey, H. T., J. Beacham, S. F. Cernosek, F. M. Finn, C. Yanaihara and K. Hofmann. 1972. *J. Am. Chem. Soc.*, 94:6170–6178.

145 Otvos, L., Jr., I. A. Tangoren, I. Elekes and V. M.-Y. Lee. 1990. "Solid-Phase Synthetic Methods Leading to Selectively Phosphorylated Neurofilament Frag-

ments," in *Innovations and Perspectives in Solid-Phase Synthesis*, R. Epton, ed., Birmingham, UK: Solid-Phase Conference Coordination, pp. 421–426.

146 Likhosterov, L. M., O. S. Novikova, V. A. Derevitskaja and N. K. Kochetkov. 1986. *Carbohydr. Res.*, 146:c1–c5.

147 Otvos, L., Jr., L. Urge, M. Hollosi, K. Wroblewski, G. Graczyk, G. D. Fasman and J. Thurin. 1990. *Tetrahedron Lett.*, 31:5889–5892.

148 Urge, L., E. Kollat, M. Hollosi, I. Laczko, K. Wroblewski, J. Thurin and L. Otvos, Jr. 1991. *Tetrahedron Lett.*, 32:3445–3448.

149 Hollosi, M., E. Kollat, I. Laczko, K. F. Medzihradszky, J. Thurin and L. Otvos, Jr. 1991. *Tetrahedron Lett.*, 32:1531–1534.

150 Chen, S.-T., L.-C. Lo, S.-H. Wu and K.-T. Wang. 1990. *Int. J. Pept. Protein Res.*, 35:52–54.

151 Sasaki, H., N. Norimichi, A. Dell and M. Fukuda. 1988. *Biochemistry*, 27:8618–8626.

152 Dua, V. K. and A. Bush. 1984. *Anal. Biochem.*, 137:33–40.

153 Folsch, G. 1955. "Synthesis of Phosphopeptides," *Acta Chim. Scand.*, 9:1039.

154 Folsch, G. 1959. "Synthesis of Phosphopeptides," *Acta Chim. Scand.*, 13:1407–1421.

155 Folsch, G. 1966. "Synthesis of Phosphopeptides," *Acta Chim. Scand.*, 20:459–473.

156 Ferrel, R. E., H. S. Olcott and H. Fraenkel-Conrat. 1948. *J. Am. Chem. Soc.*, 70:2101–2107.

157 Otvos, L., Jr., A. Tangoren, K. Wroblewski, M. Hollosi and V. M.-Y. Lee. 1990. *J. Chromatogr.*, 512:265–272.

158 Kafarski, P., B. Lejczak, P. Mastalerz, J. Szewczyk and C. Wasielewski. 1982. *Can. J. Chem.*, 60:3081–3084.

159 Pogliani, L. and D. Ziessow. 1979. *Tetrahedron*, 35:2867–2873.

160 Johns, R. B., P. F. Alewood, J. W. Perich, A. L. Chaffee and J. K. MacLeod. 1986. *Tetrahedron Lett.*, 27:4791–4794.

161 Johnson, T. B. and J. K. Coward. 1987. *J. Org. Chem.*, 52:1771–1779.

162 Bannwarth, W. and J. W. Trzeciak. 1987. *Helvetica Chim. Acta*, 70:175–186.

163 Riley, G., J. H. Turnbull and W. Wilson. 1957. *J. Chem. Soc.*, 1373–1379.

164 Atherton, F. R. 1957. "Dibenzyl Phosphochloridate," *Biochem. Prep.*, 5:1–4.

165 Alewood, P. F., J. W. Perich and R. B. Johns. 1984. *Tetrahedron Lett.*, 25:987–990.

166 Alewood, P. F., J. W. Perich and R. B. Johns. 1984. *Aust. J. Chem.*, 37:429–433.

167 Perich, J. W., P. F. Alewood and R. B. Johns. 1986. *Tetrahedron Lett.*, 27:1373–1376.

168 Schlesinger, D. H., A. Buku, H. R. Wyssbrod and D. I. Hay. 1987. *Int. J. Pept. Protein Res.*, 30:257–262.

169 Schlesinger, D. H., A. Buku, H. R. Wyssbrod and D. I. Hay. 1988. "Solution Synthesis of Phosphoseryl-Phosphoserine, a Partial Analog of Human Salivary Statherin Essential for Inhibition of Primary and Secondary Precipitation of Calcium Phosphate," in *Peptide Chemistry 1987*, T. Shiba and S. Sakakibara, eds., Osaka, Japan: Protein Research Foundation, pp. 311–314.

170 Perich, J. W. and R. B. Johns. 1988. *J. Chem. Soc. Chem. Commun.*, pp. 664–666.

171 Perich, J. W., P. F. Alewood and R. B. Johns. 1986. *Synthesis*, 572–573.

172 DeBont, H. B. A., G. H. Veenan, J. H. Van Boom and R. M. J. Liskamp. 1987. *Recl. Trav. Chim. Pays-Bas*, 106:641–642.

173 DeBont, H. B. A., R. M. J. Liskamp, C. A. O'Brian, C. Erkelens, G. H. Veeneman and J. H. Van Boom. 1989. *Int. J. Pept. Protein Res.*, 33:115–123.

174 Perich, J. W. and R. B. Johns. 1989. *J. Org. Chem.*, 54:1750–1752.

175 Otvos, L., Jr., I. Elekes and V. M.-Y. Lee. 1989. *Int. J. Pept. Protein Res.*, 34: 129–133.

176 Arendt, A., K. Palczewski, W. T. Morre, R. M. Caprioli, J. H. McDowell and P. A. Hargrave. 1989. *Int. J. Pept. Protein Res.*, 33:468–476.

177 Perich, J. W., R. M. Valerio and R. B. Johns. 1986. *Tetrahedron Lett.*, 27: 1377–1380.

178 Valerio, R. M., P. F. Alewood, R. B. Johns and B. E. Kemp. 1984. *Tetrahedron Lett.*, 25:2609–2612.

179 DeBont, H. B. A., J. H. Van Boom and R. M. J. Liskamp. 1990. *Tetrahedron Lett.*, 31:2497–2500.

180 Urge, L., L. Gorbics and L. Otvos, Jr. 1992. *Biochem. Biophys. Res. Commun.*, 184:1125–1132.

181 Laczko, I., H. Hollosi, L. Urge, K. E. Ugen, D. B. Weiner, H. H. Mantsch, J. Thurin and L. Otvos., Jr. 1992. *Biochemistry*, 31:4282–4288.

182 Larson, J. K., L. Otvos, Jr. and H. C. Ertl. 1992. (In press.) *J. Virol.*

CHAPTER 8

Design and Synthesis of Biologically Active Peptide Mimics

ROBERT M. WILLIAMS[1]

INTRODUCTION

D URING the past decade, there has been a virtual explosion of activity in the design, synthesis and biological applications of peptide mimics. The elucidation of a wide array of receptors and enzymes to which highly active small, soluble peptides bind or are substrates for has fueled a range of interesting approaches to translate the natural substrate structure into a proteolytically stable molecule that will have desirable therapeutic properties. This chapter will highlight some of the more interesting and potentially successful peptide mimic structures that have appeared in the literature. Many additional specific examples have appeared in the patent literature, but have not been reviewed. This overview is by no means exhaustive, as the literature in this area is vast. Some of the key and unique classes of inhibitors (and some representative syntheses) that followed in the wake of the discovery of pepstatin by Umezawa will be reviewed.

PEPSTATIN

Most enzymes have evolved to catalyze reactions by stabilization of the structure of the transition state. This is certainly true for the various classes of proteases that serve a wide range of important functions in the processing of protein and peptide substrates. Pepstatin (1) is a naturally occurring peptide produced by various *Streptomyces sp.* that was shown by Umezawa [1] to be a potent and general inhibitor of aspartic proteases such

[1]Department of Chemistry, Colorado State University, Fort Collins, CO 80523, U.S.A.

as, pepsin, renin and cathepsin D. Pepstatin contains the unusual amino acid statine (2) which has become the prototypical hydroxymethylene isostere of the putative tetrahedral transition state intermediate (3) for peptide bond hydrolysis [2]. The proposal that statine and the homologous hydroxyethylene isosteres to be discussed later resemble the transition state for peptide bond hydrolysis has received support from x-ray structural studies of various inhibitors complexed to aspartic proteases at the active site. In these structures, the statine or hydroxyethylene unit occupies the scissile dipeptide binding site with the (S)-hydroxyl group oriented between the two catalytic Asp carboxyl residues replacing a bound solvent water molecule.

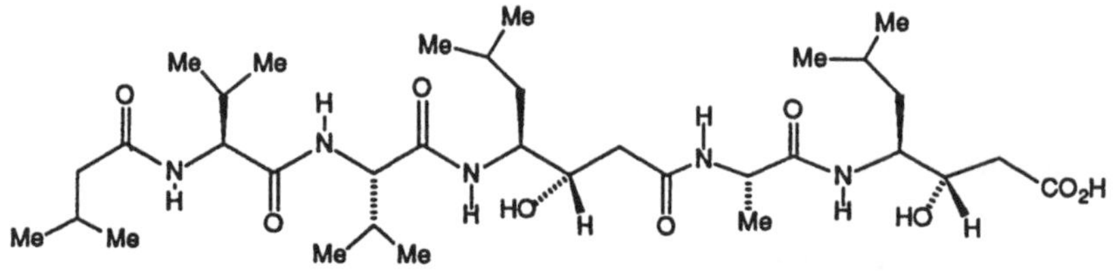

1, PEPSTATIN

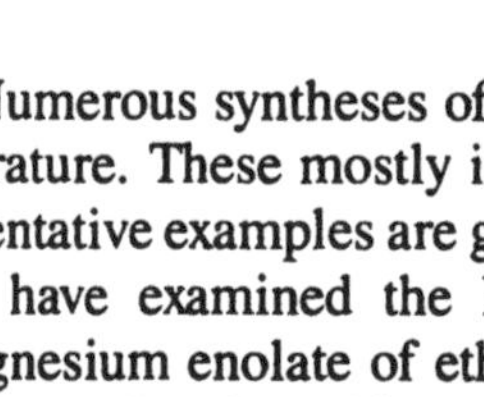

2, STATINE

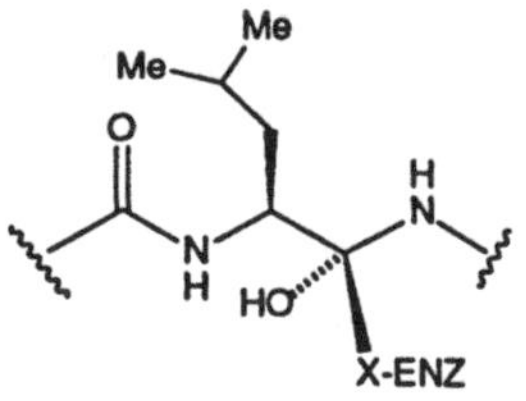

3

Numerous syntheses of statine and statine analogs have appeared in the literature. These mostly involve the homologation of isoleucine. Two representative examples are given in Schemes 8.1 and 8.2. Rich and associates [2] have examined the Brooks/Masamune condensation of the monomagnesium enolate of ethyl malonate with t-BOC–protected amino acids [Scheme 8.1 (4)] which affords the β-keto esters (5) in good yields. Subsequent reduction with sodium borohydride or K-selectride provides a mixture of the corresponding syn- (6) and anti- (7) hydroxymethylene isosteres in modest to excellent stereoselectivities. Statine is produced as a 9:1 mixture with the syn-diastereomer. After chromatographic separation of the diastereomers, the desired N-BOC amino acids were obtained in high optical purity. This procedure was also employed to prepare the corresponding phenylalanine, lysine, cysteine and histidine hydroxymethylene isosteres.

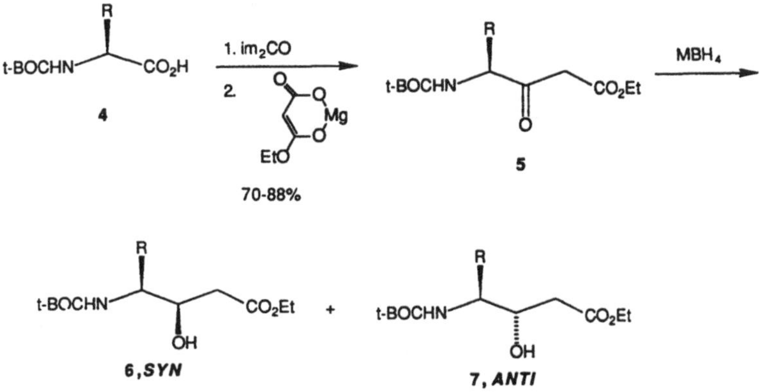

R	MBH₄	YIELD	RATIO (SYN : ANTI)
Me, Me (sec-butyl)	NaBH₄	97	61 : 39
	K-sec-Bu₃BH₄	15-20	10 : 90
cyclohexylmethyl	NaBH₄	87	83 : 17
	K-sec-Bu₃BH₄	24	4 : 96
CBzHN	NaBH₄	94	65 : 35
MeSCH₂	NaBH₄	37	58 : 42
imidazole-NTs			

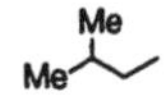

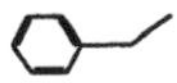

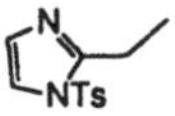

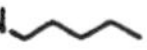

Maibaum, J.; Rich, D.H., *J.Org.Chem.* (1988) 5 3, 869

Scheme 8.1.

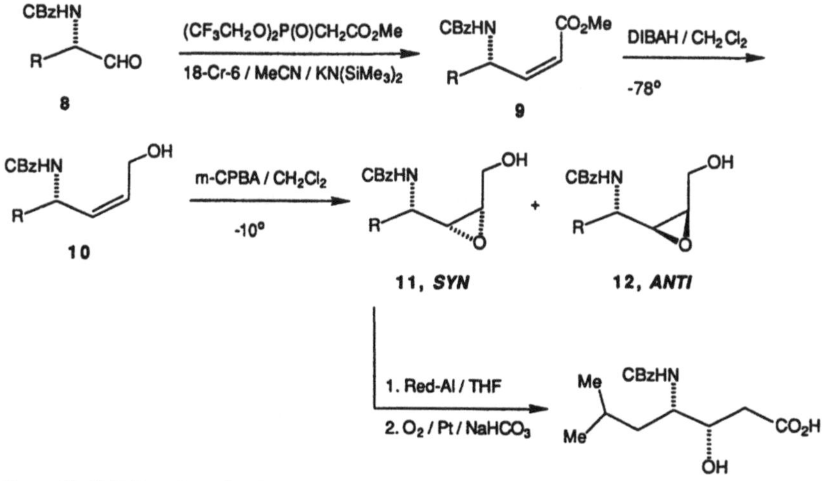

$(CF_3CH_2O)_2P(O)CH_2CO_2Me$

18-Cr-6 / MeCN / KN(SiMe$_3$)$_2$

8 → **9**

DIBAH / CH$_2$Cl$_2$

−78°

m-CPBA / CH$_2$Cl$_2$

−10°

10 → **11, SYN** + **12, ANTI**

1. Red-Al / THF
2. O$_2$ / Pt / NaHCO$_3$

13

Kogen, H.; Nishi, T., *J.Chem.Soc.Chem.Comm.* (1987) 311

R	YIELD (%9)	YIELD (%10)	YIELD (%11)	SYN : ANTI
Me	86	73	98	10 : 1
i-Pr	95	76	99	28 : 1
i-Bu	86	75	98	21 : 1
PhCH$_2$	89	86	98	21 : 1
MeCH(OTMS)CH$_2$	85	72	98	20 : 1
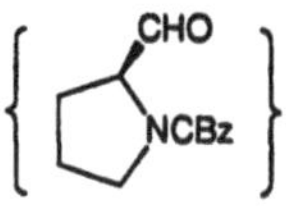 {CHO, NCBz}	79	53	98	16 : 1

Scheme 8.2.

Using the Kishi diastereoselective polyol protocol, Kogen and Nishi [3] reported an efficient synthesis of statine from the Z-protected amino aldehydes [Scheme 8.2 (8)]. Horner-Emmons condensation according to Still provided good yields of the Z-esters (9). Reduction to the allylic alcohols (10) followed by stereoselective epoxidation proceeded with high stereoselectivity to afford the syn-epoxides (11) as the major products along with the anti-isomers (12). Conversion of the epoxide into the hydroxymethylene isostere was demonstrated for statine. Thus, Red-Al reduction of the epoxide (R = isobutyl) proceeded regioselectively in 93% yield. Selective oxidation of the primary alcohol to the acid was achieved with oxygen on a platinum catalyst in 95% yield affording N-CBz–statine.

A stereocontrolled synthesis of statine and the corresponding phenylalanine derivative (3S,4S)-4-amino-3-hydroxy-5-phenyl pentanoic acid, AHPPA, (18) was recently reported by Misiti and Zappia [4] as shown in Scheme 8.3. Homologation of the aldehydes (14) with the Still phosphonate gave the Z-olefins (15) in good yield. Iodo lactonization proceeded with high facial selectivity (~98:2) to furnish the iodo urethanes (16). Reductive removal of the iodine atom and saponification furnished statine (2) and AHPPA (18) in reasonable yields.

Prasad and Rich [5] have devised a useful strategy that accesses both the statine manifold as well as the homologous hydroxyethylene isosteres as shown in Scheme 8.4. The key reaction is the stereocontrolled allyl silane addition to the α-amino aldehydes (19); the threo isomers (20) could be obtained as the major product with tin tetrachloride as the Lewis acid. The allylic adducts (20) could either be oxidatively cleaved to the statine analogs (21) and (22) or converted stepwise via hydroboration/oxidation and diastereoselective enolate alkylation into the hydroxyethylene isosteres (26) and (27).

Hiemstra, Speckamp and associates [5] have reported an interesting, stereocontrolled synthesis of statine and 4-epi-statine from (S)-malic acid

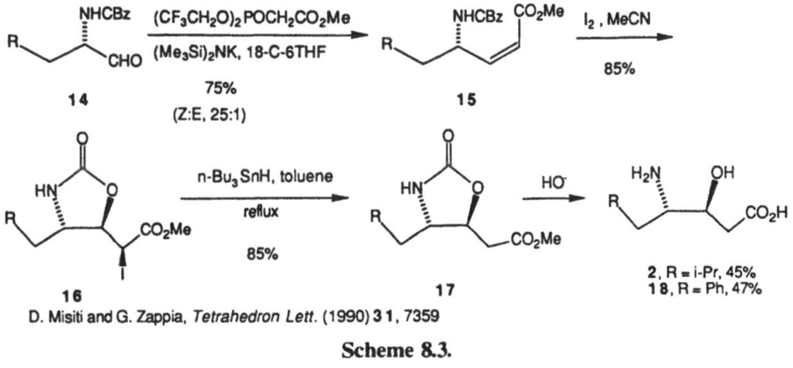

D. Misiti and G. Zappia, *Tetrahedron Lett.* (1990) 3 1, 7359

Scheme 8.3.

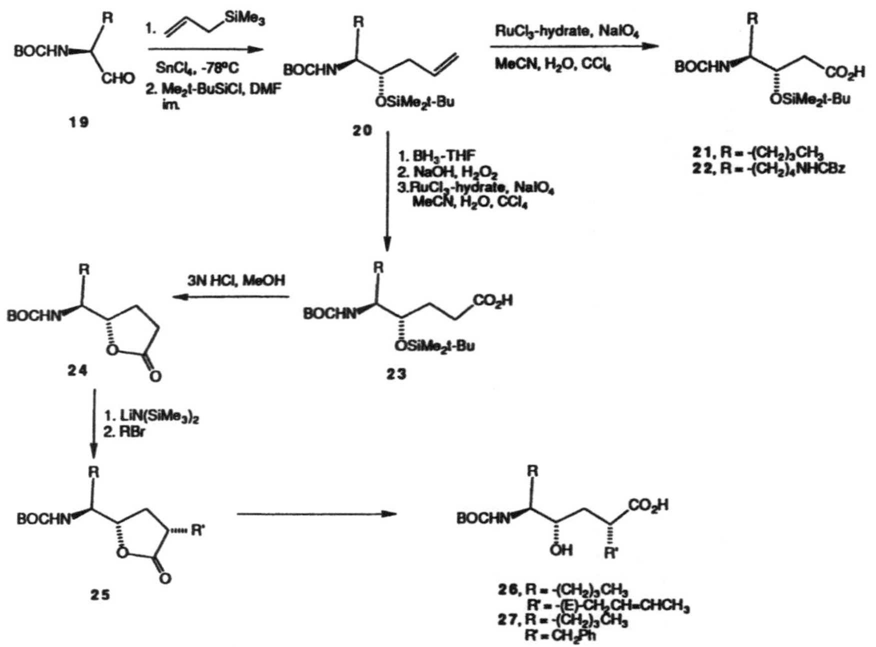

Scheme 8.4.

J.V.N. V. Prasad and D.H. Rich, *Tetrahedron Lett.* (1990) **31**, 1803

21, R = -(CH$_2$)$_2$CH$_3$
22, R = -(CH$_2$)$_4$NHCBz

26, R = -(CH$_2$)$_3$CH$_3$
R' = -(E)-CH$_2$CH=CHCH$_3$
27, R = -(CH$_2$)$_2$CH$_3$
R' = CH$_2$Ph

as shown in Scheme 8.5. The key reaction involves the intramolecular α-acylamino radical cyclization of substrate (32). Although a 3:2 mixture of epimers (33) is obtained in this reaction, subsequent desilyation affords the stereochemically pure lactam (34); further processing of this material affords statine.

A large array of statine derivatives have been prepared and incorporated into various peptides as potential protease inhibitors. For example, Rich and Maibaum [6] prepared the histidine analog (36) from which peptide (37) was prepared. This substance was a potent inhibitor of the aspartic protease penicillopepsin ($K_i = 4.5 \times 10^{-9}$ M) which is ca. ten times more potent than the corresponding statine-containing peptide and several fold more potent than the corresponding AHPPA (18) derivative; the analogous ornithine and lysine derivatives (at P1) were, however slightly better inhibitors than (36).

36

37
$K_i = 4.5 \times 10^{-9}$ M (penicillopepsin)

A systematic study of the stereochemistry of the hydroxymethylene moiety in statine on several aspartic proteases has revealed that the natural 3(S)-configuration provides significantly better inhibitors than the 3(R)-isomers (36). Incorporation of the 3-deoxy derivative (37) also results in loss of inhibitory activity emphasizing the importance of the hydroxyl group. Conversion of the 3-hydroxyl to the corresponding 3-keto derivative (38) reduces inhibition by six-fold. However, both (38) and the more sterically demanding dimethylsulfonium analog (39) provide better inhibitors than the deoxy statine system indicating that partial hydration of the keto moiety can lead to better binding. More interesting, is the success obtained with the difluoro ketone derivative (40) which has provided excellent inhibitors of renin and pepsin. Unexpectedly, the more active diastereomers of the C-3–substituted statine analogs has the 3-(R) configuration (42) rather than the 3-(S) configuration (41). This situation is also observed in the corresponding AHPPA (18) series. The 3-(S) configuration of AHPPA (18) provides better inhibitors than 3-(R) isomers (43); the corresponding 3-methyl series parallels the 3-methyl statine situation, where 3-(R) (45) provides better inhibitors than 3-(S) (44). The reasons for this apparent stereochemical anomaly have been discussed [8] in terms of a different mechanism of inhibition by the 3-methyl analogs. Rich has

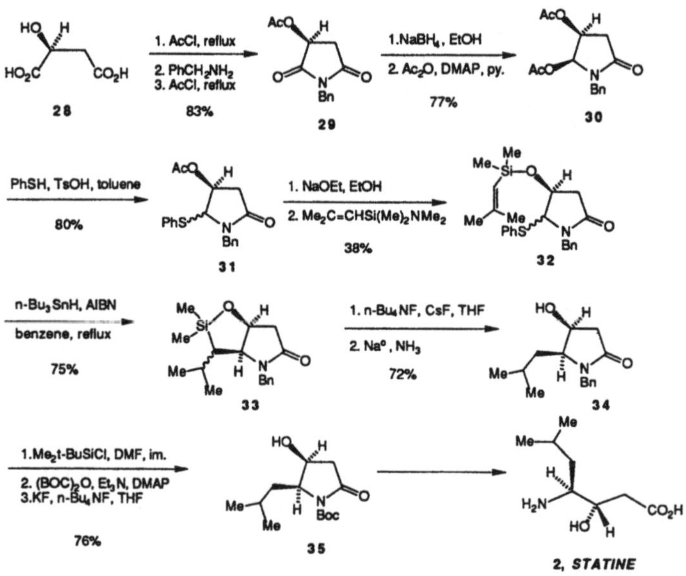

Scheme 8.5.

W~J Koot, R.van Ginkel, M. Kranenburg , H. Hiemstra, S. Louwrier, M.J. Molenaar and W.N. Speckamp *Tetrahedron Lett.* (1991) 3 2, 401

proposed a collected–substrate-inhibitor mechanism for the aspartic proteases and, with supporting NMR and x-ray structural data, argues that the
primary driving force for the tight binding of the 3-(R) methyl substrates
derives from the displacement of bound water to the bulk solvent by the
methyl group. Additional hydrogen-bonding of the 3-(R)-hydroxyl to Asp-
33 provides additional stabilization.

FLUORO KETONES

Abeles [9] has discussed the use of fluoro ketone-containing substrates
for inhibiting a variety of hydrolytic enzymes including, acetylcho-
linesterase, zinc metallo proteases, aspartyl proteases, carboxypeptidase,
and angiotensin converting enzyme (ACE). For example, the alanyl-
typtophan modeled compound (**46**) is a very potent inhibitor of ACE and
the pepstatine analog (**47**) is a nanomolar inhibitor of pepsin.

Numerous syntheses of the fluoro ketone building blocks have been reported in the literature. A representative synthesis reported by an Upjohn

group [10] is detailed in Scheme 8.6. Reformatsky coupling of α-amino aldehydes with bromodifluoro acetate furnishes the adducts (50) and (51). The reaction conditions can be varied to provide either stereoisomer exclusively (50) or diastereomeric mixtures of (50) and (51). The major isomer (50) was processed to provide several renin inhibitors the most potent of which was the difluoro ketone (57). It should also be noted that the stereogenic center adjacent to the highly electronegative ketone spontane-

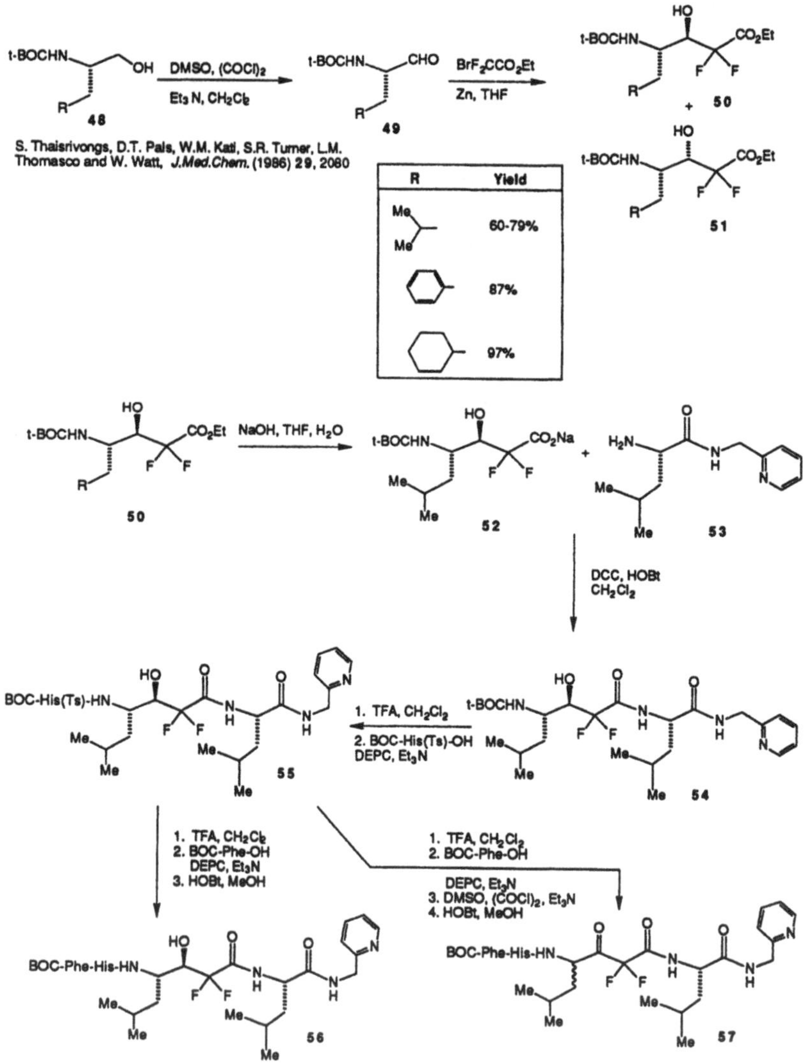

S. Thaisrivongs, D.T. Pals, W.M. Kati, S.R. Turner, L.M. Thomasco and W. Watt, *J.Med.Chem.* (1986) 29, 2080

R	Yield
Me⟍⟍Me (isopropyl)	60-79%
(phenyl)	87%
(cyclohexyl)	97%

Scheme 8.6.

ously undergoes epimerization. Comparative inhibition (IC_{50} M) of (57) with pepstatin against several proteases is presented below.

Substrate	Human Plasma Renin	Porcine Pepsin	Bovine Cathepsin D	Rabbit ACE
57	1.4×10^{-9}	4.2×10^{-5}	1.7×10^{-6}	24%
Pepstatin	6.0×10^{-6}	1.0×10^{-8}	2.8×10^{-8}	at 10^{-1}

Another interesting case involving the fluoro ketone system was reported by Meyer and associates (Scheme 8.7) [11]. The valinyl difluoro ketone moiety was constructed in similar fashion to that used previously (Scheme 8.6) involving the Reformatsky condensation reaction. Peptide (64) was constructed as shown in the scheme and was co-crystallized as a covalent adduct at the active site of porcine pancreatic elastase (1.78 angstrom resolution). The crystal structure reveals a hemiketal complex between the fluoro ketone and the catalytic Ser-195 (65). The carbonyl oxygen atom is situated in an "oxyanion hole" with hydrogen bonds to the amide nitrogens of Ser-195 and Gly-193; an additional, strong hydrogen bond between His-57 and one of the fluorine atoms provides additional stabilization of the complex. The hemiketal complex therefore structurally and chemically resembles the putative tetrahedral intermediate of a productive enzyme-ligand complex.

HYDROXYETHYLENE ISOSTERES

The successes achieved with the statine hydroxymethylene structural subunit have been extended to the hydroxyethylene homologs (67) and ketomethylene (68) systems which more closely mimics the tetrahedral intermediate for the hydrolysis of a dipeptide subunit. Many syntheses of various hydroxyethylene isostere dipeptide subunits have been reported and employed to construct an array of protease inhibitors.

66   67   68

Holladay and Rich [12] reported the preparation of hydroxyethylene and ketomethylene isosteres of Leu-Ala as shown in Scheme 8.8. Grignard condensation of (69) with leucinal (70) furnished the adducts (71) as a 4:1 di-

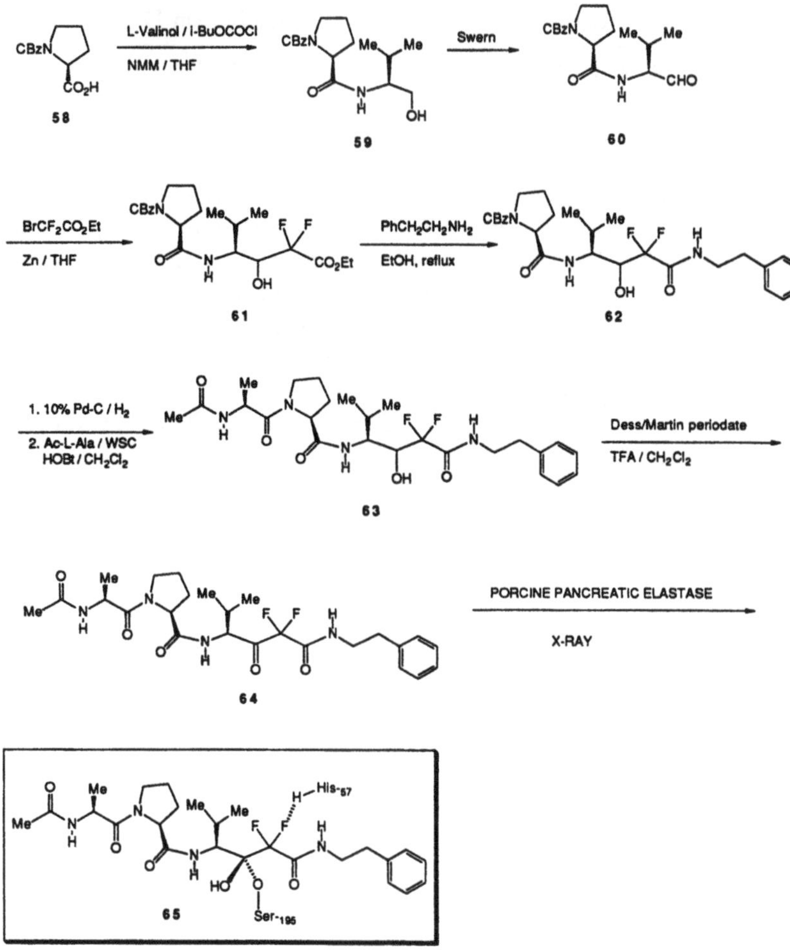

Takahashi, L.H.; Radhakrishnan, R.; Rosenfeld, R.E.; Meyer, E.F.; Trainor, D.A., *J.Am.Chem.Soc.* (1989) 1 1 1, 3368

Scheme 8.7.

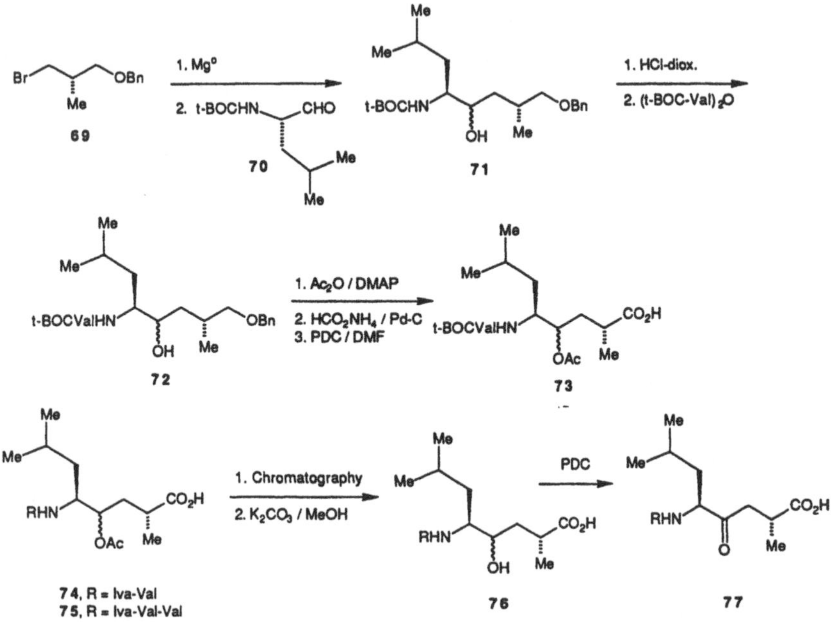

Holladay, M.W.; Rich, D.H., *Tetrahedron Lett.* (1983) 24, 4401.

Scheme 8.8.

astereomeric mixture in 67% combined yield. The benzyloxymethyl group (72) could be converted into the carboxyl group (73) by debenzylation and PDC oxidation. The secondary alcohol (76) could be similarly oxidized to the ketomethylene systems (77) with PDC in 60–70% yield.

Two closely related natural products arphamenine A (78) and B (79) were recently isolated by Umezawa and associates [13] from the bacterium *Chromobacterium violaceum* and shown to be potent inhibitors of aminopeptidase B. These substances are composed of the Arg-Phe and Arg-Tyr ketomethylene dipeptide isosteres. Harbeson and Rich [12] have prepared

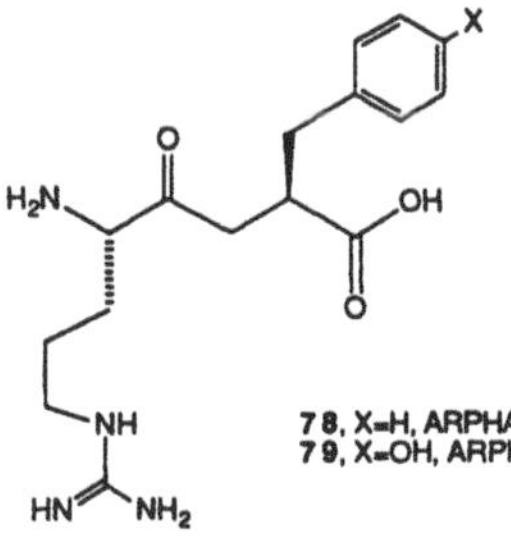

78, X=H, ARPHAMENINE A K_i= 2.5 nM (aminopeptidase B)
79, X=OH, ARPHAMENINE B K_i= 0.84 nM (aminopeptidase B)

a variety of ketomethylene dipeptide isotere-containing substrates and have evaluated these as inhibitors of leucine aminopeptidase; aminopeptidase M and aminopeptidase B (see Table 8.1). All of these proved to be relatively weak inhibitors of all three enzymes with the exception of the Lys-Phe ketomethylene isostere which inhibited aminopeptidase M at 4 nanomolar

TABLE 8.1.

Structure	Leucine Aminopeptidase	Aminopeptidase M	Aminopeptidase B
(structure 1)	Competitive $K_{is} = 57.0 \pm 5$ uM	Non-competitive $K_{is} = 79.0 \pm 12$ uM $_i = 0.26 \pm 0.04$ mM	Competitive $K_i 0.17 \pm 0.01$ uM
(structure 2)	Competitive $K_{is} = 0.24 \pm 0.02$ mM	$_{50} > 0.8$ mM	Competitive $K_i 0.77 \pm 0.05$ uM
(structure 3)	Competitive $K_{is} = 1.1 \pm 0.1$ mM	Non-competitive $K_{is} = 0.66 \pm 0.1$ mM $_i = 0.94 \pm 0.1$ mM	Competitive $K_i 0.13 \pm 0.02$ mM
(structure 4)	Competitive $K_{is} = 0.35 \pm 0.03$ mM	Competitive $K_{is} = 0.13 \pm 0.01$ mM	$_{50} > 0.4$ mM
(structure 5)	Competitive $K_{is} = 25.0 \pm 0.8$ uM	Competitive $K_{is} = 8.3 \pm 0.4$ uM	Competitive $K_i 36.0 \pm 6$ uM
(structure 6)	$IC_{50} > 1.0$ mM	$_{50} > 0.2$ mM	Competitive $K_{is} = 2.0 \pm 0.2$ uM
(structure 7)	$IC_{50} > 0.5$ mM	Competitive $K_{is} = 0.21 \pm 0.02$ mM	Non-competitive $K = 8.8 \pm 0.7$ uM $_i = 2.0 \pm 0.6$ uM
(structure 8)	$IC_{50} > 0.6$ mM	$_{50} > 0.9$ mM	Competitive $K_{is} = 4.0 \pm 0.7$ nM

which is close to that of the natural products (78) and (79). The authors note that the synthesis of the corresponding free hydroxyethylene isosteres is complicated by γ-lactone formation. This problem is evident in other reported syntheses [14] of hydroxyethylene isostere building blocks. For example, a Ciba-Geigy group [15] reported the synthesis of several inhibitors of renin utilizing the hydroxyethylene isostere (2S,4S,5S)-5-amino-4-hydroxy-2-isopropyl-6-cyclohexanoic acid as shown in Scheme 8.9. To obviate lactone formation, the secondary hydroxyl group is protected as an isopropylidene ketal with the amino group. After conversion of the carboxyl group (83) into an n-butyl amide (84), the secondary hydroxyl can be unmasked. The final peptide (87), proved to be a good renin inhibitor ($IC_{50} = 2 \times 10^{-9}$ M) and also possessed good oral activity (in salt-depleted marmosets, (87) inhibited plasma renin and lowered blood pressure up to 2 h after oral administration at a dose of 10 mg/kg) which has been a difficult property to engineer into active inhibitors.

Metternich and Ludi [16] have reported the preparation of α-allyloxy hydroxyethylene isosteres and utilize the γ-lactone (93) as an active ester for formation of the requisite C-terminal amide residues (Scheme 8.10). Compounds (96) and (97) are reported to be potent inhibitors of human renin ($IC_{50} = 30$ nM and 38 nM, respectively).

The hydroxymethylene and hydroxyethylene isosteres (2R,3S)-3-amino-4-cyclohexyl-2-hydroxybutanoic acid (98) and (3S,4S)-4-amino-5-cyclohexyl-3-hydroxypentanoic acid (99) have become very important building blocks for a variety of protease inhibitors. Their syntheses have thus become very important issues, particularly for large-scale production. In addition to the synthetic approaches described above, recent efficient syntheses of these compounds have been developed [18]; a representative example for the synthesis of (98) is presented in Scheme 8.11.

which is close to that of the natural products (78) and (79). The authors

Terashima and associates [17] have utilized mandelic acid as the basic starting material to prepare (98) as shown in Scheme 8.11. Reduction of methyl mandelate (100) followed by imine formation and ketene-imine cycloaddition provides β-lactam (102) as a 12:1 mixture of diastereomers. Ring-opening and reductive processing provides the isopropyl ester (104) of (98). The overall yield for this eight-step procedure is reported as 44%.

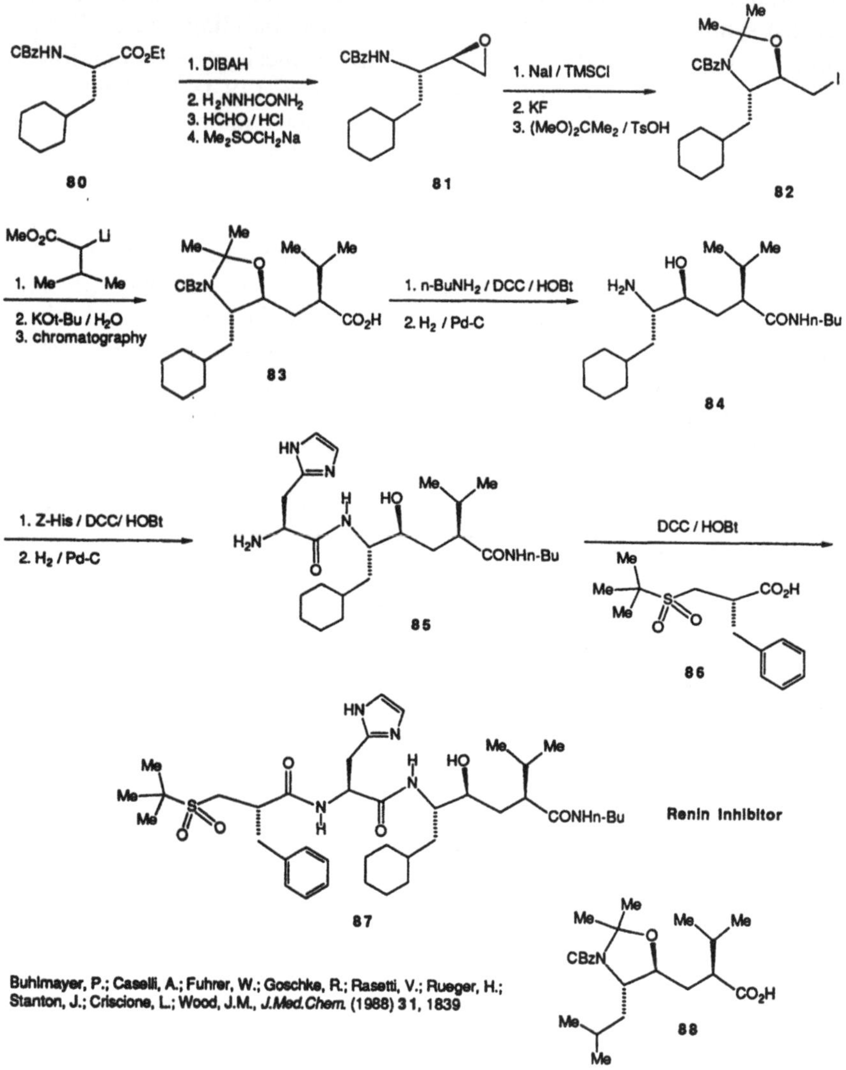

Scheme 8.9.

Buhlmayer, P.; Caselli, A.; Fuhrer, W.; Goschke, R.; Rasetti, V.; Rueger, H.; Stanton, J.; Criscione, L.; Wood, J.M., *J.Med.Chem.* (1988) 31, 1839

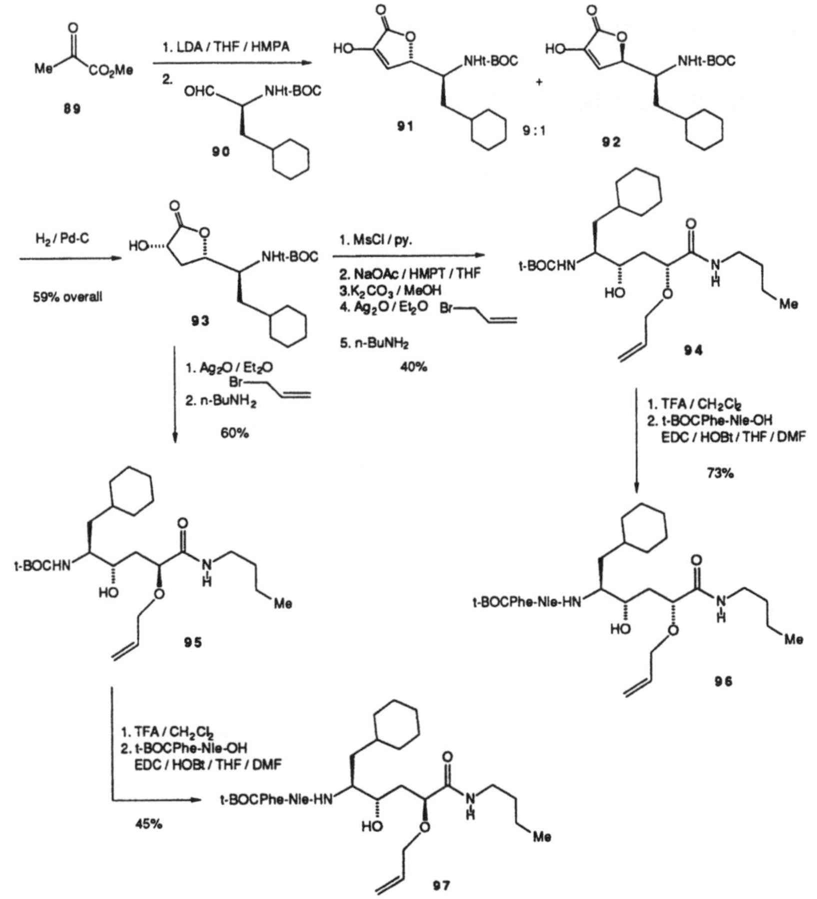

1. LDA / THF / HMPA
2.

89

90

91   9:1   **92**

H₂ / Pd-C

59% overall

93

1. MsCl / py.
2. NaOAc / HMPT / THF
3. K₂CO₃ / MeOH
4. Ag₂O / Et₂O   Br
5. n-BuNH₂

40%

94

1. Ag₂O / Et₂O
   Br
2. n-BuNH₂

60%

95

1. TFA / CH₂Cl₂
2. t-BOCPhe-Nle-OH
   EDC / HOBt / THF / DMF

73%

96

1. TFA / CH₂Cl₂
2. t-BOCPhe-Nle-OH
   EDC / HOBt / THF / DMF

45%

97

Metternich, R.; Ludi, W., *Tetrahedron Lett.* (1988) **29**, 3923

Scheme 8.10.

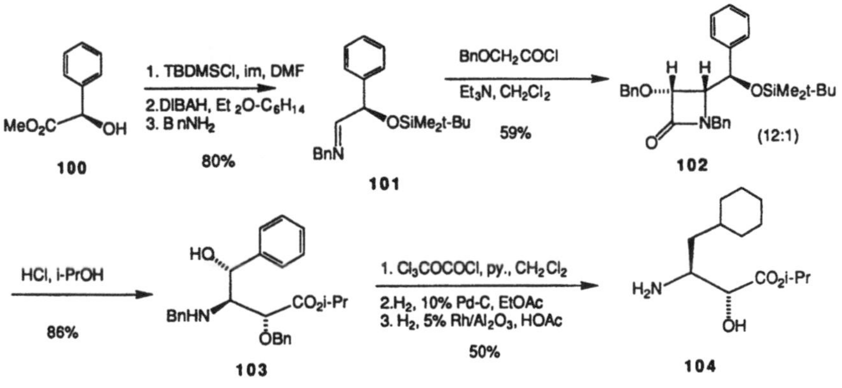

1. TBDMSCl, im, DMF
2. DIBAH, Et₂O-C₆H₁₄
3. BnNH₂

80%

100

101

BnOCH₂COCl

Et₃N, CH₂Cl₂

59%

102   (12:1)

HCl, i-PrOH

86%

103

1. Cl₃COCOCl, py., CH₂Cl₂
2. H₂, 10% Pd-C, EtOAc
3. H₂, 5% Rh/Al₂O₃, HOAc

50%

104

Y. Kobayashi, Y. Takemoto, Y. Ito and S. Terashima, *Tetrahedron Lett.* (1990) **31**, 3031

Scheme 8.11.

HIV PROTEASE INHIBITORS

The fairly general successes realized with the statine core substructure for constructing protease inhibitors has been vigorously applied to the development of HIV-1 protease inhibitors. The HIV-1 protease is required for cleaving the polyproteins encoded by the gag and pol genes into mature virion proteins and enzymes essential for HIV replication. The HIV protease is the smallest member of the aspartyl proteases that is catalytically active as a homodimer. The HIV protease is distinguished by its specificity for cleaving the Phe-Pro and Tyr-Pro sequences found in the gag and gag-pol gene products. This structural specificity has been recently exploited by a number of groups in designing nonhydrolyzable surrogates of the scissile peptide moiety.

An Upjohn group [19] reported the synthesis and activity of U-81749 (105) which inhibited recombinant HIV-1 protease *in vitro* (K_i 70 nM) and significantly, inhibited HIV-1 replication *in vivo* (IC_{50} 0.1 ~ 1 uM).

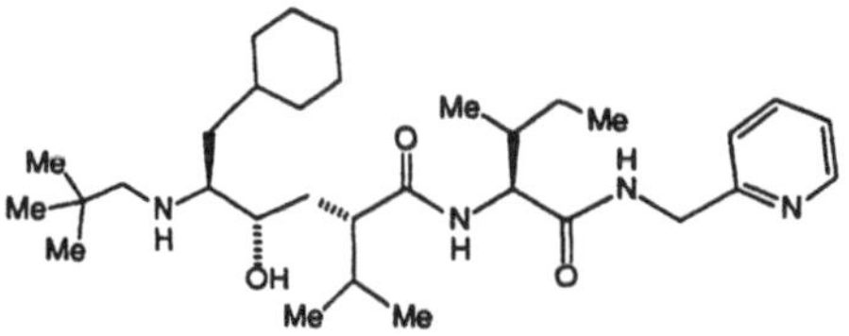

105, U-81749

Dreyer et al. [20], have examined a large variety of substrate analogs containing various amide bond replacements (see Table 8.2) (106)–(119). A variety of Phe-Pro isosteres were prepared (110)–(112), (115), (118), and (119) and were shown to have inhibitory activity in the micromolar range. Surprisingly, substrates containing the simple hydroxyethylene isostere of Phe-Gly or Tyr-Gly (107), (108), and (113) were the most potent inhibitors with one derivative (113) exhibiting a K_i = 0.018 uM.

In a parallel study published contemporaneously, the same group [21], prepared the hydroxymethylene-containing (AHPPA) substrate (120) and the reduced amide surrogates (121) and (122) and examined these for inhibition of HIV-1 protease. All three compounds proved to be inhibitors of the enzyme, but only in the micromolar range.

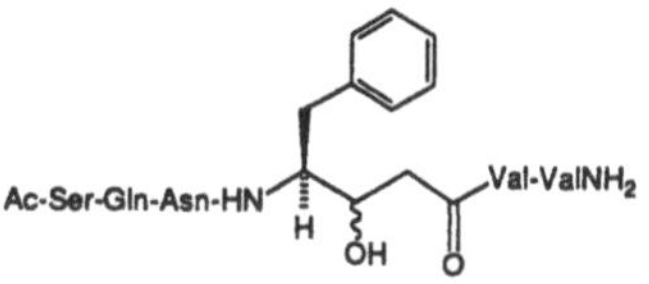

120, K_i = 39 ± 6

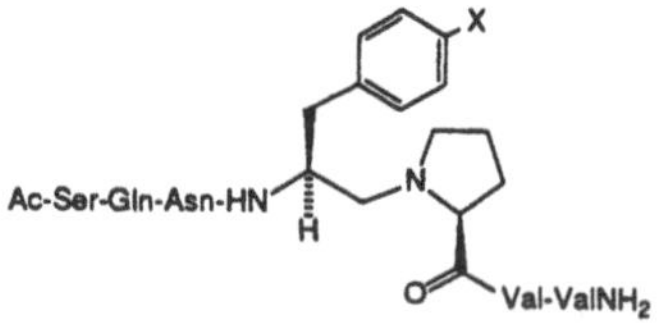

121, X = OH, K_i = 13 ± 1
122, X = H, K_i = 14 ± /2

TABLE 8.2.

Ser-Ala-Ala-HN—...—Val-Val-OMe
106, $K_i = 0.81$ uM

Ser-Ala-Ala-HN—...—Val-Val-OMe
107, $K_i = 0.062$ uM

Ser-Ala-Ala-HN—...—Val-Val-OMe
108, $K_i = 0.079$ uM

Ser-Ala-Ala-HN—...—Val-Val-OMe
109, $K_i = 4.9$ uM

Ser-Ala-Ala-HN—...—Val-Val-OMe
110, $K_i = 0.5$ uM

Ser-Ala-Ala-HN—...—Val-Val-OMe
111, $K_i = 28$ uM

Boc-Ser-Ala-Ala-HN—...—Val-Val-OMe
112, $K_i = 30$ uM

Ala-Ala-HN—...—Val-Val-OMe
113, $K_i = 0.018$ uM

Boc-Ser-Ala-Ala-HN—...—Val-Val-OMe
114, $K_i = 1.6$ uM

Ser-Ala-Ala-HN—...—Val-Val-OMe
115, $K_i = 4$ uM

Ser-Ala-Ala-HN—...—Val-Val-OMe
116, $K_i = 4.4$ uM

Ser-Ala-Ala-HN—...—Val-Val-OMe
117, $K_i = 4.5$ uM

Ac-Ser-Ala-Ala-HN—...—Val-Val-NH₂
118, $K_i = 38$ uM

Boc-Ser-Ala-Ala-HN—...—Val-Val-OMe
119, $K_i = 40$ uM

Dreyer, et.al., *Proc.Natl.Acad.Sci. USA* (1989) **86**, 9752

In a very provocative recent study, Roberts et al. [22] have prepared a series of peptide derivatives based on the Phe[167]-Pro[168] sequence and found the potent and selective HIV protease inhibitor (123). This substance had an $IC_{50} < 0.4$ nM against HIV-1 protease and an $IC_{50} < 0.8$ nM against HIV-2 protease. Significantly, the authors point out that (123) caused less than 50% inhibition of other human aspartic proteases such as renin, pepsin, gastricsin, cathepsin D and cathepsin E at a concentration of 10 micromolar. This compound also had no effect on proteases of the cysteine, serine, or metallo-classes at 10 micromolar. Proteolytic cleavage of the gag polyprotein (p55) to p24 was inhibited in chronically infected CEM cells. Furthermore, compound (123) showed good antiviral activity in the nanomolar range and cytotoxicity (TD_{50}) at least 2000 fold above the concentrations required for antiviral activity. One unusual feature of this compound is that the stereochemistry of the secondary hydroxyl group is (R)- rather than the usual (S)-stereochemistry of the statine and related hydroxyethylene isosteres that typically display better inhibitory activities.

123, IC_{50}, 0.4 nM (HIV-I)

Rich et al. [23], have attempted to address the anomalous stereochemical divergence of the highly active (R)-inhibitor (123) with that of other HIV protease inhibitors containing hydroxyethylene or hydroxymethylene isosteric replacements. By carrying out highly stereoselective syntheses of hydroxyethylamines derived from Phe-Pro (Schemes 8.12 and 8.13), a careful stereochemical/activity study was undertaken. These authors had previously synthesized JG-365 as an R,S diastereomeric mixture [24] and crystallized the (S)-isomer with HIV-1 protease for which an x-ray crystal analysis was secured [25]. These apparently contrasting observations meant that either the weaker-binding isomer of JG-365 had crystallized with the protease or that (123) and the (S)-isomer of JG-365 [Scheme 8.12 (128)], were binding to the enzyme in significantly different ways. The stereoselective syntheses provided data that confirmed that the (S)-isomer (128) was ca. 80 fold more potent than the (R)-isomer (132). Other substrates prepared that lacked the P3' substituent showed better activity with the (R)-configuration which is consistent with the observation of

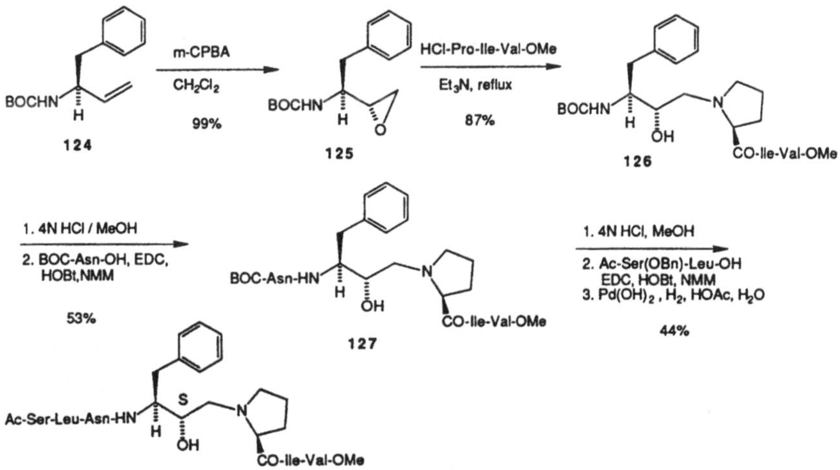

124 → m-CPBA, CH$_2$Cl$_2$, 99% → **125**

BOCHN

125 → HCl-Pro-Ile-Val-OMe, Et$_3$N, reflux, 87% → **126**

BOCHN ... OH ... CO-Ile-Val-OMe

1. 4N HCl / MeOH
2. BOC-Asn-OH, EDC, HOBt, NMM
53%

BOC-Asn-HN ... OH ... CO-Ile-Val-OMe
127

1. 4N HCl, MeOH
2. Ac-Ser(OBn)-Leu-OH, EDC, HOBt, NMM
3. Pd(OH)$_2$, H$_2$, HOAc, H$_2$O
44%

Ac-Ser-Leu-Asn-HN ... S ... OH ... CO-Ile-Val-OMe
128

D.H. Rich, et.al, *J.Med.Chem* (1991) 3 4,1222

SUBSTRATE	IC$_{50}$ nM
Ac-Ser-Leu-Asn-Phe-HEA(RS)-Pro-Ile-Val-OMe	9 (Ki= 0.6 nM)
Ac-Ser-Leu-Asn-Phe-HEA(S)-Pro-Ile-Val-OMe	3.4 (Ki= 0.24 nM)
Ac-Ser-Leu-Asn-Phe-HEA(R)-Pro-Ile-Val-OMe	65 (Ki= 20 nM)
BOC-Asn-Phe-HEA(S)-Pro-Ile-Val-OMe	16
BOC-Asn-Phe-HEA(R)-Pro-Ile-Val-OMe	850
CBz-Asn-Phe-HEA(S)-Pro-O-t-Bu	450
CBz-Asn-Phe-HEA(R)-Pro-O-t-Bu	51
Ac-Ser-Leu-Asn-Phe-HEA(S)-Pro-O-t-Bu	14
Ac-Ser-Leu-Asn-Phe-HEA(R)-Pro-O-t-Bu	14
CBz-Asn-Phe-HEA(S)-Pro-Ile-Phe-OMe	4
Qua-Asn-Phe-HEA(S)-Pro-Ile-Phe-OMe	2.3

Qua = quinoline-2-carboxylic acid

Scheme 8.12.

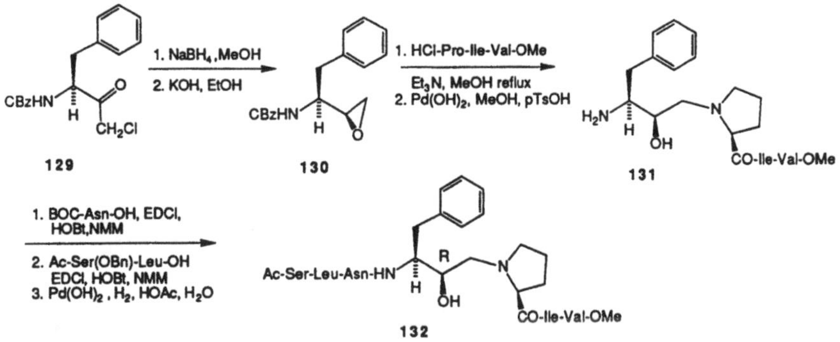

129 (CBzHN ... CH$_2$Cl) → 1. NaBH$_4$, MeOH; 2. KOH, EtOH → **130** (CBzHN, epoxide)

130 → 1. HCl-Pro-Ile-Val-OMe, Et$_3$N, MeOH reflux; 2. Pd(OH)$_2$, MeOH, pTsOH → **131**

H$_2$N ... OH ... CO-Ile-Val-OMe
131

1. BOC-Asn-OH, EDCl, HOBt, NMM
2. Ac-Ser(OBn)-Leu-OH, EDCl, HOBt, NMM
3. Pd(OH)$_2$, H$_2$, HOAc, H$_2$O

Ac-Ser-Leu-Asn-HN ... R ... OH ... CO-Ile-Val-OMe
132

Scheme 8.13.

Roberts with inhibitor (123). These results demonstrate that the configuration of the hydroxyl group necessary for maximal inhibitory activity is dependent on the size and nature of the peptide framework.

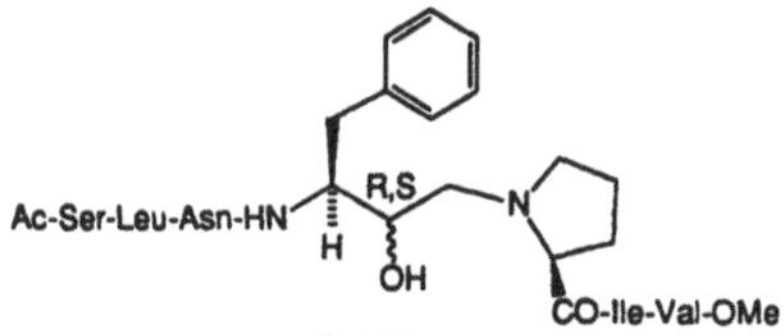

JG-365

An extremely interesting and provocative set of HIV protease inhibitors was recently communicated by Kempf et al. [26]. The recent crystallographic structure determination of the HIV protease demonstrates that the enzyme functions as a C_2 symmetric homodimer. Based on this symmetry consideration, this group designed and synthesized a series of C_2 symmetric and C_2 pseudosymmetric amide bond replacements and derived some very potent inhibitors as shown in Schemes 8.14 and 8.15. The authors state that these substances, which are inherently less peptide-like than structures based on the pepstatin model, should be considerably more stable to proteolytic degradation *in vivo* and concomitantly exhibit greater specificity towards the HIV protease. The design exercise utilized deletes the P' subsite due to the greater importance of the P subsites in renin inhibitors. The symmetry axis was placed on or near the carbonyl carbon undergoing cleavage. The structures arrived at include peptides of (144) and (145). In both instances, nanomolar inhibitors were produced. The three CBz-Val derivatives of (145) blocked the spread of HIV infection in two immortalized human T-lymphocytic cell lines at concentrations of 20–60 nM. A

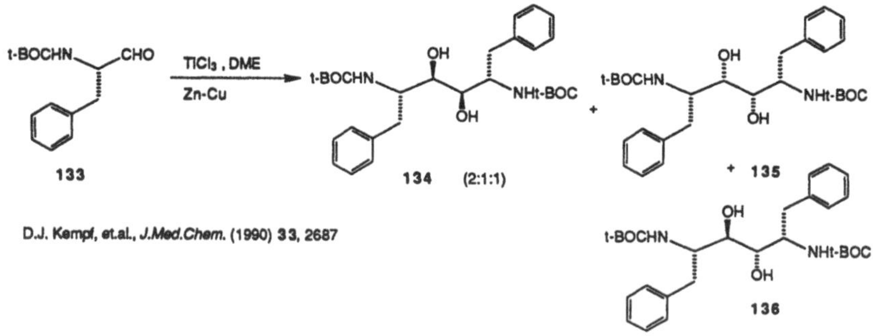

D.J. Kempf, et.al., J.Med.Chem. (1990) **33**, 2687

Scheme 8.14.

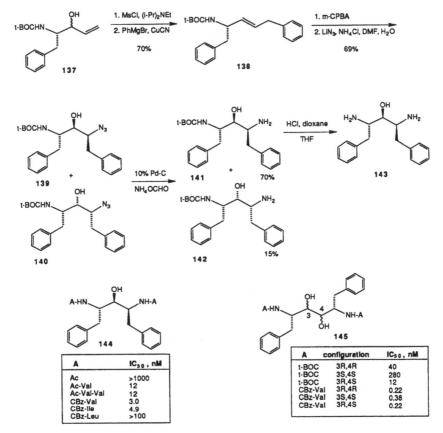

Scheme 8.15.

crystal structure of the CBz-Val derivative of (144) complexed to the active site of recombinant HIV-1 protease revealed that the inhibitor (IC$_{50}$ = 3 nM) binds to the enzyme in a highly symmetrical fashion.

INVERTED AMINES

In a preliminary disclosure, an Abbott group [27] has reported on a series of "inverted amines" exemplified by (146) and (147) as potent renin inhibitors. Compound (146) is reported to have an IC$_{50}$ of 8.2 nM *in vitro* and compounds in the (147) series also inhibit human plasma renin in the nanomolar concentration range. The authors also note that these potent inhibitors were effective in reducing mean arterial pressure in experimental animals and exhibit improved oral bioavailability.

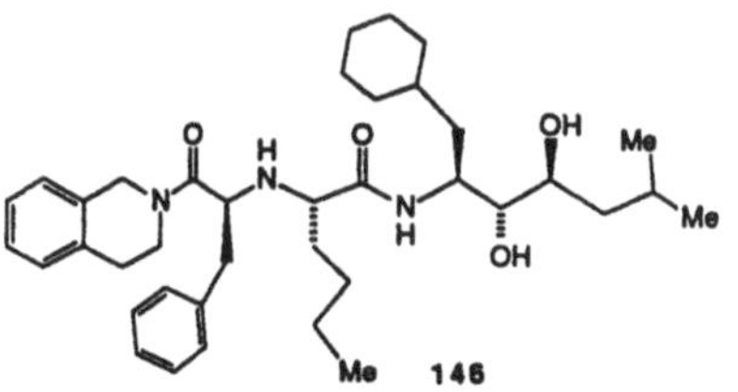

PHOSPHOROUS ANALOGS

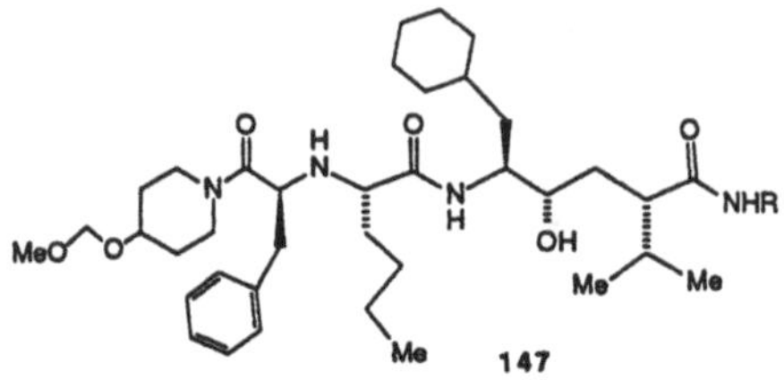

Bartlett and Kezer [28] have reported on the synthesis and inhibitory activity of phosphinic acid dipeptide analogs and has prepared the phosphorous-containing analog of statine (Scheme 8.16). The peptide

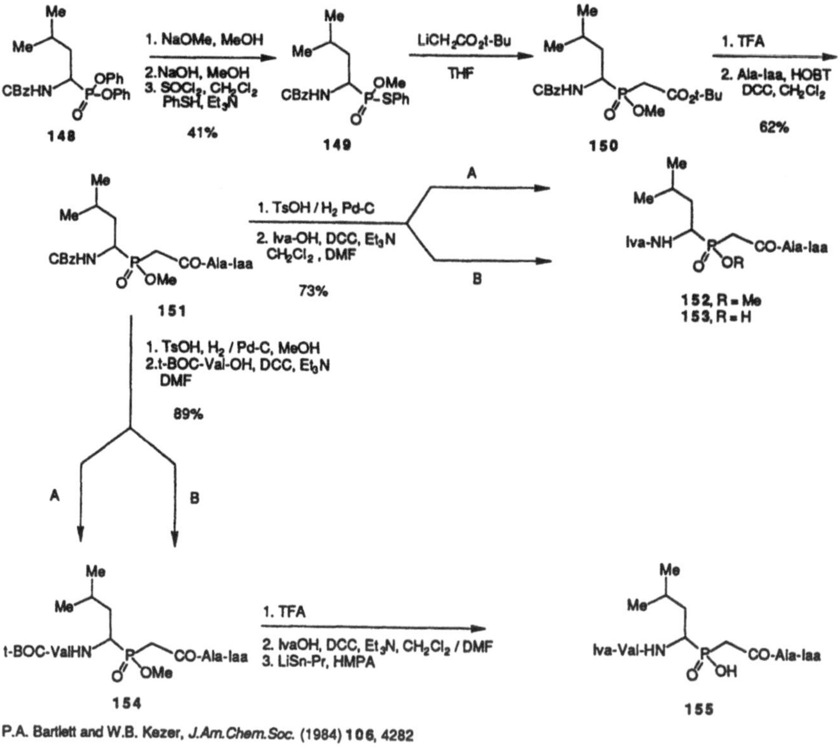

P.A. Bartlett and W.B. Kezer, *J.Am.Chem.Soc.* (1984) 106, 4282

Scheme 8.16.

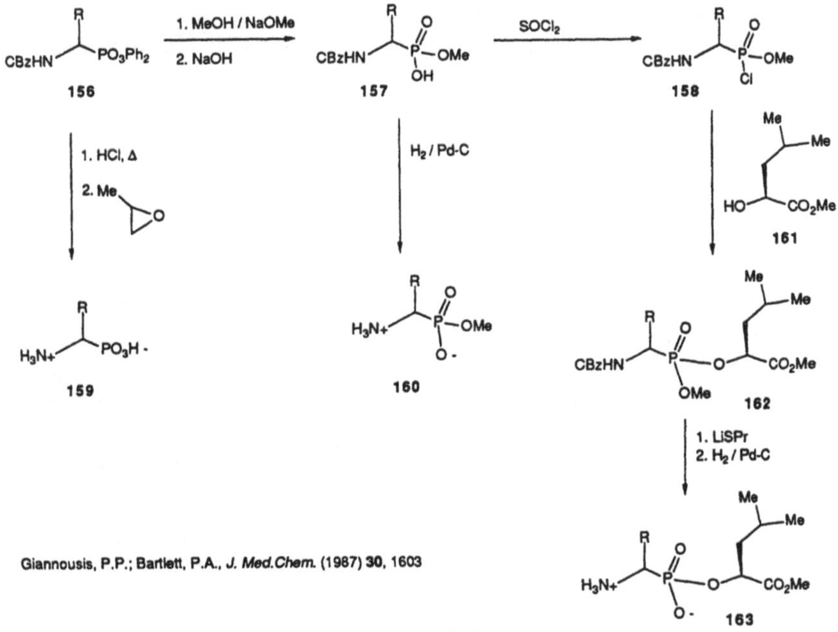

Giannousis, P.P.; Bartlett, P.A., *J. Med.Chem.* (1987) **30**, 1603

Scheme 8.17.

(155) containing the L-configured phosphorous analog of statine, was a sub-nanomolar slow-binding inhibitor of pepsin.

In a related study, Bartlett and Giannousis [29] prepared the two interesting phosphorous-containing dipeptide analogs [Schemes 8.17 and 8.18 (163) and (169)]. Both series exhibited micromolar inhibition of leucine aminopeptidase which belongs to a family of zinc-containing exopeptidases with specificity for cleavage at the N-terminus of peptides.

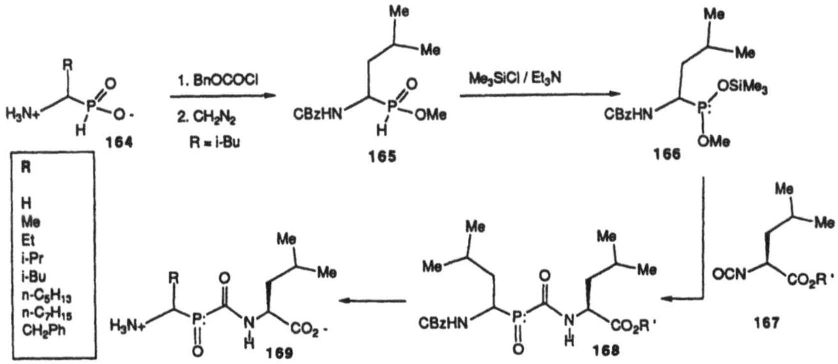

Scheme 8.18.

Many additional examples of phosphorous-containing amide mimics have been reported; the reader is referred to papers cited in the previous examples [28,29].

The rapidly accumulating body of knowledge on the energetics and structural details of how peptidomimetics bind to various families of proteases such as the HIV-1 protease and the renin-angiotensin [30] system, and fundamental knowledge of enzyme structure and catalytic mechanisms, will surely continue to stimulate significant advances in the design and production of many therapeutically useful drugs. As the above overview should have made clear, the isolation of the lead structure pepstatin obtained from natural sources has played a key role in opening a large and important area of drug design and development. Ultimately, the ability to access structures designed and targeted for a specific application rely on the ability of available synthetic technology to make such substances available in stereochemically pure form. Rapidly advancing synthetic technologies [31] to access nonproteinogenic amino acids will undoubtedly serve a critical role in providing the raw materials for preparing a vast array of new structural and functional group families of peptide mimics.

ABBREVIATIONS

AcCl	acetyl chloride
Ac_2O	acetic anhydride
AIBN	azo-(bis)-isobutyronitrile
Bn	benzyl
n-Bu	normal-butyl
$(BOC)_2O$	di-tert-butyl dicarbonate
t-BOC	tert-butyloxycarbonyl (or BOC)
CBz	benzyloxycarbonyl
18-C-6	18-crown-6 ether
DCC	N,N'-dicyclohexyl carbodiimide
DEPC	diethyl phosphorocyanidate
DIBAH	diisobutyl aluminum hydride
diox.	dioxane
DMAP	N,N-dimethylamino pyridine
DME	dimethoxyethane
DMF	N,N-dimethyl formamide
DMSO	dimethyl sulfoxide
EDC	1-(3-dimethylaminopropyl)-3-ethylcarbodiimide (also WSC)
Et	ethyl
Et_2O	diethyl ether
Et_3N	triethyl amine

EtOH	ethanol
HEA	hydroxyethylene isostere
HMPA	hexamethylphosphoramide
HMPT	hexamethylphosphorous triamide
HOAc	acetic acid
HOBT	N-hydroxybenzotriazole
Iaa	statine
im.	imidazole
im₂CO	carbonyl diimidazole
Iva	isovaleryl
IvaOH	isovaleric acid
LDA	lithium diisopropylamide
m-CPBA	meta-chloroperoxybenzoic acid
Me	methyl
MeCN	acetonitrile
MeOH	methanol
MsCl	methane sulfonyl chloride (mesylchloride)
NaOAc	sodium acetate
NMM	N-methyl morpholine
Ts	tosylate
PDC	pryridinium dichromate
Ph	phenyl
Pr	propyl
py	pyridine
Red-Al	sodium bis(2-methoxy-ethoxy)aluminum hydride in toluene
SWERN	oxidation using DMSO, oxalyl chloride and Et₃N
TBDMSCI	tert-butyldimethylsilyl chloride
TFA	trifluoro acetic acid
THF	tetrahydrofuran
TMSCl	trimethylsilyl chloride
TsOH	para-toluene sulfonic acid (or p-TsOH)
WSC	water-soluble carbodiimide 1-(3-dimethylamino)propyl-3-ethylcarbodiimide hydrochloride (also EDC)

REFERENCES

1 Umezawa, H., T. Aoyagi, H. Morishima, M. Matzuzaki, M. Hamada and T. Takeuchi. 1970. *J. Antibiotics*, 23:259.

2 Rich, D. H. 1985. *J. Med. Chem.*, 28:263; Maibaum, J. and D. H. Rich. 1988. *J. Org. Chem.*, 53:869 and references cited therein; Schuda, P. F., W. J. Greenlee, P. K. Chakravarty and P. Eskola, 1988. *J. Org. Chem.*, 53:873.

3 Kogen, H. and T. Nishi. 1987. *J. Chem. Soc. Chem. Comm.*, pp. 311.

4 Misiti, D. and G. Zappia. 1990. *Tetrahedron Lett.*, 31:7359.

5 Koot, W.-J., R. van Ginkel, M. Kranenburg, H. Hiemstra, S. Louwrier, M. J. Moolenaar and W. N. Speckamp. 1991. *Tetrahedron Lett.*, 32:401; Ohta, T., S. Shiokawa, R. Sakamoto and S. Nozoe. 1990. *Tetrahedron Lett.*, 31:7329.

6 Maibaum, J. and D. H. Rich. 1989. *J. Med. Chem.*, 32:1571.

7 Agarwal, N. S. and D. H. Rich. 1986. *J. Med. Chem.*, 29:2519.

8 Rich, D. H., M. S. Bernatowicz, N. S. Agarwal, M. Kawai, F. G. Salituro and P. G. Schmidt. 1985. *Biochemistry*, 24:3165.

9 Gelb, M. H., J. P. Svaren and R. H. Abeles. 1985. *Biochemistry*, 24:1813.

10 Thaisrivongs, S., D. T. Pals, W. M. Kati, S. R. Turner, L. M. Thomasco and W. Watt. 1986. *J. Med. Chem.*, 29:2080.

11 Takahashi, L. H., R. Radhakrishnan, R. E. Rosenfeld, E. F. Meyer and D. A. Trainor. 1989. *J. Am. Chem. Soc.*, 111:3368.

12 Holladay, M. W. and D. H. Rich. 1983. *Tetrahedron Lett.*, 24:4401; Harbeson, S. L. and D. H. Rich. 1989. *J. Med. Chem.*, 32:1378.

13 Umezawa, H., T. Aoyagi, S. Ohuchi, A. Okuyama, H. Suda, T. Takita, M. Hamada and T. Takeuchi. 1983. *J. Antibiotics*, 36:1572; Ohuchi, S., H. Suda, H. Naganawa, T. Takita, T. Aoyagi, H. Umezawa, H. Nakamura and Y. Iitaka. 1983. *J. Antibiotics*, 36:1576.

14 Bradbury, R. H., J. M. Revill, J. E. Rivett and D. Waterson. 1989. *Tetrahedron Lett.*, 30:3845; Fray, A. H., R. L. Kaye and E. F. Kleinman. 1986. *J. Org. Chem.*, 51:4828.

15 Buhlmayer, P., A. Caselli, W. Fuhrer, R. Goschke, V. Rasetti, H. Rueger, J. L. Stanton, L. Criscione and J. M. Wood. 1988. *J. Med. Chem.*, 31:1839.

16 Metternich, R. and W. Ludi. 1988. *Tetrahedron Lett.*, 29:3923.

17 Kobayashi, Y., Y. Takemoto, Y. Ito and S. Terashima. 1990. *Tetrahedron Lett.*, 31:3031; Matsuda, F., T. Matsumoto, M. Ohsaki, Y. Ito and S. Terashima. 1990. *Chemistry Lett.*, p. 723; Matsumoto, T., Y. Kobayashi, Y. Takemoto, Y. Ito, T. Kamijo, H. Harada and S. Terashima. 1990. *Tetrahedron Lett.*, 31:4175; Kobayashi, Y., Y. Takemoto, Y. Ito and S. Terashima. 1990. *Tetrahedron Lett.*, 31:3031.

18 Kempf, D. J. 1986. *J. Org. Chem.*, 51:3921; Wuts, P. G. M., S. R. Putt and A. R. Ritter. 1988. *J. Org. Chem.*, 53:4503; Herold, P., R. Duthaler, G. Rihs and C. Angst. 1989. *J. Org. Chem.*, 54:1178; Rosenberg, S. H., K. W. Woods, H. D. Kleinert, H. Stein, H. N. Nellans, D. J. Hoffman, S. G. Spanton, R. A. Pyter, J. Cohen, D. A. Egan, J. J. Plattner and T. J. Perun. 1989. *J. Med. Chem.*, 32:1371.

19 McQuade, T. J., A. G. Tomasselli, L. Liu, V. Karacostas, B. Moss, T. K. Sawyer, R. L. Heinrikson and W. G. Tarpley. 1990. *Science*, 247:454.

20 Dreyer, G. B., B. W. Metcalf, T. A. Tomaszek, T. J. Carr, A. C. Chandler, L. J. Hyland, S. A. Fakhoury, V. A. Magaard, M. L. Moore, J. E. Strickler, C. Debouck and T. D. Meck. 1989. *Proc. Natl. Acad. Sci. USA*, 86:9752; Meek, T. D., D. M. Lambert, G. B. Dreyer, T. J. Carr, T. A. Tomaszek, M. L. Moore, J. E. Strickler, C. Debouck, L. J. Hyland, T. J. Matthews, B. W. Metcalf and S. R. Petteway. 1990. *Nature*, 343:90.

21 Moore, M. L., W. M. Bryan, S. A. Fakhoury, V. W. Magaard, W. F. Huffman, B. D. Dayton, T. D. Meek, L. J. Hyland, G. B. Dreyer, B. W. Metcalf, J. E. Strickler, J. G. Gorniak and C. Debouck. 1989. *Biochem. Biophys. Res. Comm.*, 159:420.

22 Roberts, N. A., J. A. Martin, D. Kinchington, A. V. Broadhurst, J. C. Craig, I. B. Duncan, S. A. Galpin, B. K. Handa, J. Kay, A. Krohn, R. W. Lambert, J. H. Merrett, J. S. Mills, K. E. B. Parkes, S. Redshaw, A. J. Ritchie, D. L. Taylor, G. J. Thomas and P. J. Machin. 1990. *Science*, 248:358.

23 Rich, D. H., C.-Q Sun, J. V. N. Vara Prasad, A. Pathiasseril, M. V. Toth, G. R. Marshall, M. Clare, R. A. Mueller and K. Houseman. 1991. *J. Med. Chem.*, 34:1222.

24 Rich, D. H., J. Green, M. V. Toth, G. R. Marshall and S. B. H. Kent. 1990. *J. Med. Chem.*, 33:1285.

25 Swain, A. L., M. M. Miller, J. Green, D. H. Rich, S. B. H. Kent and A. Wlodawer. 1990. *Proc. Natl. Acad. Sci. USA*, 87:8805.

26 Kempf, D. J., D. W. Norbeck, L. M. Codacovi, X. C. Wang, W. E. Kohlbrenner, N. E. Wideburg, D. A. Paul, M. F. Knigge, S. Vasavanonda, A. Craig-Kennard, A. Saldivar, W. Rosenbrook, J. J. Clement, J. J. Plattner and J. Erikson. 1990. *J. Med. Chem.*, 33:2687; Erikson, J., D. J. Neidhart, J. VanDrie, D. J. Kempf, X. C. Wang, D. W. Norbeck, J. J. Plattner, J. W. Rittenhouse, M. Turon, N. Wideburg, W. E. Kohlbrenner, R. Simmer, R. Helfrich, D. A. Paul and M. Knigge. 1990. *Science*, 249:527; Chenera, B., J. C. Boehm and G. B. Dreyer. 1991. *Bioorganic and Med. Chem. Lett.*, 1:219.

27 Boyd, S. A., A. K. L. Fung, W. R. Baker, R. A. Mantei, Y.-L. Armiger, H. H. Stein, J. Cohen, D. A. Egan, J. L. Barlow, V. Klinghofer, H. D. Kleinert, K. M. Verburg, D. L. Martin, G. A. Young, J. S. Polakowski, D. J. Hoffman, K. W. Garren and T. J. Perun. 1991. *Abstracts of Papers, 201st ACS National Meeting, Atlanta, GA*, Washington, DC: American Chemical Society, MEDI 53; Fung, A. K. L., W. R. Baker, H. H. Stein, H. D. Kleinert, J. J. Plattner, Y.-L. Armiger, S. L. Condon, J. Cohen, D. A. Egan, J. L. Barlow, K. M. Verburg, D. L. Martin, G. A. Young, J. S. Polakowski and T. J. Perun. 1991. *Abstracts of Papers, 201st ACS National Meeting, Atlanta, GA*, Washington, DC: American Chemical Society, MEDI 54; Boyd, S. A., R. A. Mantei, C.-N. Hsiao and W. R. Baker. 1991. *J. Org. Chem.*, 56:438.

28 Bartlett, P. A. and W. B. Kezer. 1984. *J. Am. Chem. Soc.*, 106:4282 and references cited therein.

29 Giannousis, P. P. and P. A. Bartlett. 1987. *J. Med. Chem.*, 30:1603.

30 Ondetti, M. A. and D. W. Cushman. 1981. *J. Med. Chem.*, 24:355; Andrews, P. R., J. M. Carson, A. Caselli, M. J. Spark and R. Woods. 1985. *J. Med. Chem.*, 28:393; Godfrey, J. D., E. M. Gordon, D. Von Langen, J. Engebrecht and J. Plusec. 1986. *J. Org. Chem.*, 51:3073; Flynn, G. A., E. L. Giroux and R. C. Dage. 1987. *J. Am. Chem. Soc.*, 109:7914.

31 Williams, R. M. 1989. *Synthesis of Optically Active α-Amino Acids*. Oxford: Pergamon Press.

UTILIZATION OF
BIOACTIVE PEPTIDES

Synthetic Peptide-Based Vaccines and Antiviral Agents Including HIV/AIDS as a Model System

DAVID N. LEVY[1]
DAVID B. WEINER[1]

INTRODUCTION

VACCINATION, including vaccination against viral disease, has been one of the great triumphs of medicine in the past 200 years. Today, equipped with a maturing knowledge of immunity and of virus-host interactions and with modern analytical tools of biochemistry and molecular and cell biology we face the challenge of developing preventive therapies that are safer, less expensive, easier to prepare and store, and are more effective than their earlier counterparts. In addition, new vaccines are under development for other viral diseases, for diseases which we are only now recognizing as virally based, and for diseases with which mankind has only recently been confronted, such as AIDS.

This review will focus on the development of synthetic peptides as vaccines and as post-exposure antiviral agents. Such peptide sequences are derived from knowledge of the structures of proteins of viral or immune system origin. We will focus on the theoretical and practical considerations for developing peptide-based therapies and use specific model systems, mostly HIV/AIDS, to illustrate these points. The first section will deal with peptides as vaccines and the second section will deal with the budding field of peptides as inhibitors of virus infection or spread at the level of virus-receptor interaction. A separate chapter in this volume deals with peptides as inhibitors of viral functions within the host cell.

This work was supported in part by grants from AMFAR, the M. L. Smith Charitable Trust and the NIH.

[1]University of Pennsylvania School of Medicine and the Wistar Institute Biotechnology Center, Philadelphia, PA 19104, U.S.A.

The motivation for this chapter is not primarily the development of an anti-AIDS vaccine, nor is it to exhaustively review the immunology of the virus; the purpose is to discuss issues relating to the use of peptides in antiviral vaccines. Since many of the important current developments in vaccine design have used HIV as a model, much of this chapter is devoted to discussion of HIV and the immune response to it. With its ability to change rapidly, to destroy the immune system either directly or through trickery, to hide out in a dormant state in cell lineages, and to induce the destruction of nerve cells in the brain, HIV presents one of the most formidable challenge researchers have yet faced. With the demonstration that protective immunity against HIV is possible, at least in an animal model, the outlook for the development of an AIDS vaccine is more hopeful than anytime since the discovery of the disease. Peptide immunotherapy may play a role in any future AIDS vaccine. The lessons learned and yet to be learned in this system should have broad application to all aspects of vaccine development.

THE IMMUNE RESPONSE

In the early 1960s using Tobacco Mosaic Virus, Anderer first demonstrated that antibodies to a peptide fragment of a viral protein could neutralize infectivity of the virus [1]. In 1986 Townsend et al. [2], using influenza nucleoprotein, showed that antigen presenting cells incubated with small peptides can act as targets for T cell recognition, that in effect these peptides represent the minimal determinants for T cell recognition. They further demonstrated that a series of overlapping peptides can be used to map the T cell epitopes on the antigen. The T epitopes on many antigens [2,3] have been mapped using this procedure and this stands as an important advance in the understanding of immune response.

All vaccination strategies rely on a fundamental property of the immune system called immunologic memory. Upon reexposure to an antigen the memory, or anamnestic response, is swifter and stronger than the response produced by the initial challenge. This is characteristic of both the cellular and the antibody response. It is the augmented strength and rapidity of a memory response which protects us from diseases against which we have been vaccinated.

ANTIGEN PRESENTATION

Many of the recent advances in vaccine research have been based on an expanding understanding of the ways antigens are processed and recognized within the immune system. Antigens (Ag) are presented as processed protein fragments (peptides) in association with highly polymorphic major histocompatibility complex (MHC) molecules. Antigen presenting cells (APCs) display these MHC molecules in association with peptide Ag on their cell surface. T lymphocytes, which display clonal T cell receptors (TCRs) on their surface, recognize and bind specific Ag-MHC combinations. This recognition/binding event, the phenotype of the T cell activated (helper versus suppressor versus cytotoxic), and the antigen specificity of antibody binding are the keys to the specificity of the immune response.

The binding of the T cell with its cognate partner, the Ag-MHC-APC complex, sets in motion a cascade of subsequent immunologic functions performed by the T cell. These functions include the clonal expansion of the T cells, direct killing of virally infected cells by CD8$^+$ MHC class I restricted cytolytic T cells, and the induction of T cell help by CD4$^+$ MHC class II restricted T cells. Cytokine release by these T cells influences other immune cells, activating them and recruiting them into regions of inflammation.

There is a physical association of the peptide antigen with the MHC molecule. Class II molecules, (which are normally restricted in their expression to cells that specialize in antigen presentation such as B cells, macrophages and dendritic cells), generally present antigen that originates outside the cells. These exogenous antigens (such as protein-carrier complexes) are taken up by APCs, degraded in endocytic vesicles, and presented to CD4$^+$ T cells in association with class II molecules. Class II molecules but not class I molecules have been demonstrated to intersect with endocytic vesicles following biosynthesis within a lymphoblastoid cell line [4,5]. T cells displaying the CD4 antigen are generally of the T helper subset required for the maturation of effector populations such as antibody producing B cells and cytotoxic T lymphocytes (CTL). CD8$^+$ T cells, which generally carry cytotoxic or suppressor function, recognize antigen in the context of class I MHC molecules. Class I MHC molecules are found on most cells in the body and their function is mainly to present antigens made within the cell such as viral proteins. CD8$^+$ cytotoxic cells (CTL) rid the body of intracellular parasites by killing the antigen-tagged infected cells directly.

Antibody responses are due to B lymphocytes. Mature resting B cells bear surface immunoglobulin (sIg) molecules. A B cell binds its cognate antigen via sIg, internalizes the Ag-sIg complex, processes the antigen, and presents Ag-MHC (class I and class II) complexes on its surface. If the B cell is a memory cell then the antigen binding event is sufficient to generate production of immunoglobulin-secreting plasma cells. The generation of a primary B cell response leading to antibody secretion requires the induction of specific T cell help. T cell help is induced by the presentation of antigen to CD4⁺ T cells and the subsequent activation and expansion of them. This original presentation of Ag to the T cells may or may not be performed by the B cells themselves. In general, for an Ag to elicit an antibody response, it must possess both a B cell epitope (for surface Ig binding) and a T cell epitope (recognized as the Ag in the APC-Ag-MHC complex).

CONSIDERATIONS FOR VACCINE DESIGN

A vaccine should elicit a response from both the humoral (antibody) and cellular (cytotoxic T cell) arms of the immune system. Protective humoral immunity should include antibody responses which block vital functions (neutralize) and which target free virus and virally infected cells for destruction by the effector arms of the immune system including cytotoxic cells (CTL). One inherent disadvantage of many vaccine strategies that do not use live infectious virus as the immune stimulant is their relatively poor ability to elicit a cell mediated cytotoxic response. A soluble antigen coupled to one of the traditional carrier moieties can usually evoke a strong antibody response to the antigen, but under most circumstances cytotoxic cells will not be produced. This is believed to be due to the inability of free antigen normally to enter the class I presentation pathway. This failing has hindered the development of peptide-based vaccines for diseases in which a cytotoxic response is necessary for adequate protection. Recent developments in carrier and adjuvant design (discussed in a later section) suggest that these limitations may soon be overcome.

WHY PEPTIDES?

The use of peptides for prophylactic immunotherapy has been made practical by recent advances in immunology and biochemistry. First, the invention of solid-phase peptide synthesis by Merrifield [6] has allowed the wide scale use of peptides to map both T and B epitopes and the synthesis of the vaccines themselves. Second, the technology to molecularly clone and sequence genes and the ability to predict their protein sequence and even their structure in the absence of the protein itself has enabled the rapid determination of candidate epitopes. Third, the most recent discoveries of methods for increasing the antigenicity of peptides and for eliciting cytotoxic cellular responses with exogenous antigens has promised the development in the near future of peptide vaccines that are as effective as whole virus vaccines but carry an increased measure of safety.

Why bother with a peptide based vaccine (which is noninfectious and thus is "seen" as exogenous antigen) if *de novo* protein synthesis is necessary for the stimulation of class I restricted T cells? As the biological rules governing antigen presentation are becoming more clearly understood they are seen to be somewhat less absolute. Strategies are being developed to target antigens directly into the presentation pathway of choice, particularly to deliver exogenous antigens to the class I presentation pathway. The most important advantage of synthetic vaccines has to do with the opportunity to tailor the immune response. One can include in a vaccine extremely small and specific antigenic epitopes that elicit strong protective immune responses and not include other epitopes present in a live inoculum which might yield responses not useful or even detrimental to the vaccinated host. Inclusion of peptides representing regions conserved among many strains (regions which are perhaps not ordinarily very immunogenic) may confer broad protective immunity which would be impossible to induce with whole protein or virus.

Peptide based vaccines offer implicit safety. A virus-based vaccine must be grown as live virus in culture, a laborious, expensive, and potentially hazardous process. If live virus is used to immunize, then there are risks to the recipient associated with the resulting infection. The Sabin polio vaccine has occasionally caused the disease in the individuals it was designed to protect. During the 1970s the swine flu vaccine caused disease in some who were inoculated with it. Furthermore, a whole-virus vaccine preparation can carry antigens from the culture or animal strain in which it was grown. Cross-reactive immune responses induced by such preparations can have severe consequences for a subset of the vaccinated population. One side effect of the live rubella vaccine is the occasional occurrence of a rheumatoid arthritis–like syndrome observed in a small percentage of vaccinated women.

Despite these occasional outcomes, live attenuated vaccines have generally proven to be safe and effective in the population at large. But the use of vaccines which contain no live pathogen obviates all the hazards of infection with that organism. A peptide-based vaccine can be synthesized chemically, avoiding the necessity of viral culture. As a chemical rather than biological product a peptide-based vaccine can be made to great purity without such contaminants as DNA and other viral or cellular debris.

Peptide vaccines do suffer from some inherent disadvantages. A native protein molecule has a complex three-dimensional structure, often held together by intramolecular bonds and often covalently or noncovalently linked to other polypeptides. This secondary, tertiary, and quaternary structure may not be reproduced by small linear peptides. Antibody binding and the uptake of antigen by cells for presentation to immune cells is often dependent on these higher-order features of a protein. Thus a peptide is not always a good substitute for the authentic protein. Creating peptide immunogens that possess the characteristics of the native protein is not always an easy task, although the potential rewards are high.

PEPTIDES AS ANTIGENS AND IMMUNOGENS

ANTIGENICITY VERSUS IMMUNOGENICITY

Immunogenicity is the ability of an antigen to elicit a primary response in an animal and induce the production of memory cells. Antigenicity is the ability of an antigen to elicit a secondary response *in vitro* or *in vivo*. A vaccine must be immunogenic, i.e., elicit an immune response, for it to be protective.

CARRIERS

There have been reports where peptides in the absence of a carrier protein elicited antibody responses *in vivo* [7–12], but this is more the exception than the rule. In some cases it has been demonstrated that the peptide contained a T helper epitope which functioned as a carrier [8]. To render them immunogenic, peptides are typically coupled to a carrier molecule such as keyhole limpet hemocyanin (KLH) or tetanus toxoid (TT). The use of such strong immunogens as KLH is not practical in a human vaccine because repeated exposure to them may induce hyperimmunity. Antigens such as tetanus toxoid have been used in humans as carriers but here prior exposure to TT may reduce response to the peptide epitope (hapten) in a phenomenon called carrier induced suppression (7,13–17). Alternatively in some cases the strong antigenicity of the carrier can overwhelm the response to the hapten and the memory response is only to the carrier [18]. More importantly, when true pathogen exposure were to occur, the pathogen might not elicit a T cell response, as the carrier protein which elicited the original T cell response would not be present. Many other carrier moieties have been used, including T independent antigens such as Ficoll and synthetic polypeptides such as poly-(L-lysine). It has been shown that immunization first with free peptide followed by immunization with whole protein can induce a high level of response [18–20]. For a single administration antiviral vaccine the best strategy is to find T helper epitopes in viral proteins and include them in the vaccine.

Targeting antigen specifically to antigen presenting cells increases their antigenicity. Anti-Ig [21] and anti-class II [22] coupled to antigens have been shown by several groups to greatly improve the immunogenicity and/or antigenicity of various proteins. Less specific targeting methods for improving the response to antigens include the adjuvants. The use of adjuvants will not be discussed here in great detail as there have been several excellent reviews in the recent past [23–27], but there have been advances that are worth mentioning. Foremost among these can be broadly classified as the lipid micellar category. They include lipid micelles, liposomes, virosomes and so-called immune stimulating complexes or ISCOMs. Each has shown potential for increasing the antigenicity and immunogenicity of peptides *in vivo*. ISCOMs have received the greatest attention lately and are discussed in detail in a later section. The induction of class I restricted CTL is only the most recent success for ISCOMs, as they have been used in a variety of systems to increase both cellular and antibody responses.

MULTIMERIZATION

The size of a protein is a factor in determining its antigenicity and immunogenicity. Covalently linking peptides into multimeric structures has been used by several groups to increase their antigenicity [28]. The increased antigenicity may be the result of an increased ability of antigen presenting cells to "see" the multimeric structures. Antigen presenting cells such as macrophages may be better able to phagocytose and thus present peptides derived from large versus small molecules.

An elaborate system for multimerization of peptides is the multiple antigen peptide system (MAP) created by Tam [29,30]. The MAP is created by solid phase peptide synthesis. Trifunctional amino acids allow branched peptide structures; the number of peptides added is doubled by each additional level added. Antibodies generated using MAP antigen in mice and rabbits cross-reacted with native protein.

Multimerization allows the inclusion of separate epitopes for T and B cells on one structure. The inclusion of T helper epitopes increases the immunogenicity of the B epitopes without the need for a classical carrier. The presence of B epitopes probably in turn increases the antigenicity for T cells because antigen specific B cells are able to take up and present cognate antigen extremely efficiently. The invention of methods, discussed later in this chapter, for inducing class I restricted CTL with exogenous antigen *in vivo* makes practical the inclusion of CTL epitopes (Figure 9.1).

So far only the copolymerization of B with T helper epitopes has been reported [30–35] and in each case in which it was examined the antibody response to the antigen was stronger than to the B peptide alone. In some cases the response to copolymerized T and B epitopes was reported to be stronger than the response to the B peptide coupled to a classical carrier such as KLH [33]. In one report [32] the synthetic immunogen acquired a novel T epitope not present on either peptide. The production of new epitopes (T or B) by the combining of peptides from different regions of a protein or even different proteins may pose a problem for the usefulness of copolymerization of peptides. If these new epitopes are immunodominant over the genuine viral epitopes then the synthetic vaccine may have little or no advantage over the native protein. Cross-reactivity of the novel epi-

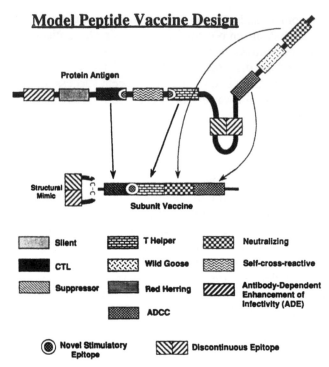

Figure 9.1 "Peptide vaccine design"—different types of antigenic determinants are represented by variously patterned boxes. Highly stylized protein shows all epitopes as separate regions, however in a real protein different types of epitopes often overlap. T epitopes: CTL, suppressor and T helper, must be linear epitopes, i.e., sequential or continuous. The remaining epitopes which are B cell epitopes, can be linear or discontinuous. The novel epitope is a linear epitope made of parts of two previously separate epitopes brought together in the vaccine. The subunit vaccine can, of course, be composed of sequences from different proteins.

topes with host proteins may induce autoimmunity. Another result that could foil the use of this technique would be the induction of novel T suppressor epitopes which might reduce response to the vaccine. Such potential consequences indicate that the combining of peptides should be a strategy that is adequately tested before use.

VIRAL STRATEGIES

Every virus has evolved strategies to avoid elimination by the immune system. These mechanisms are formidable obstacles to the development of antiviral vaccines. A nonexhaustive list would include the following (another list with additional categories can be found in Reference [36]): (1) infection via cell-cell contact, (2) latency, (3) epitope-dependent avoidance, and (4) immune modulation. Every virus probably employs one or several of these strategies (Table 9.1). Some viruses, including HIV, can spread from cell to cell directly via contact between the cellular membranes of the infected and uninfected cells. Cell-cell infection is much less vulnerable to inhibition by antibodies which neutralize free virus. Cell-cell infection by HIV appears immune from neutralizing antibody [37]. Viruses such as HIV and Epstein Barr Virus (EBV) can enter a latent phase of infection, expressing reduced levels of viral antigens in the infected cells, making immune surveillance more difficult.

The epitope-dependent avoidance tactics include:

a. Mutational evolution of viral proteins which are targets of neutralizing antibodies and of T cell responses. The natural variation in a virus can have a profound effect on the usefulness of a given epitope as an immune target. If there is a great diversity in a given region, no matter how well that epitope immunizes against one variant, antibody to it may be inneffective against others. Viruses such as HIV can mutate their antigenic proteins rapidly during infection and avoid defenses already in place. A neutralizing epitope that is immunogenic is under selective pressure by the immune system. If the neutralizing domain on the protein can withstand alterations in sequence and still yield viable virus then it can behave as a region of hypervariability. The immune

TABLE 9.1. "Viral Strategies"—Partial List of Strategies Viruses Are Known or Believed to Employ in Order to Avoid Elimination by the Host's Immune System. Those Strategies Known or Believed to Be Employed by HIV Are Preceded by a √.

Used by HIV:	
√	1. Infection via cell-cell contact
√	2. Latency
	3. Epitope-dependent avoidance
√	A. "Wild geese": mutational evolution
?	B. "Red herrings": immunodominant, nonneutralizing
?	C. "Canyons": sequestration of neutralizing epitopes
√	D. "Original antigenic sin"
√	E. "Redirection prevention"
	4. Immune Modulation
?	A. T suppression induction
√	B. Direct cytopathicity
√	C. Autoimmune and bystander killing
	D. Immune cell functional disruption
√	I) signalling via cell surface receptors
√	II) disruption of intracellular signaling
√	III) transacting disregulation

system may devote its efforts to an elusive target, a "wild goose" that can outrun the immune system through mutational evolution.

b. Display of immunodominant epitopes which are nonneutralizing. This kind can be called a "red herring" because responding to it provides no benefits to the host and may divert "attention" away from neutralizing epitopes.

c. Sequestration of neutralizing epitopes within pockets on the surface of viral proteins so that antibodies cannot bind them. The rhinovirus receptor-binding site is located in a pocket or "canyon" [38], which may allow a region with inherent structural constraints to avoid immune selective pressure.

d. "Original antigenic sin" [36,39], a paradoxical theory, in which a primary antibody response to a "wild goose" epitope prevents a neutralizing response to mutated versions of the neutralizing epitope.

e. "Redirection prevention" of the neutralizing response. Animals immunized with peptides from a region of the HIV-1 envelope called V3 (discussed later in this chapter) make antibodies which cross-react with other regions of the HIV-1 envelope [40] that do not mutate during infection at the high rate at which the V3 region does. In a theory related to the "original sin" model, continuous stimulation of B cells specific for V3, during infection with HIV, by these unchanging, nonneutralizing, cross-reactive regions "locks" the humoral response to the early specificities, preventing a redirected response to the emergent viruses' novel V3 sequences. This theory remains to be tested.

Among the immune modulatory strategies viruses have devised are: (a) viral epitopes that induce T suppressor cells; (b) infection and direct killing of immune cells; (c) induction of autoimmune and bystander killing of immune cells; and (d) modulation of immune cell function through various mechanisms. Immune modulatory mechanisms include: (1) modulation of cell proliferation through virus interaction with cell surface receptors; (2) interference with intracellular signaling pathways; and (3) genetic regulation of host gene expression such as class I expression, as has been demonstrated *in vitro* for HIV-infected fibroblasts [41]. What role each of these plays in the natural history of a given pathogen must be considered when designing strategies to interfere with the virus life cycle.

Where there is strain diversity it may be necessary to include in a vaccine sequences representing each variant. Whether the immune system makes a protective response against all epitopes included in a vaccine or whether some epitopes become immunodominant may have to be determined for each case. The precedent for this however is the Sabin polio vaccine where three strains are represented in one vaccine and together they induce complete protection.

B CELL RESPONSES

ROLE OF IMMUNOGLOBULIN

Antibodies have been considered the first line of defense against viruses. Antibody alone is sufficient to protect animals and humans from many viral diseases including polio in humans, murine leukemia virus induced leukemia in mice, and rabies in humans. Antibodies can protect from virus infection and virus-induced pathology by several mechanisms including blockade of virus entry, antibody-induced conformational changes in virus proteins required for infectivity, interference with proteins that exert pathogenic or immune suppressive effects, interference with virus maturation and budding, opsonization of viral particles for phagocytosis by macrophages and neutrophils, and antibody-dependent complement-mediated lysis and targeting for antibody dependent cellular cytotoxicity (ADCC) (role in HIV reviewed in Reference [42]) by T cells and natural killer (NK) cells. Different isotypes of antibodies mediate these effector functions and the ability of a given peptide and immunization protocol to induce the desired isotype classes must be determined experimentally. However, if a systemic IgG or IgM response is desired systemic immunization is required; if secretory IgA is desired for mucosal immunity local immunization is necessary. For the induction of an oral IgA response peptides incorporated into liposomes have shown some promise [43].

PREDICTION OF B CELL EPITOPES

There are theoretically three kinds of structures of B cell epitopes: sequential, continuous, and discontinuous. A sequential epitope is a contiguous series of amino acids recognized by antibody as a linear sequence. That is, only the primary structure of the protein is important for the response. A continuous epitope is one that is made up of a contiguous stretch of amino acids but is recognized by antibody in a conformation-dependent manner. A discontinuous epitope is constituted of amino acids from different regions of the protein which are brought together by the folding of the polypeptide chain or by the association of separate polypeptide chains. Most B cell epitopes on native proteins are not sequential but are dependent on conformation and are therefore continuous or discontinuous. In fact, evidence suggests that there may be no such thing as a purely sequential B cell epitope [44]. This creates a problem for the design of peptide-based immunization strategies since small peptides are not very good at mimicking three-dimensional structures, especially ones made up of bits from here and there in the native protein. However, a mixture of flexible linear immunogens would be expected to include some subset of the peptides in conformations similar to the native antigen. Importantly, many anti-sera and a significant proportion of antibodies to synthetic peptides cross-react with the native protein [45,46], though many possess lower affinity as compared with B cell responses to the native protein immunogen [47].

B cells produce antibodies to native (unprocessed) antigen and the primary requirement for a B epitope is that it be physically accessible to the antibody on the native protein. A protein in solution assumes many conformations and a given epitope may only need to be accessible for a fraction of the time for an antibody to bind there effectively. The various methods for predicting B cell antigenic sites has been reviewed elsewhere [47]. Briefly, estimation of surface accessibility [48] is one of the better predictors of B cell antigenicity. Several other methods of predicting B cell epitopes are just alternative ways of estimating how likely a portion of the protein resides on the outer surface. Polypeptide chain termini are often found on the outside of soluble proteins as are hydrophilic stretches. The method of Hopp and Woods [49] uses averages of hydrophilicity over discrete regions to predict primary antigenic sites using only primary sequence data.

Estimations of segment mobility have been used to predict B cell epitopes [50–52]. Though predictions of segmental mobility are restricted to proteins for which much structural data is already known [47], Tainer et al. have noted that peptides derived from regions with a high mobility coefficient were exceptionally good at inducing antibodies that cross-reacted with the native protein in solution [51,52]. Others have concluded that while mobility can predict cross-reactivity it is not a measure of antigenicity per se [47]. In practice the natural B cell epitopes of a protein are often determined empirically in antibody binding assays (ELISA or RIA) against immune sera with the use of overlapping peptides that span most or protein. The theoretical and empirical methods outlined above only account for sequential epitopes or continuous epitopes or ones with large areas that are dependent on contiguous residues; they do not locate discontinuous epitopes. For the identification of discontinuous epitopes, mutation studies and x-ray crystallography are necessary. As studies by Westof et al. [50] and Berzofsky and colleagues [53,54] point out, antibodies that bind protein subunits represent only a fraction of those made against the whole protein, underlining the importance of tertiary and quaternary structure for high affinity antibody reactivity.

The practical and theoretical considerations involved in designing peptides which elicit antibodies that cross-react with the native protein have been extensively reviewed elsewhere (for example, References [45,55]) and will only be discussed briefly here. Most importantly the peptide must be soluble in aqueous solution and so should contain hydrophilic polar residues [46]. Such regions of the protein are also likely to be on the surface and accessible to antibodies. Proline residues located in such hydrophilic stretches form kinks or corners which are likely to be exposed at the surface of the protein. The imide bonds of proline residues allow the local conformation to be more rigidly fixed than usual and this may contribute to enhanced cross-reactivity between peptide and native protein.

The peptide must be at least of a minimal length which has been found to be on the order of six residues [46] in some instances and 15 to 20 in others [47]. Longer peptides are usually at least as good as shorter peptides at eliciting antibodies that react with the native protein [46]. Even though peptides of 20 or so residues are not able to completely adopt tertiary structures, they may assume partial or local character, and this may be the reason for increased antibody reactivity of longer peptides. Longer peptides can often include a T helper cell epitope that is near or overlaps a B cell epitope, as in the HIV envelope, and Influenza Virus H5 Hemagglutinin [56], or as is the case for Hepatitis B core antigen. T cell epitopes for different MHC haplotypes may themselves overlap [57]. As discussed above, inclusion of viral-derived helper epitopes would eliminate the need for a classical carrier molecule [30–34,57] and allow the development of specific memory T responses to the virus.

It has historically been the practice to find antigenic regions of a viral protein and assume these are the best candidates for a vaccine. This may not always be the best approach. Highly immunogenic sites can be missed when screening with short peptides, and those found may be nonneutralizing or highly variable. Other sites which are less immunogenic on the native protein might confer protection if they can be rendered antigenic through immunization strategies. Highly conserved stretches are likely to possess functionally important domains such as receptor binding sites or structural framework regions. Blocking or disrupting such sites with antibodies can have profound effects on viral functions. The ability of functionally important sites to remain relatively or absolutely unchanged among isolates despite immune responses to the protein as a whole may indicate that these sites are not highly immunogenic on the native protein to B or to T cells, or are otherwise sheltered from the immune response.

The fact that antibodies are usually not made to a particular region of a native protein does not mean that a response to that region can not be induced if it is presented to the immune system in a proper form and context. It has been demonstrated that there is a hierarchy of immunodominance among B cell epitopes such that if the major immunodominant epitope of a protein is removed antibodies are then made to regions that had previously been immunorecessive. What this implies for vaccine design is that memory cells elicited by a peptide mimic of a recessive region may be able to respond to that region on the native protein, and by extension, the virus. Memory B cells require less stimulation to produce immunoglobulin than virgin B cells. Whether such antibodies are able to function *in vivo* as mediators of an antiviral response can only be known empirically on a case by case basis. If the immune system can be "redirected" to a neutralizing but normally immunosilent region then broad protective immunity to the pathogen might be achieved.

Examples of such redirection are provided by immunogenicity studies of HIV-1. Rabbit serum against a synthetic peptide to an immunosilent region of the HIV-1 envelope protein gp120 spanning amino acids 254 to 274 has been reported to neutralize virus infectivity at fairly high titer (1:64 to 1:256) and to "mediate ADCC against HIV coated cells" [58]. While this region would provide a rigorous test of the theory that a neutralizing antibody response can be redirected to immunosilent domains, recently the ability of peptides to this region to induce neutralizing antibody, or even antibody that reacts with native envelope protein, has been questioned [59].

A potential variation on the above theory is provided by a region of HIV-1 gp120 that is believed to be the region of contact with the cognate receptor for HIV-1, the CD4 molecule. Antibodies to this region have been alternatively reported to inhibit CD4 binding [60,61] and to neutralize divergent strains [60] or to not neutralize [62]. The latter case involves serum raised against a peptide and so the failure of the antibody to neutralize might be explained by a possible inability of the particular peptide to generate antibody with sufficiently high affinity to neutralize. The relative affinity of this serum was not examined. While this region of the envelope does in fact induce an antibody response in infected individuals, the neutralizing antibody present in HIV positive individuals is largely directed to the hypervariable V3 loop. If an anti-peptide response can elicit neutralizing antibodies to the 120-CD4 contact region, immunization with the peptide might redirect the secondary immune response such that upon challenge with virus *in vivo*, neutralizing rather than nonneutralizing antibody to this region would be produced.

MODIFICATION OF PEPTIDES TO ENHANCE B CELL RESPONSES

Peptides which cover only part of an antibody contact region often can bind anti-whole protein antibodies to that region. This may be due in part to the ability of antibodies specific for a given tertiary structure to "fold" an unconstrained short peptide into a binding conformation. If short peptides are used to map *in vivo* B cell responses to the virus the full extent of the genuine epitope might be missed. The antibodies are likely to bind the native protein with higher affinity than the peptide. The converse is usually true: antibodies against peptides may bind with low affinity to the native protein, but this is for a different reason. That reason has to do with the fact that peptides in solution are less constrained than the native protein. They may assume many conformations which do not represent the appearance of the native protein. Antisera made against these peptides may have highest affinity for conformations not assumed by the native protein and thus have low neutralizing titers. Thus, the ability of a peptide to react with immune sera against the native protein or whole virus is not a reliable predictor that antibodies raised against the peptide will bind the native protein. Each peptide must be tested for its ability to induce Ab that cross-react with high affinity with the intact virus or viral protein.

Attempts to increase the cross-reactivity of peptide and virus have focused on two broad strategies: stabilizing the peptide structure through intramolecular bonds and producing conformational mimics through structural analysis and comparative model building [14].

Bidart et al. [63] report success in immunizing against a conformational epitope present on human choriogonadotropin (hCG) with a synthetic peptide. (The goal is to make an anti-fertility vaccine.) This epitope was defined by an hCG specific monoclonal antibody whose binding site was a discontinuous (quarternary structural) epitope covering amino acids on both the α and β subunits of hCG. Synthetic peptides were constructed whose linear sequence was composed of amino acids from the α subunit on the amino end and sequence from the β subunit on the carboxyl end of the peptide (ex. hCGα(43–49)-hCGβ(110–116)-tetanus toxoid). When immunized into rabbits antibody resulted that did not cross-react with the structurally related hormone human leutropin but did bind native hCG.

A discussion of the use of antibody hypervariable regions as templates for the design of structurally constrained peptides is found in Chapter 3 of this volume [64].

VIRUS NEUTRALIZATION: HIV-1 V3 DOMAIN

Effective neutralizing antibodies for HIV-1 are directed against the envelope proteins [61,65–68]. The protein product of the env gene of HIV-1, gp160, is cleaved to form the two mature viral envelope proteins: gp41, the transmembrane glycoprotein, and gp120, the external glycoprotein (Figures 9.2 and 9.3). In the mature retroviral particle, gp120 is noncovalently attached to gp41. HIV-1 gp120 contains the binding domain for the CD4 molecule, the primary cellular receptor for HIV [69]. Most antibodies which neutralize HIV-1 infectivity map to a region of gp120 between amino acid residues 301 and 341 called the V3 loop or major neutralizing determinant (MND) [70,71]. The V3 domain is a loop formed by bonded cysteines. It is a region of significant diversity, up to 50% variation [72] in

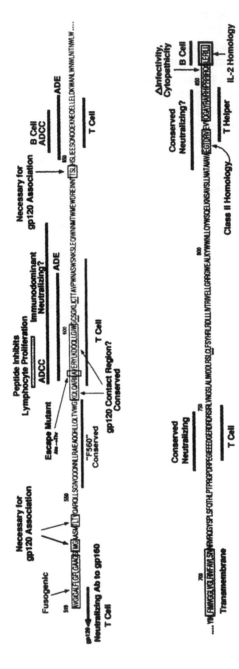

Figure 9.2 "HIV-1 gp120 epitopes" — linear amino acid sequence of HIV-1 external protein gp120 with mapped antibody and T cell responses represented with solid lines. These data represent *in vivo* responses to infection with HIV-1 and/or envelope protein(s) alone in various species. Regions of gp120 with known or putative function are labeled. Amino acid numbers are in small type next to sequence. ADCC: antibody-dependent cellular cytotoxicity. CTL cytotoxic T lymphocyte epitope.

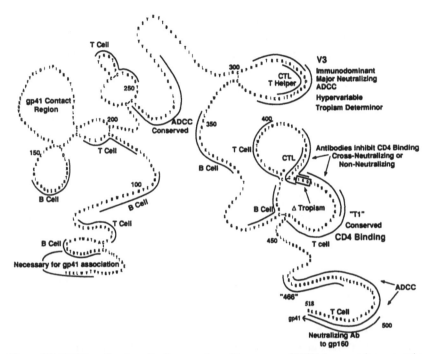

Figure 9.3 "HIV-1 gp41 epitopes"—linear amino acid sequence of HIV-1 transmembrane protein gp41 with mapped antibody and T cell responses represented with solid horizontal bars above and below the sequence, respectively. These data represent *in vivo* responses to infection with HIV-1 and/or envelope protein(s) alone in various species. Very long indicator lines represent compilation of data from several studies. Regions of gp41 with known or putative function are shown with boxes around the amino acid sequence. Amino acid numbers are in small type above sequence. ADE: antibody-dependent enhancement of infection. ADCC: antibody-dependent cellular cytotoxicity. Disulfide structure of gp120 was derived by C. K. Leonard and colleagues [225].

amino acid sequence between isolates, though recent studies have demonstrated a somewhat more constrained diversity among most isolates [73]. Neutralizing antibodies to the V3 domain inhibit syncytium formation and virus fusion but do not inhibit CD4-gp120 binding [74]. The CD4 binding domain on gp120 resides elsewhere, roughly between amino acids 420 and 450 [61,75]. Mutation studies have confirmed a requirement for an intact V3 loop in fusion events but not virus binding [76,77]. The exact role the V3 loop plays in infection is unknown; it appears to function in determining cell tropism of HIV-1 isolates [78]. It has been postulated that the loop may be directly or indirectly involved in fusion with the cell membrane [76]. It also has been shown that the V3 loop may be the target of a cellular protease [79–81]. In this model cleavage of the V3 loop induces a conformational change in the envelope protein which facilitates virus entry. These two models are not, of course, mutually exclusive.

There is intense interest in the role of anti-V3 antibodies in the course of HIV infection and disease progression. Following infection of humans and chimps, concomitant with the reduction in viremia, early antibodies that neutralize virus possess high type-specific activity against the V3 region. Over the course of infection variants mutated in the V3 region appear. The ability of the virus to escape early immune responses may hinge on mutations which reduce neutralization by antibodies to the MND [82]. The demonstration that changes in sequence outside the V3 loop can abrogate V3-dependent neutralization [82,83] suggests a conformational dependence for the antibody recognition. Within the first one or two years following infection more broadly neutralizing antibodies appear which are generally of lower titer than the early antibodies.

Since anti-V3 antibodies can neutralize both cell-free infection [71] and syncytium formation [71,84] (the latter assay taken as an indirect, though imperfect [77], measure of the potential for direct cell-cell spread of infection), the potential benefits of a strong anti-V3 response are high. Type-specific neutralizing antibodies can be elicited in animals using synthetic peptides from the MND [33,62,67,71,84–88]. One notable report [33] demonstrates that neutralizing antibodies can be made in goats inoculated with a polyvalent immunogen comprised of peptides of the MND and the T helper site T1. A memory T cell proliferative response to the native gp120 protein was induced with this peptide.

An important caveat was reported by Berman et al. [89] who protected chimpanzees from infection with HIV-1 by immunizing them with HIV-1 gp120. Chimpanzees were immunized with recombinant gp120 or recombinant gp160 in aluminum hydroxide adjuvant. The animals receiving gp120 or gp160 made antibody responses that neutralized infectivity of the immunizing strain *in vitro*, though the neutralizing titer and the titer of antibodies to the V3 loop from the gp120 recipients was significantly higher than that from the gp160 recipients. All animals had lymphoproliferative responses to gp120 *in vitro*. After three immunizations the gp120 recipients (but not the gp160 recipients) were protected from infection with the immunizing strain of HIV-1. The correlation between anti-V3 titer and protection is highlighted by the observation that one gp120 recipient with a low anti-gp120 titer nevertheless had the highest anti-V3 response and was protected from infection.

The inability of gp160 to protect the chimpanzees from infection may or may not be due to the relative inability to induce an anti-V3 response. As the authors suggest "it is possible that the neutralizing antibodies elicited by gp160 are protective, but that a second factor abrogates their effect." The authors suggest that antibodies to other regions of the envelope (such as gp41) might interfere with the ability to generate neutralizing antibodies to the V3 loop through antigenic competition with immunodominant regions in gp41. Such competing regions might be simply much more antigenic or they might be in close proximity to the neutralizing epitope(s), in which case antibody bind to the nonneutralizing region might sterically hinder binding to the neutralizing epitope, as has been shown to happen in another viral system [90]. Another possibility is that anti-gp41 antibodies might enhance infection *in vivo*, as has been demonstrated *in vitro* for HIV-1 in general [91,92], or for HIV-1 gp41 specifically [93]. (For a review of antibody enhancement of viral infection see Reference [94].) Finally, protection may be in part or wholly dependent on cellular immunity.

The implications for peptide-based vaccines (and anti-HIV vaccines in general) are several. First, protective immunity is possible against HIV, at least against a homologous strain in a nonhuman animal model. Second, protection against a retrovirus was induced by a subunit vaccine; live or killed whole virus was not necessary. Third, the related observations that gp120 but not gp160 was able to elicit protection and that anti-V3 titer correlated with protection underscores the fact that the context in which an immunogenic determinant is presented to the immune system can be vital to the success of the vaccination. Since gp120 is a subunit of gp160 and not vice versa, something present in gp160 inhibited the protection inducing epitope(s) in gp120 from inducing protection against infection *in vivo*. If that something is an epitope that induces counterproductive antibodies or effector cells, then such an epitope should be excluded from a vaccine.

The major dilemma with including the V3 region in a vaccine concerns its great sequence diversity among isolates from different individuals and among separate isolates from single HIV positive individuals. Antibodies against one V3 region rarely neutralize other virus isolates. (In the chimp study discussed above, there was no demonstration that the animals were protected from infection with divergent strains of virus. But there was also no conclusive demonstration that anti-V3 antibodies were important in protection from infection *in vivo*.) There has been shown to be very high conservation of a small region at the tip of the loop consisting of the β-turn sequence GPGR, but antibody binding to this region can be abrogated by alterations in primary sequence outside the GPGR region [82,83,95,96].

Recently it was reported that diverse isolates of HIV-1 can be neutralized by sera from guinea pigs immunized with V3-derived peptides [88]. Antibody binding was found to be directed to a six amino acid region — GPGRAF — that is conserved among those isolates neutralized by the antisera. Neutralization was not affected by sequences outside this region. So far this is the only demonstration that a dominant response can be made to such a small and conserved region within an otherwise highly variable landscape. Whether this fortunate outcome is a result of the use of guinea pigs rather than some other animal model such as mice or rabbits (or monkeys, chimps, or humans) is not clear but seems possible. An important implication of this work is that if an antibody response can be directed to the small relatively conserved sequence GPGRAF using a peptide vaccine containing this sequence, then a human host might be effectively immunized against a wide variety of HIV-1 strains. It must be added, however, that many natural isolates of HIV-1 do not carry the GPGRAF determinant and would not be neutralized by such antibodies. Extensive studies of the natural variation in the MND found *in vivo* [73] have confirmed that while there is great variation in the V3 loop, there is a prevalence of certain sequences *in vivo* that were not reflected by earlier *in vitro* studies. This includes a wide prevalence of the GPGRAF sequence in naturally occurring isolates. However, any truly universal vaccine is likely to carry multiple determinants representing several HIV-1 types [97].

There is a high (ca. 60–80%) seroreactivity among patients to the MN strain of HIV-1 (which contains the GPGRAF epitope) [98]. Some studies [99] have suggested that fast replicating types (such as MN) *in vivo* are responsible for early seroconversion while other variants are responsible for viral escape from neutralization. According to one scenario [99], in an infected individual antibodies to the V3 region of these MN-like types successfully neutralize the virus during the early stages of infection. In this scheme, escape mutants than come to predominate but are slow growing or latent and do not cause much overt pathology [100]. The mechanism(s) of the immune destruction are still not well understood (reviewed in References [100–103]) but may result at least in part through autoimmune ([104] and references therein) and bystander killing of uninfected cells [105,106] and direct cytopathicity [101–103] by the virus. When the antibody titer and cellular immunity are sufficiently weakened, the virus is free to produce fast replicating MN-like types and expand again. At this point the second acute or terminal phase begins. If this scenario proves correct then it will be important to define the exact mechanisms of viral escape, to see if there are prevalences among these escape variants as there have been shown to be among the fast replicating types and to incorporate epitopes from them in a vaccine.

OTHER HIV B CELL EPITOPES

There are several other regions on HIV-1 gp160 that are targets of B cell responses (reviewed in References [107–109]). Only a limited number have been demonstrated to induce anti-viral immunity. Ab that bind at or near the putative CD4 contact region (ca. 415–440) have been reported to inhibit [60,61,110] or not to inhibit [60,111,112] gp120-CD4 binding. Antibodies that block gp120-CD4 attachment do not always neutralize infectivity

[60,110]. Reports of neutralizing antibody to this region show neutralization across types due to the sequence conservation within this functional region. Peptides to the CD4 binding site are prime candidates for inclusion in a vaccine, particularly since a T helper epitope (TI) has been found at this site [33]. This region is not easily mimicked by small linear peptides. Back et al. [113] found that antibodies that inhibit HIV-1 gp160-CD4 binding could not be mapped with synthetic peptides.

It is important to point out that, as for other proteins [44], many epitopes (such as the CD4 binding region [113]) on HIV proteins are likely to be conformation-dependent, and not well mimicked by small linear peptides. Most studies mapping the antigenicity of HIV envelope have used small peptides. These studies are likely to be at least partially misleading as to the true nature of the immune response to the envelope during infection and as to the potential antigenicity and neutralization capacity of conformation-dependent epitopes. This issue is particularly important given the extreme diversity in linear sequence observed in some regions of gp160, for this diversity may be hiding possible conservation of structural conformations important for preservation of function (such as interactions with other proteins). Constraints on function leading to conservation of epitopes may lead to antibodies with broad neutralization potential. To this point, Steimer et al. [114] and Ho et al. [115] have described human antibodies directed to conformational epitopes with HIV-1 gp120 that neutralize infection by diverse HIV-1 isolates. The use of such epitopes, or of peptides conformationally constrained to mimic such epitopes, in a vaccine might induce an antibody response which neutralizes many isolates and also reduces the chances of immune escape by the virus.

Weiner, Kieber-Emmons, and colleagues [116,117] have analyzed the humoral immune response of HIV-1 infected individuals to long peptides (20 + a.a. average length). Several epitopes were found to be preferentially recognized in patients with high anti-syncytial, high neutralizing activity. A synthetic peptide ("466") induced neutralizing antibodies and antisyncytial activity against several isolates. Structural studies demonstrated that the 466 epitope can fold into a reverse β-turn structure. Fine mapping of the turn region demonstrates that the response is chiefly to the top of the loop. Such conformation-dependent epitopes have clear importance in vaccine design.

The benefits of inducing responses to multiple epitopes is demonstrated by the studies of this group [118]. They found that anti-syncytial activity was greatly enhanced by combining the reactivities to different peptides within gp120 and gp41. Anti-466 sera in combination with anti-V3 peptide sera yielded an antisyncytial activity synergistically greater than that observed with either alone. A peptide to gp41 ("560") induced antibodies that had no anti-viral activity alone, but in combination with anti-V3 peptide sera gave increased anti-syncytial and neutralizing activity.

HIV-1 gp41 shows additional promise for vaccine strategies. At least four distinct neutralizing or ADCC epitopes have been mapped on the molecule and each significantly overlaps a reported T epitope [107,119]. This phenomenon of coincidence T and B epitopes has also been observed for other proteins including myoglobin [120] and Foot and Mouth Disease Virus protein VP1 [8,121]. The significance of this phenomenon remains to be determined. The segment of gp41 adjacent to the F560 epitope described above, corresponding to amino acids ca. 580–600, is particularly interesting. The epitope is relatively conserved and overlaps a known T cell epitope. Gallaher et al. [122] show that this region is likely to form an amphipathic α-helix. gp41 580–630 constitutes the immunodominant epitope of gp41 [123]. It has been reported that there is a correlation between the presence of antibodies to the immunodominant epitope on gp41 and lack of clinical disease symptoms [124], although this finding has been disputed [125]. Human monoclonal antibodies to this region have been reported to enhance HIV-1 infection *in vitro* via their complement receptors [93].

A series of studies describes an antibody-neutralization escape mutant with a single amino acid change within this domain (ala^{582} to thr^{582}) [126–128]. Based on their recent studies the authors suggest that the region surrounding this sequence is not the binding site for neutralizing antibodies [128]. Because of the inability of anti-peptide sera to this region to neutralize, the failure of these peptides to block infectivity or syncytium inhibition by neutralizing antibodies, and the fact that other mutations in this region produced noninfectious virus, they postulate that the 582 A → T mutation affects the conformation of a neutralizing structural epitope distal to the mutation. Because it is not shown whether antibodies to these peptides are capable of binding the gp41 with high affinity, it is possible that short linear peptides do not reflect the conformational structure present on the native molecule sufficiently to yield conclusive results about the neutralization capacity of antibodies to this region. In fact, their studies indicate that the 580–600 epitope is highly conformation-dependent [128].

Clearly, this conserved epitope represents an area of functional significance for the virus. There is sequence similarity in this region with the transmembrane proteins of other retroviruses. Peptides to this region from various retroviruses, including HIV-1, inhibit lymphoproliferation. One group has demonstrated that a peptide from this region binds CD4$^+$ cells, suggesting that this domain may be a receptor for a non-CD4 cellular protein [129]. For inclusion in a vaccine this epitope is obviously problematic. If it truly is a neutralization target it may be so only in combination with other specificities [128], as is the contiguous F560 region. Suggestively, F560 and the 582 region are predicted to be part of the same α-helical structure on gp41 [122].

An area of the gp41 molecule that might elicit antibodies detrimental to the host is found at the carboxyl terminus (a.a. 837–844 EGTDRVI) that has homology with a portion of the β-chain of all human class II molecules (NGTERVR) [130]. It has been reported that about one-third of HIV seropositive patients make antibodies to this region of gp41 [130,131]. Murine antibodies to this peptide inhibit class II-dependent T cell responses. The murine sera and peptide-reactive patient sera could mediate ADCC against class II-expressing cells. This epitope is a good candidate for exclusion from any anti-viral vaccine. Another region of class II similarity has been reported within gp120 [132].

T CELL RESPONSES

The induction of class II restricted T cell help can be achieved with classical carrier moieties or by including in the immunizing complex T helper epitopes from other proteins, including those of the pathogen itself. It is of utility to include epitopes derived from T cell epitopes elicited by natural infection. Predicting such immunodominant T cell epitopes would therefore be useful.

PREDICTION OF T EPITOPES

There are several factors governing which regions of a protein serve as T cell epitopes. These include: (1) the composition of the peptides produced by proteolytic cleavage within the cell, (2) how the protein and the peptide fragments are directed within the cellular trafficking system: whether the peptide fragment and MHC pathways converge, (3) the ability of the peptide to bind the MHC molecule for presentation to T cells, and (4) the repertoire of T cells in the body: there must be a T cell with a receptor that binds the peptide-MHC ligand.

Since the T epitope is a proteolytic fragment of an antigen (a peptide), it need not come from the protein's exposed surface but can be derived from residues anywhere on the protein. Likewise, the protein need not appear on the surface of the pathogen but can come from within it. T epitopes are sequential, since they must survive the reducing conditions of intracellular processing. T cell receptors bind the dual complex of the processed antigen (peptide) bound to MHC molecules. Based on x-ray crystallographic studies of class I molecules it is widely accepted that the peptide lies in a pocket or groove on the apical end of the MHC molecule. In theory, detailed knowledge of the structure of this peptide receptacle [133] might allow predictions, in an MHC allele-specific manner, of regions of a protein likely to fit. This would allow predictions of sites on proteins likely to function as T epitopes.

Outbred populations such as humans carry different alleles of the MHC class I and II molecules with varying affinities for any given peptide. Using HIV gag and pol peptides Frelinger and colleagues examined the ability of 102 peptides to bind purified human class I proteins [134]. They found that most of the gag or pol peptides did not bind any class I proteins but that all five of five known gag peptides could bind at least one class I protein. They also found that those peptides that bound one class I molecule were likely to bind others as well, though analysis of peptide binding to MHC *in vitro* is not necessarily a predictor of successful MHC-restricted presentation by cells [135]. It can be the case that a peptide that can be presented by one MHC haplotype may not be presented well by another MHC haplotype; thus a peptide can be a T cell epitope for one haplotype and not for another [136]. This phenomenon must be reckoned with when designing peptide-based vaccines for use in outbred populations such as humans. If T cell epitopes cannot be found that are used by many MHC haplotypes then several T cell epitopes should be incorporated in the vaccine.

Though T cell epitopes can be derived from regions of a protein that do not lie on the surface of the native structure, not all regions of the protein possess the required characteristics for successful presentation to, and stimulation of, T cells. On those proteins which have been extensively mapped, not only does there seem to be a very limited number of T cell epitopes [137], but there is to date no evidence that a peptide can prime for a secondary response to a previously silent area. To the contrary, the literature indicates that peptides from regions that are not T epitopes on the native protein cannot prime for a T cell response [137,138]. The use of peptides is thus an even more useful and important tool for determining T epitopes than for determining B epitopes.

Townsend et al. [2] first demonstrated that CTL epitopes can be located using target cells incubated with synthetic peptides, and this has become the method of choice for CTL epitope mapping. Mapping of CTL epitopes is done in much the same way as for T helper cell epitopes but with the experimental readout being target cell killing instead of proliferation or cytokine release. The CTL response is usually class I restricted.

Berzofsky and De Lisi [139] have made the observation that many T cell epitopes come from regions of a protein that have a high theoretical probability of forming amphipathic helices. These regions are stretches of amino acids that are predicted to form α-helices with predominately hydrophilic residues on one face and predominately hydrophobic residues on the other. They reason that these structures are suited to interact with the MHC molecule. They have used this observation to predict with fairly good success where T epitopes will be found in several proteins [34,140], including HIV gp120 [141].

Rothbard and Taylor [142] has developed a method for predicting T epitopes that look for the sequence motif of "C or G/H/H/C or P" where C = charged, G = Glycine, H = Hydrophobic, and P = polar. Bastin et al. [3] have used this method to predict CTL epitopes within the influenza nucleoprotein. There are clearly limitations to these predictive algorithms as there are cases where T cell epitopes reside in areas not predicted by the methods of Berzofsky and of Rothbard. However, these algorithms serve as useful tools for investigating T cell immunity [143].

Two other methods for predicting T epitopes have been applied to the HIV proteins. Claverie et al. [144] have predicted HIV-1 gag epitopes by finding tetrapeptide clusters within gag that are not found within a set of known host proteins. Choppin, J. P. Levy and colleagues have employed a technique called the peptide binding assay [145] to evaluate the binding of synthetic peptides from HIV protein sequences to MHC molecules *in vitro*. By this method they have successfully predicted the known epitopes for several HIV proteins [146,147]. Since MHC binding is a necessary but not sufficient condition for antigen presentation, only a subset (though rather large subset) of peptides which are found to bind MHC molecules in this assay are known to be genuine T epitopes [135]. However, it appears that few actual T epitopes are missed by such analysis [146,147]. This method may prove useful in determining novel T epitopes for inclusion in peptide vaccines.

CLASS I PRIMING

MHC class II restricted T (helper) cell epitopes are generally derived from exogenous antigens which are endocytosed into endosomal compartments for processing and association with class II molecules. In contrast, MHC class I restricted epitopes typically arise from endogenously synthesized antigens. When a class I restricted CTL response is sought, not only must the proper target antigen be used, but provision must be made for its ending up in the class I presentation pathway. The use of peptide vaccines to stimulate class I restricted CTL is contingent on an ability to prime *in vivo* for class I presentation with exogenous antigen. Presentation of free peptides on class I molecules *in vitro* does not require intracellular processing and the association with MHC molecules can occur at the cell surface. *In vivo*, however, concentrations of antigen are not high enough to demonstrate direct binding to MHC for stimulation of T cells.

Proteins are synthesized in the endoplasmic reticulum. Association of peptide fragments of newly synthesized proteins with class I molecules is believed to occur in the endoplasmic reticulum [148]. Moore et al. [149]

and Yewdell and colleagues [150,151] has shown that exogenous proteins may be presented to class I restricted T cells if the antigen can gain access to the cytosolic compartment of the cell. The technologies for delivering vaccine antigen to the class I presentation pathway will be discussed later in the chapter.

It is the general case that free antigens fail to elicit *in vivo* any CTL response. However, there have been reports of exogenous antigens (including peptides) being presented by class I molecules *in vivo* [151–155]. A recent report describes the ability of antigen-specific B cells to present HBenvAg to class I restricted CTL [156]. Whether this capability is inherent to some B cells or is a factor intrinsic to the antigen is not known. Barnaba et al. [156] point out that HBenvAg is synthesized as a transmembrane protein and contains membrane lipid, which they believe may facilitate fusion of antigen with the target cell membrane. Thus the authors postulate that antigen-specific B cells may focus the antigen with their immunoglobulin receptors at the cell surface where the lipid on the antigen can mediate entry into the cell cytoplasm.

Researchers have demonstrated that certain antigens are capable of inducing CTL *in vivo*. Aichele et al. [138] describes the priming of class I restricted CD8+ CTL *in vivo* by a free synthetic peptide of *Lymphocytic Choriomeningitis* Virus (LCMV) in mice. Using chicken ovalbumin (OVA), Carbone and Bevan [157] have demonstrated that native chicken ovalbumin can prime *in vivo* for OVA-specific CTL when introduced in a cell-associated form. Chicken ovalbumin contains a putative targeting sequence which may play a role in directing ovalbumin to an intracellular pathway convergent with the class I presentation pathway. Indeed, an OVA tryptic digest can prime CTL *in vivo* [155,157], though free native ovalbumin fails to do so. In one case [157] it was shown that the minimal sequence necessary to induce CTL contained the putative targeting sequence.

Previous work from Bevan [158], and others [13], indicates that cell-associated antigens can prime *in vivo* class I restricted responses, perhaps by being presented by APC that have phagocytosed *in vivo* the cells that contain the antigen in question. The work of Bevan and Carbone also demonstrated [157,159] that the ability of a peptide to induce primed CTL response *in vitro* is not a predictor of whether that peptide can prime *in vivo*. This situation is analogous to that for B cells. But the inability of a peptide to prime *in vivo* for CTL recognition may simply reflect an inability of the naked peptide to reach the class I presentation pathway. The inclusion of a protein trafficking signal sequence in a peptide might in theory target the antigen to the class I presentation pathway.

Attempts to create a vaccine that can prime CTL *in vivo* have focused on coupling peptides to other moieties that presumably direct the immunogen to an intracellular destination where it can be presented to class I restricted cells. The exact method of action of these conjugates are not known, however. Deres et al. [160] have generated class I restricted CTL *in vivo* against influenza nucleoprotein using a synthetic lipoprotein construct. The vaccine consisted of a synthetic influenza peptide conjugated to a lipoprotein (P3CSS or Braun's lipoprotein) derived from *E. coli* bacteria. P3CSS directs attachment to cell membranes and is believed to mediate entry of the antigen into the cytoplasm of the antigen presenting cell. The peptide-lipoprotein construct was preincubated with syngeneic spleen cells *in vitro* and injected into mice. A control influenza peptide unconjugated to lipoprotein did not elicit a response. This indicates it is possible to prime an antiviral CTL response *in vivo* with synthetic peptide.

When the immunogen of Deres et al. [160] can prime *in vivo* when injected in a cell-free form was not addressed. It is possible that the phenomenon they report is similar to the one Carbone and Bevan observed using cells incubated *in vitro* with chicken ovalbumin. Whether the antigen is targeted to the class I presentation pathway of the *in vitro* APC which then presents *in vivo* to class I restricted T cells or whether the *in vitro* targets act as vesicles that are phagocytosed by other APC *in vivo* is not clear.

A strategy for increasing the antigenicity of proteins has proven capable of priming CD8$^+$ CTL *in vivo*. Immunostimulating complexes (ISCOMs) [161–165] are microspheres of the adjuvant glycoside Quil A surrounding the antigenic protein. Takahashi and colleagues have demonstrated that a single subcutaneous immunization with ISCOMs containing either HIV-1 envelope or influenza hemagglutinin can prime mice for a class I restricted CTL response *in vitro* [168]. Complement depletion experiments demonstrated that primed CD8$^+$ cells are required for the *in vitro* response, indicating that the response is not due to primary *in vitro* induction of CD8$^+$ cells with *in vivo*-primed CD4$^+$ T cell help.

Because of their demonstrated ability to elicit MHC class II restricted T cell responses, as well as class I restricted CTL responses *in vivo*, ISCOMs and lipopeptide conjugates show much promise for use in future peptide antiviral vaccines. Why they work is not clear, but one mode of action may be protection and prolongation of the life of the antigen *in vivo*. ISCOMs, lipopeptide conjugates, and liposomes all contain large fractions of lipid and this may be the most important factor in their activity. Lipid can mediate the attachment of these vesicles to cell surfaces. Liposomes can fuse with the cell surface and deliver their contents to the cytoplasmic compartment where the antigen can enter the class I or class II [166] processing pathways. It has been reported [167] that the protein content of ISCOMs is unimportant for their function and that the lipid Quill A is the only requisite ingredient. Takahashi et al. [168] suggest that ISCOMs, though they do not fuse with cell membranes, may nevertheless be capable of entering cells and dispensing their contents to the class I pathway.

Watari et al. [169] describe a synthetic peptide, derived from the amino terminus of Herpes Simplex Virus 2 glycoprotein D, that, when coupled to palmitic acid, inserted into liposomes and injected into the foot pads, confers resistance to Herpes Simplex Virus 2 in mice. Induction of immunity required acylated peptide, liposome, and adjuvant. The protection appears due to cellular immunity in as much as transfer of T cells confers resistance to naive mice, while serum does not. There is indirect evidence that T suppressor cells may be the mediators of the protection.

HIV CTL

Cytotoxic T lymphocytes have been shown to be important mediators of antiviral defense in other systems [170–173]. Instances have been reported where viral clearance is achieved in the absence of an antibody response [170–174]. Hom et al. [175] found that effective defense against a retrovirus in mice required both $CD8^+$ and $CD4^+$ T cells. Against a virus such as HIV, that can infect cells via cell-cell contact, elimination of infected cells via the cellular arm of the immune system is particularly important. There is evidence that MHC-restricted CTL in long-term asymptomatic seropositive individuals correlates with health [176].

Virus-specific CTL have also been implicated as a cause of disease pathogenesis and thus in some instances it may prove to be disadvantageous to include CTL epitopes in a vaccine. For example, there is a report of class I restricted CTL killing of Hepatitis B virus envelope-specific B cells [156]. It was hypothesized that if this phenomenon occurs *in vivo* it may be a mechanism for suppression of an antibody response to the virus. In the case of hepatitis, at least, immunization against such CTL epitopes may not be desirable. It has been also speculated that the CTL response to HIV-infected lung cells such as alveolar macrophages [177] may contribute [178,179] to alveolitis which is a chronic problem for many AIDS patients ([178] and reference therein). If a cytotoxic response can help clear the virus before infection of the lung can occur then this problem will not arise. However, any post-infection vaccination strategy must take the possible role of CTL in AIDS morbidity into account. Whether NK cells can mediate bystander killing of uninfected cell is not known.

While it is likely that a cytotoxic response will be important for protection from HIV infection, there is no guarantee that during infection a CTL response will do more good than harm. CTL have been implicated in the immune destruction that is the hallmark of the progression of AIDS. Siliciano et al. [105,106] have shown that gp120, through its interaction with CD4 on T cells, can flag uninfected cells *in vitro* for killing by class II restricted cytotoxic cells or by ADCC and that such cells can be elicited in humans immunized with recombinant gp160 (Science [105]). It has been shown by others that gp120 can be taken into human T cells via endocytosis of the gp120-CD4 complex, processed, then presented in association with class II molecules [180]. In the work of Siliciano and coworkers these recombinant gp160-class II complexes are presented to class II restricted CTL which lyse them. Whether this bystander killing functions *in vivo* is not known. Since it is estimated that only about 1 in 10^4 CD4$^+$ T cells is actually infected with HIV at any one time, some explanation other than direct killing by the virus is needed to account for the cell loss. At any rate the inclusion of gp120 CTL epitopes in an HIV vaccine will have to be weighed carefully against the potential for harm to the immune system such bystander killing might cause during actual infection with HIV. The above discussion is only meant as a caveat to the inclusion of HIV CTL epitopes in a vaccine, not as advocacy against their utilization.

Several groups (reviewed in References [181,182]) have found CTL in infected individuals specific for the gag polypeptide [134,144,183–186], reverse transcriptase [187], nef [185,188–190], vif [185], rev [191], and the envelope proteins (reviewed in Reference [182]). Also, Riviere and colleagues [185] report that env-specific cytolytic activity from fresh blood cells of HIV-1 seropositive patients was not MHC restricted and not mediated by T lymphocytes. They propose that natural killer cells (NK) may be mediating the observed cytolytic activity.

In addition to its being the major neutralizing epitope, the V3 domain of HIV-1 gp120 is immunodominant for CTL in mice [136]. CTL recognition can be altered by changes in single amino acids in this region [192]. Takahashi et al. [136] have found that mouse CTL to env peptide 308–322 are restricted to H-2^d such that strains not expressing this allele are nonresponders to env for CTL production. These findings indicate that if the V3 loop is represented in a vaccine it may be necessary to include, if they can be found, peptides from several strains that act as T epitopes for diverse HLA types.

Epitopes for CTL that can lyse targets expressing proteins other than the envelope may be extremely useful in an HIV vaccine. These proteins' amino acid sequences are conserved to a much greater extent than that of the envelope and in addition should not elicit a bystander killing response as has been described for gp120.

PEPTIDES AS VIRAL ANTAGONISTS

Agents that block infectivity at the level of virus binding are called receptor antagonists. Use of such antagonists following exposure to the virus might prevent infection. As with traditional immunization therapy, prevention of disease might be accomplished without actually preventing infection. Following infection the course of the disease might be checked through the inhibition of both virus spread and of viral cytopathological effects, such as syncytium formation. In addition, an agent that binds to a virus or to viral protein expressed on cell might be used to deliver agents that disrupt viral or cellular functions important to the virus life cycle.

Just as neutralizing antibodies can bind either the virus or its cellular receptor, peptide analogs of either molecule potentially can block infectivity. Whereas the repertoire of antibodies to be tested for inhibition can be generated *in vivo*, without knowledge of protein structure, the design of peptide antagonists is based on detailed knowledge at the molecular level of the virus-receptor interaction. At the very least, primary sequence information is required. An understanding of the contact sites between the viral protein(s) and the host receptors(s) is useful in order to limit the number of peptides to be tested for activity.

A potential advantage peptide-based antagonists are likely to have over antibody-based neutralization (either passive or active immunization) is less sensitivity to the variability of the virus. Peptides can be directed to the conserved binding domains of the virus or host receptors and potentially block all strains that require a particular host receptor. Antibodies that bind the virus at or near the receptor combining site can nevertheless be dependent on variable and type-specific target amino acids which are not part of the virus-cell interface. Such antibodies are likely be type-specific in their neutralizing capability despite the fact that they bind at or near the conserved receptor-combining site. A receptor analog, on the other hand, mimics either the virus or the cellular receptor protein and should interact with all proteins capable of binding that receptor epitope.

In considering peptides for therapeutic use *in vivo*, the effects of the peptide on cellular and systems function must be accounted for. In addition to possible direct pharmacologic activity, the potential antigenicity of the peptide is a factor in the selection. It might be wise to avoid any peptide containing regions to which detrimental immune responses have been demonstrated. If a virus-derived peptide is to be used, any known influences of the natural protein on cellular function might suggest regions to be avoided. For example it has been well documented that native transmembrane proteins, (including HIV [193]) or peptides derived from them are capable of inhibiting lymphoproliferation [194–198]. A synthetic peptide with homology to various retroviral transmembrane proteins has been linked to inhibition of monocyte-mediated killing [199], perhaps via inhibition of IL-1 [199]. gp120 has been implicated in inhibition of chemotactic functions of peripheral blood monocytes in AIDS patients [200], and also in neuron death [201]. Whether these latter putative functions of the

HIV envelope protein can be replicated by peptide analogs is not known. The other possibility is that these detrimental effects might be blocked by such or similar peptides.

VIRUS-RECEPTOR ANALOGS

Many known viral pathogens have been molecularly cloned and their DNA and predicted protein sequences derived. However, few viral receptor proteins have been identified; the list of known human virus receptors is short: HIV gp120-CD4, EBV-CR2 (the receptor for the 3d component of complement, C3d), rhinovirus-ICAM-1 [202,203] and ICAM-2, poliovirus and its novel receptor protein [204], and recently, echovirus 1-Integrin VLA-2 [224]. Influenza virus binds carbohydrate sialic acid residues. Of the viruses with proteinaceous receptors, only for HIV has an extensive analysis of the residues critical for binding been done.

The gp120 residues most likely to contact CD4 are found near the carboxyl terminus of gp120 [61,75,205–207]. However there are other distal regions critical for CD4 binding ability such that mutating or eliminating these destroys this binding [207]. It thus appears that for gp120 to bind CD4, fairly large areas of teritary structure are involved, suggesting that small peptide molecules are unlikely to reconstitute high affinity binding. Indeed no peptide fragments of gp120 smaller than 25 kd [201] have been reported to bind CD4 or block infection.

CD4/sCD4 AND THEIR PEPTIDE ANALOGS

The CD4 molecule possesses four extracellular immunoglobulin-like domains. Expression, through recombinant technology, of a truncated molecule lacking the transmembrane or cytoplasmic regions yields a secreted molecule (recombinant soluble CD4 or sCD4) that has the same affinity for gp120 as the complete receptor. Extensive studies have been performed and are continuing on the bioactivity of sCD4 and its derivatives. sCD4 at nanamolar to micromolar concentrations can inhibit virus binding and infection by HIV-1 and SIV and syncytium formation by HIV-1 of CD4+ cells [208–212] and to a lesser extent of myelomonocytic cells (monocytes and macrophages) [208]. Prevention of HIV-2 infection *in vitro* requires 25 times the amount of sCD4 than does HIV-1 [208]. In one report [213] prevention of HIV-2 induced syncytium formation was not achieved by sCD4, but hybrid CD4-immunoglobulin molecules were able to block syncytium formation. Inhibition of infection by HIV of glioma and rhabdomyosarcoma cells was not achievable with sCD4 or anti-CD4 antibodies [213]. Hussey et al. [210] demonstrated that sCD4 does not interfere with class II interactions *in vitro*.

In addition to these relatively large CD4 derivatives, the use of small CD4 peptides as inhibitors has been investigated. Chief among these are benzylated derivatives of peptides containing residues 81–92 of CD4 [214,215]. These peptide derivatives inhibit binding, infection, and cell fusion induced by a variety of HIV-1 isolates and by SIV. Complete inhibition of virus infection required the addition of peptide at the time of inoculation, but significant reduction in *in vitro* virus spread was observed when peptide was added as late as 48 hours following exposure. The authors believe that their peptide derivative may be entering the infected cells and inhibiting virus spread at the source of virus production itself by interfering with virus maturation and/or budding. They base this argument on the fact that the peptide is hydrophilic, that washing the treated cells did not eliminate the effect of peptide that was added 48 hours after infection, and an observed decrease in p24 gag antigen released into the medium following addition of peptide.

Hayashi et al. [216] demonstrate that a peptide spanning amino acids 70–132 inhibited HIV-1 replication and HIV-1-induced syncytium formation. Neither the benzylated peptides nor the 70–132 peptide spans the region (a.a. 18–51) shown in studies [217] using monoclonal antibodies to CD4 as critical for gp120 binding. Hayashi et al. [216] showed that a peptide covering this region (18–69) does not inhibit HIV-1 replication or syncytium formation. The authors suggest that the reason for this may be due to an insolubility in culture medium of the contact region peptide.

Finberg et al. [218] report on the anti-HIV activity of derivatives of the dipeptide prolyphenylalanine. These small molecules were created and tested based on their observation [218] that CD4 binding to gp120 could be abolished by a substitution of leucine for phenylalanine at a.a. 43 in CD4. The authors reasoned that small phenylalanine containing molecules might bind gp120 and prevent gp120-CD4 binding. The compounds reported on bound gp120 and could inhibit binding of gp120 to CD4 and HIV infection by free virus or T cells infected with viral clones. The molecules did not inhibit CD4-class II interactions and were able to inhibit the gp120 mediated interference in CD4-class II interactions.

All of the original experiments demonstrating the promise of CD4-based therapeutics for HIV infection were performed *in vitro* on strains of HIV that have been grown for many passages in laboratory culture. The initial results from *in vivo* studies have not been so encouraging. Daar et al. [219] report that patients receiving sCD4 at 30 mg/day (mean steady state sCD4 of 156 ng/ml in serum) showed no decrease in HIV-1 titer. Virus in plasma samples from these patients showed considerable resistance to neutralization by sCD4. When they examined the amount of sCD4 required to neutralize primary isolates from patients, that is isolates that had been passaged once *in vitro* on peripheral blood mononuclear cells (PBMC), they found a 200–2700 fold increase in the level of sCD4 required as compared with tissue culture strains of HIV-1 or HIV-2. The neutralization of laboratory strains was unaffected by the target cell type used for infection, including PBMCs, however a primary isolate that was cultured *in vitro* for one year on a T lymphoblastoid clone showed increased susceptibility to neutralization by sCD4. Finally, there does not appear to be a CD4-independent mechanism of infection operating in the primary isolates insofar as the anti-CD4 antibody Leu3a effectively neutralized infection by them.

The implications of this study [219] are significant for the use of sCD4 for treatment of HIV infected patients. The use of oligomeric or multimeric CD4 structures such as CD4-immunoglobulin hybrids seem unlikely to overcome the problems demonstrated, and, as the authors point out, it will be more important in the future to examine the anti-HIV efficacy of any pharmaceutical on primary or unselected HIV populations.

ICAM-1 AND ICAM-2

The lymphocyte adhesion molecules ICAM-1 and ICAM-2 have been identified [202,203] as the cellular receptors necessary for binding and infection by the vast majority (80–90%) of serotypes of rhinovirus, a picornavirus that is the causative agent for the common cold in humans. The crystal structure of a rhinovirus serotype (HRV14) that binds this receptor has been accomplished [220] and this revealed a protein capsid structure consisting of deep valleys or "canyons" surrounded by prominent, variable, immunodominant peptide loops. The canyons are believed to be the receptor combining sites. They are too narrow to allow entry and binding of a (potentially neutralizing) antibody molecule. The exposed loops are thought of as "wild geese" whose hypervariability provides immune escape. The "canyon hypothesis" [38] has lead many investigators to search for agents that directly and specifically interdict in the virus-receptor interaction by interacting with the canyon in a specific manner. Staunton et al. suggest that soluble ICAM-1 molecules might have been used to inhibit rhinovirus binding and infection. The WIN series of hydrophobic isoxazoles are prominent among these [221]. These compounds [222] bind picornavirus (including rhinovirus) capsids in the hydrophobic crevice of the β-barrel fold [223].

CONCLUSION

As we enter the age of "rational" drug and vaccine design, we are reminded of how much, but also of how little we really understand about the biological mechanisms which govern our lives. We know something about the way a virus such as HIV exploits the weaknesses in our natural defenses to gain access to the cellular machinery vital to its reproduction. We know quite a lot about our own immune system, and we are learning fast. But we really understand very little about why the body, after millions of years of evolution, fails every time to rid itself of certain parasites and why it instead succumbs to the destructive effects of the infection. Our knowledge of the strategies the virus employs to subvert the very defenses on which we rely is incomplete at best. Our best theories are just that, theories, our knowledge is often merely circumstantial.

On the other hand, humankind, as a thinking animal, has a short but illustrious history of successfully managing, even eradicating, plagues by immunizing populations against the infections. These campaigns have relied on one very profound bit of knowledge: prior exposure to an agent that evokes a response from the immune system promotes protection to reexposure to that or other infectious agents which sufficiently resemble it. Today we can apply that principle in combination with a battery of other, no less profound bits of wisdom pertaining to our immunity and the properties of the viral enemy.

The prospects for controlling viral diseases improve constantly as we gain new knowledge. The application of these insights will be necessary in the design of agents against so far intractable illnesses. But time is passing; the desire to rationalize every aspect of vaccine design in order to protect ourselves and those we are responsible to from potential missteps must not lead to a stagnation in the testing and application of these diverse strategies. We are challenged to find the right compromise between caution and initiative, for our goal is a practical one: produce vaccines that protects from disease.

REFERENCES

1 Anderer, F. A. 1963. "Versuche zur Bestimmung der Serologisch Determinanten Gruppen des Tabakmosaikvirus," Z. Naturforsch., 18b:1010.

2 Townsend, A. R. M., J. Rothbard, F. M. Gotch, G. Bahadur, D. Wraith and A. J. McMichael. 1986. "The Epitopes of Influenza Nucleoprotein Recognized by Cytotoxic T Lymphocytes Can Be Defined with Short Synthetic Peptides," Cell, 44:959.

3 Bastin, J., J. Rothbard, J. Davey, I. Jones and A. Townsend. 1987. "Use of Synthetic Peptides of Influenza Nucleoprotein to Define Epitopes Recognized by Class I-Restricted Cytotoxic T Lymphocytes," J. Exp. Med. 165:1508.

4 Neefjes, J. J., V. Stollorz, P. J. Peters, H. J. Geuze and H. L. Ploegh. 1990. "The Biosynthetic Pathway of MHC Class II but Not Class I Molecules Intersects the Endocytic Route," Cell, 61:171.

5 Guagliardi, L. E., B. Koppelman, J. S. Blum, M. S. Marks, P. Cresswell and F. M. Brodsky. 1990. "Co-Localization of Molecules Involved in Antigen Processing and Presentation in an Early Endocytic Compartment," *Nature*, 343:133.

6 Merrifield, R. B. 1964. "Solid Phase Peptide Synthesis. II. The Synthesis of Bradikinin," *J. Am. Chem. Soc.*, 86:304.

7 Sela, M. 1987. "The Choice of Carrier," *Synthetic Vaccines*, I:83.

8 Francis, M. J., C. M. Fry, D. J. Rowlands, J. L. Bittle, R. A. Houghten, R. A. Lerner and F. Brown. 1987. "Immune Response to Uncoupled Peptides of Foot-and-Mouth Disease Virus," *Immunology*, 61:1.

9 Atassi, M. Z. and R. G. Webster. 1983. "Localization, Synthesis and Activity of an Antigenic Site on Influenza Virus Hemagglutinin," *PNAS*, 82:840.

10 Ermini, E. A., B. A. Jameson and E. Wimmer. 1983. "Priming for and Induction of Anti-Poliovirus Neutralizing Antibodies by Synthetic Peptides," *Nature*, 304:699.

11 Dreesman, G. R., Y. Sanchez, I. Ionescu-Matiu, J. T. Sparrow, H. R. Six, D. L. Peterson, F. B. Hollinger and J. L. Melnick. 1982. "Antibody to Hepatitis B Surface Antigen after a Single Innoculation of Uncoupled Synthetic HBsAg Peptides," *Nature*, 295:158.

12 Chow, M., R. Yabrow, J. Bittle, J. Hogle and D. Baltimore. 1985. "Synthetic Peptides from Four Separate Regions of the Poliovirus Type 1 Capsid Protein VP1 Induce Neutralizing Antibodies," *Proc. Natl. Acad. Sci. USA*, 82:910.

13 Gooding, L. R. and C. B. Edwards. 1980. "H-2 Antigen Requirements in the *in vitro* Induction of SV40-Specific Cytotoxic T Lymphocytes," *J. Immunol.*, 124:1258.

14 Schutze, M.-P., C. LeClerc, M. Jolivet, F. Audibert and L. Chedid. 1985. "Carrier-Induced Epitopic Suppression, a Major Issue for Future Synthetic Vaccines," *J. Immunol.*, 135:2319.

15 Jacob, C. O., R. Arnon and M. Sela. 1985. "Effect of Carrier on the Immunogenic Capacity of Synthetic Cholera Vaccine," *Mol. Immunol.*, 22:1333.

16 Jacob, C. O., S. Grossfeld, M. Sela and R. Arnon. 1986. "Priming Immune Response to Cholera Toxin Induced by Synthetic Peptides," *Eur. J. Immunol.*, 16:1057.

17 Herzenberg, L. A., T. Tokuhira and L. A. Herzenberg. 1980. "Carrier-Priming Leads to Hapten-Specific Suppression," *Nature*, 285:664.

18 Audibert, F. 1986. "Carriers and Adjuvants for the Development of Synthetic Vaccines," *Synthetic Peptides as Viral Vaccines*, 137E:514.

19 Emini, E. A., B. A. Jameson and E. Wimmer. 1983. "Priming for and Induction of Anti-Poliovirus Neutralizing Antibodies by Synthetic Peptides," *Nature*, 304:699.

20 Jolivet, M., F. Audibert, E. H. Beachy, A. Tartar, H. Gras-Masse and L. Chedid. 1983. *Biochem. Biophys. Res. Commun.*, 117:359.

21 Kawamura, H. and J. A. Berzofsky. 1986. "Enhancement of Antigenic Potency *in vitro* and Immunogenicity *in vivo* by Coupling the Antigen to Anti-Immunoglobulin," *J. Immunol.*, 136:58.

22 Carayanniotis, G., E. Vizi, J. M. R. Parker, R. S. Hodges and B. H. Barber. 1988. "Delivery of Synthetic Peptides by Anti-Class II MHC Monoclonal Antibodies Induces Specific Adjuvant-Free IgG Responses *in Vivo*," *Molec. Immunol.*, 25:907.

23 Warren, H. S., F. R. Vogel and L. A. Chedid. 1986. "Current Status of Immunological Adjuvants," *Annu. Rev. Immunol.*, 4:369.

24 Gregoriadis, G. 1990. "Immunological Adjuvants: A Role for Liposomes," *Immunol. Today*, 11:89.

25 Warren, H. S. and L. A. Chedid. 1988. "Future Prospects for Vaccine Adjuvants," *Crit. Rev. Immunol.*, 8:83.

26 Lederer, E. 1986. "New Developments in the Field of Synthetic Muramyl Peptides, Especially as Adjuvants for Synthetic Vaccines," *Drugs Exp. Clin. Res.*, 12:429.

27 Chedid, L. 1987. "Use of Adjuvants for Synthetic Vaccines," *Synthetic Vaccines*, 1:93.

28 Chedid, L., C. Carelli and F. Audibert. 1986. *Veterinary Biologics*, p. 48.

29 Tam, J. P. 1988. "Synthetic Peptide Vaccine Design: Synthesis and Properties of a High-Density Multiple Antigenic Peptide System," *Proc. Natl. Acad. Sci. USA*, 85:5409.

30 Tam, J. P. and Y.-A. Lu. 1989. "Vaccine Engineering: Enhancement of Immunogenicity of Synthetic Peptide Vaccines Related to Hepatitis in Chemically Defined Models Consisting of T- and B-Cell Epitopes," *Proc. Natl. Acad. Sci. USA*, 86: 9084.

31 Palker, T. J., M. E. Tanner, R. M. Scearce, A. Langlois, T. J. Matthews, D. P. Bolognesi and B. F. Haynes. 1988. "Neutralization of 2 Human Immunodeficiency Virus (HIV) Isolates with a Bivalent Anti-Synthetic Peptide Antiserum to Neutralizing Determinants of gp120," *Clin. Res.*, 36:465.

32 Leclerc, C., G. Przewlocki, M.-P. Schutze and L. Chedid. 1987. "A Synthetic Vaccine Constructed by Copolymerization of B and T Cell Determinants," *Eur. J. Immunol.*, 17:269.

33 Palker, T. J., T. J. Matthews, A. Langlois, M. E. Tanner, M. E. Martin, R. M. Scearce, J. E. Kim, J. A. Berzofsky, D. P. Bolognesi and B. F. Haynes. 1989. "Polyvalent Human Immunodeficiency Virus Synthetic Immunogen Comprised of Envelope gp120 T Helper Cell Sites and B Cell Neutralization Epitopes," *J. Immunol.*, 142:3612.

34 Good, M. F., W. L. Maloy, M. N. Lunde, H. Margalit, J. L. Cornette, G. L. Smith, B. Moss, L. H. Miller and J. A. Berzofsky. 1987. "Construction of Synthetic Immunogen: Use of New T-Helper Epitope on Malaria Circumsporozoite Protein," *Science*, 235:1059.

35 Kingsman, S. M. and A. J. Kingsman. 1988. "Polyvalent Recombinant Antigens: A New Vaccine Strategy," *Vaccine*, 6:304.

36 Nara, P. L., R. R. Garrity and J. Goudsmit. 1991. "Neutralization of HIV-1: A Paradox of Humoral Proportions," *FASEB J.*, 5:2437.

37 Gupta, P., R. Balachandran, M. Ho, A. Enrico and C. Rinaldo. 1989. "Cell-to-Cell Transmission of Human Immunodeficiency Virus Type 1 in the Presence of Azidothymidine and Neutralizing Antibody," *J. Virol.*, 63:2361.

38 Rossmann, M. G. 1989. "The Canyon Hypothesis. Hiding the Host Cell Receptor Attachment Site on a Viral Surface from Immune Surveillance," *J. Biol. Chem.*, 264:14587.

39 Nara, P. L. and J. Goudsmit. 1991. "Clonal Dominance of the Neutralizing Response to the HIV-1 V3 Epitope: Evidence for 'Original Antigenic Sin' during Vaccination and Infection in Animals, Including Humans," *Vaccines*, 91:37.

40 Weiner, D. B., T. Kieber-Emmons and W. V. Williams. Unpublished observations.

41 Kerkau, T., R. Schmitt-Landgraf, A. Schimpl and E. Wecker. 1989. "Down-regulation of HLA Class I Antigens in HIV-1–Infected Cells," *AIDS Res. Human Retrovir.*, 5:613.

42 Tyler, D. S., H. K. Lyerly and K. J. Weinhold. 1989. "Minireview: Anti-HIV-1 ADCC," *AIDS Res. Human Retrovir.*,5:557.

43 Michalek, S. M., N. K. Childers, J. Katz, F. R. Denys, A. K. Berry, J. H. Eldridge, J. R. McGhee and R. Curtiss, III. 1989. "Liposomes as Oral Adjuvants," *Curr. Topics Microbiol. Immunol.*, 146:51.

44 Barlow, D. J., M. S. Edwards and J. M. Thornton. 1986. "Continuous and Discontinuous Protein Antigenic Determinants," *Nature*, 322:747.

45 Shinnick, T. M., J. G. Sutcliffe, N. Green and R. A. Lerner. 1983. "Synthetic Peptide Immunogens as Vaccines," *Ann. Rev. Microbiol.*, 37:425.

46 Sutcliffe, J. G., T. M. Shinnick, N. Green and R. A. Lerner. 1983. "Antibodies that React with Predetermined Sites on Protiens," *Science*, 219:660.

47 Berzofsky, J. A. 1985. "Intrinsic and Extrinsic Factors in Protein Antigenic Structure," *Science*, 229:932.

48 Connolly, M. L. 1983. "Solvent-Accessible Surfaces of Proteins and Nucleic Acids," *Science*, 221:709.

49 Hopp, T. P. and K. R. Woods. 1981. "Prediction of Protein Antigenic Determinants from Amino Acid Sequences," *Proc. Natl. Acad. Sci. USA*, 78:3824.

50 Westhof, E., D. Altschuh, D. Moras, A. C. Bloomer, A. Mondragon, A. Klug and M. H. V. Van Regenmortel. 1984. "Corrlation between Segmental Mobility and the Location of Antigenic Determinants in Proteins," *Nature*, 311:123.

51 Tainer, J. A., E. D. Getzoff, H. Alexander, R. A. Houghten, A. J. Olson and R. A. Lerner. 1984. "The Reactivity of Anti-Peptide Antibodies Is a Function of the Atomic Mobility of Sites in a Protein," *Nature*, 312:127.

52 Tainer, J. A., E. D. Getzoff, Y. Paterson, A. J. Olson and R. A. Lerner. 1985. "The Atomic Mobility Component of Protein Antigenicity," *Ann. Rev. Immunol.*, 3:501.

53 Lando, G., J. A. Berzofsky and M. Reichlin. 1982. "Antigenic Structure of Sperm Whale Myoglobin. I. Partition of Specificities between Antibodies Reactive with Peptides and Native Protein," *J. Immunol.*, 129:206.

54 Berzofsky, J. A. and I. J. Berkower. 1989. "Fundamental Immunology," in *Fundamental Immunology*, p. 169.

55 Arnon, R. 1987. *Synthetic Vaccines Vol. 1 and 2.*

56 Hioe, C. E., N. Dybdahl-Sissoko, M. Philpott and V. S. Hinshaw. 1990. "Overlapping Cytotoxic T-Lymphocyte and B-Cell Antigenic Sites on the Influenza Virus H5 Hemagglutinin," *J. Virol.*, 64:6246.

57 Milich, D. R., J. L. Hughes, A. McLachlan, G. B. Thornton and A. Moriarty. 1988. "Hepatitis B Synthetic Immunogen Comprised of Nucleocapsid T-Cell Sites and an Envelope B-Cell Epitope," *Proc. Natl. Acad. Sci. USA*, 85:1610.

58 Ho, D. D., J. C. Kaplan, I. E. Rackauskas and M. E. Gurney. 1988. "Second Conserved Domain of gp120 Is Important for HIV Infectivity and Antibody Neutralization," *Science*, 239:1021.

59 Ronco, J., A. Charbit, J.-F. Dedieu, M. Mancini, M.-L. Michel, Y. Henin, D.

O'Callaghan, M. Kaczorek, M. Girard and M. Hofnung. 1991. "Is There a Neutralization Epitope in the Second Conserved Domain of HIV-1 Envelope Protein?" *AIDS Res. Human Retrovir.*, 7:1.

60 Sun, N.-C., D. D. Ho, C. R. Y. Sun, R.-S. Liou, W. Gordon, M. S. C. Fung, X. L. Li, R. C. Ting, T.-H. Lee, N. T. Chang and T.-S. Chang. 1989. "Generation and Characterization of Monoclonal Antibodies to the Putative CD4 Binding Domain of Human Immunodeficiency Virus Type 1 gp120," *J. Virol.*, 63:3579.

61 Lasky, L. A., G. Nakamura, D. H. Smith, C. Fennie, C. Shimasaki, E. Patzer, P. Berman, T. Gregory and D. J. Capon. 1987. "Delineation of a Region of the Human Immunodeficiency Virus Type 1 gp120 Glycoprotein Critical for Interaction with the CD4 Receptor," *Cell*, 50:975.

62 Kenealy, W. R., T. J. Matthews, M.-C. Ganfield, A. J. Langlois, D. M. Waselefsky and S. R. Petteway, Jr. 1989. "Antibodies from Human Immunodeficiency Virus–Infected Individuals Bind to a Short Amino Acid Sequence that Elicits Neutralizing Antibodies in Animals," *AIDS Res. Human Retrovir.*, 5:173.

63 Bidart, J.-M., F. Troalen, P. Ghillani, N. Rouas, A. Razafindratsita, C. Bohuon and D. Bellet. 1990. "Peptide Immunogen Mimicry of a Protein-Specific Structural Epitope on Human Choriogonadotropin," *Science*, 248:736.

64 Von Feldt, J. M., K. E. Ugen, T. Kieber-Emmons and W. V. Williams. 1992. "Bioactive Peptide Design Based on Antibody Structure," Chapter 3 in *Biologically Active Peptides: Design, Synthesis, and Utilization*. Lancaster, PA: Technomic Publishing Co., Inc.

65 Robey, W. G., L. O. Arthur, T. J. Matthews, A. Langlois, T. D. Copeland, N. W. Lerche, S. Oroszlan, D. P. Bolognesi, R. V. Gilden and P. J. Fischinger. 1986. "Prospect for Prevention of Human Immunodeficiency Virus Infection: Purified 120-kDa Envelope Glycoprotein Induces Neutralizing Antibidy," *Proc. Natl. Acad. Sci. USA*, 83:7023.

66 Putney, S. D., T. J. Matthews, W. G. Robey, D. L. Lynn, M. Robert-Guroff, W. T. Mueller, A. J. Langlois, J. Ghrayeb, S. R. J. Petteway, K. J. Weinhold, P. J. Fischinger, F. Wong-Staal, R. C. Gallo and D. P. Bolognesi. 1986. "HTLV-III/LAV-1 Neutralizing Antibodies to an *E. coli*–Produced Fragment of the Virus Envelope," *Science*, 234:1392.

67 Rusche, J. R., K. Javaherian, C. McDanal, J. Petro, D. L. Lynn, R. Grimaila, A. Langlois, R. C. Gallo, L. O. Arthur, P. J. Fischinger, D. P. Bolognesi, S. D. Putney and T. J. Matthews. 1988. "Antibodies that Inhibit Fusion of Human Immunodeficiency Virus–Infected Cells Bind a 24 Amino Acid Sequence of the Viral Envelope, gp120," *Proc. Natl. Acad. Sci. USA*, 85:3198.

68 Veronese, F. D., A. L. DeVico, T. D. Copland, S. Oroszian, R. C. Gallo and M. G. Sarngadharan. 1985. "Characterization of gp41 as the Transmembrane Protein Coded by the HTLV-III/LAV Envelope Gene," *Science*, 229:1402.

69 Sattentau, Q. J. and R. A. Weiss. 1988. "The CD4 Antigen: Physiological Ligand and HIV Receptor," *Cell*, 42:631.

70 Goudsmit, J., C. A. B. Boucher, R. H. Meloen, L. G. Epstein, L. Smit, L. van der Hoek and M. Bakker. 1988. "Human Antibody Responses to a Strain Specific HIV gp120 Epitope Associated with Cell Fusion Inhibition," *AIDS*, 2:157.

71 Javaherian, K., A. J. Langlois, C. McDanal, K. L. Ross, L. I. Eckler, C. L. Jellis, A. T. Profy, J. R. Rusche, D. P. Bolognesi, S. D. Putney and T. J. Matthews. 1989. "Principal Neutralizing Domain of the Human Immunodeficiency Virus Type 1 Envelope Protein," *Proc. Natl. Acad. Sci. USA*, 86:6768.

72 Myers, G., B. Korber, J. A. Berzofsky, R. F. Smith and G. N. Pavlakis. 1991. *Human Retroviruses and AIDS.* Los Alamos, NM: Los Alamos National Laboratory, p. 6.

73 LaRosa, G. J., J. P. Davide, K. Weinhold, J. A. Waterbury, A. T. Profy, J. A. Lewis, A. J. Langlois, G. R. Dreesman, R. N. Boswell, P. Shadduck, L. H. Holly, M. Karplus, D. P. Bolognesi, T. J. Matthews, E. A. Emini and S. D. Putney. 1990. "Conserved Sequence and Structural Elements in the HIV-1 Principal Neutralizing Determinant," *Science,* 249:932.

74 Skinner, M. A., A. J. Langlois, C. B. McDanal, J. S. McDougal, D. P. Bolognesi and T. J. Matthews. 1988. "Neutralizing Antibodies to an Immunodominant Envelope Sequence Do Not Prevent gp120 Binding to CD4," *J. Virol.,* 42:4195.

75 Olshevsky, U., E. Helseth, C. Furman, J. Li, W. Haseltine and J. Sodroski. 1990. "Identification of Individual Human Immunodeficiency Virus Type 1 gp120 Amino Acids Important for CD4 Receptor Binding," *J. Virol.,* 64:5701.

76 Freed, E. O., D. M. Myers and R. Risser. 1991. "Identification of the Principal Neutralizing Determinant of Human Immunodeficiency Virus Type 1 as a Fusion Domain," *J. Virol.,* 65:190.

77 Helseth, E., M. Kowalski, D. Gabuzda, U. Olshevsky, W. Haseltine and J. Sodroski. 1990. "Rapid Complementation Assays Measuring Replicative Potential of Human Immunodeficiency Virus Type 1 Envelope Glycoprotein Mutants," *J. Virol.,* 64:2416.

78 Hwang, S. S., T. J. Boyle, K. Lyerly and B. R. Cullen. 1991. "Identification of the Envelope V3 Loop as the Primary Determinant of Cell Tropism in HIV-1," *Science,* 253:71.

79 Stephens, P. E., G. J. Clements and G. T. Yarranton. 1990. "A Chink in HIV's Armour?" (letter), *Nature,* 343:219.

80 Clements, G. J., M. J. Price-Jones, P. E. Stephens, C. Sutton, T. F. Schulz, P. R. Clapham, J. A. McKeating, M. O. McClure, S. Thomson, M. Marsh, J. Kay, R. A. Weiss and J. P. Moore. 1991. "The V3 Loops of the HIV-1 and HIV-2 Surface Glycoproteins Contain Proteolytic Cleavage Sites: A Possible Function in Viral Fusion?" *AIDS Res. Human Retrovir.,* 7:3.

81 Hattori, T., A. Kioto, K. Takatsuki, H. Kido and N. Katunuma. 1989. *FEBS Lett.,* 248:48.

82 Nara, P. L., L. Smit, W. Hatch, M. Merges, D. Waters, J. Kelliher, R. C. Gallo, P. J. Fischinger and J. Goudsmit. 1990. "Emergence of Viruses Resistant to Neutralization by V3-Specific Antibodies in Experimental Human Immunodeficiency Virus Type 1 Infection of Chimpanzees," *J. Virol.,* 64:3779.

83 McKeating, J. A., J. Gow, J. Goudsmit, C. Mulder, J. McClure and R. Weiss. 1988. "Monoclonal Antibody Selection of HIV Neutralization Resistant Mutants," in *Retroviruses of Human AIDS and Related Animal Diseases,* p. 159.

84 Goudsmit, J., C. DeBouck, R. H. Meloen, L. Smit, M. Bakker, D. M. Asher, A. V. Wolff, C. J. J. Gibbs and D. C. Gajdusek. 1988. "Human Immunodeficiency Virus Type 1 Neutralization Epitope with Conserved Architecture Elicits Early Type-Specific Antibodies in Experimentally Infected Chimpanzees," *Proc. Natl. Acad. Sci. USA,* 85:4478.

85 Kennedy, R. C., G. R. Dreesman, T. C. Chanh, R. N. Boswell, J. S. Allan, T.-H. Lee, M. Essex, J. T. Sparrown, D. D. Ho and P. Kanda. 1987. "Use of a Resin-Bound Synthetic Peptide for Identifying a Neutralizing Antigenic Determinant

Associated with the Human Immunodeficiency Virus Envelope," *J. Biol. Chem.*, 262:5769.

86 Palker, T. J., M. E. Clark, A. G. Langlois, T. J. Matthews, K. J. Weinhold, R. R. Randall, D. P. Bolognesi and B. F. Haynes. 1988. "Type-Specific Neutralization of the Human Immunodeficiency Virus with Antibodies to Env-Encoded Synthetic Peptides," *Proc. Natl. Acad. Sci. USA*, 85:1932.

87 Ho, D. D., M. G. Sarngadharan, M. S. Hirsch, R. T. Schooley, T. R. Rota, R. C. Kennedy, T. C. Chanh and V. L. Sato. 1987. "Human Immunodeficiency Virus Neutralizing Antibodies Recognize Several Conserved Domains on the Envelope Glycoproteins," *J. Virol.*, 61:2024.

88 Javaherian, K., A. J. Langlois, G. J. LaRosa, A. T. Profy, D. P. Bolognesi, W. C. Herlihy, S. D. Putney and T. J. Matthews. 1990. "Broadly Neutralizing Antibodies Elicited by the Hypervariable Neutralizing Determinant of HIV-1," *Science*, 250:1590.

89 Berman, P. W., T. J. Gregory, L. Riddle, G. R. Nakamura, M. A. Champe, J. P. Porter, F. M. Wurm, R. D. Hershberg, E. K. Cobb and J. W. Eichberg. 1990. "Protection of Chimpanzees from Infection by HIV-1 after Vaccination with Recombinant Glycoprotein gp120 but Not gp160," *Nature*, 345:622.

90 Massey, R. J. and G. Schochetman. 1981. "Viral Epitopes and Monoclonal Antibodies: Isolation of Blocking Antibodies that Inhibit Virus Neutralization," *Science*, 213:447.

91 Homsy, J., M. Meyer, M. Tateno, S. Clarkson and J. A. Levy. 1989. "The Fc and Not CD4 Receptor Mediates Antibody Enhancement of HIV Infection in Human Cells," *Science*, 244:1357.

92 Robinson, J. W. E., D. C. Montefiori and W. M. Mitchell. 1988. "Antibody-Dependent Enhancement of Human Immunodeficiency Virus Type 1 Infection," *Lancet*, 1:790.

93 Robinson, J. W. E., T. Kawamura, M. K. Gorny, D. Lakes, J.-Y. Xu, Y. Matsumoto, T. Sugano, Y. Masuho, W. M. Mitchell, E. Hersh and S. Zolla-Pazner. 1990. "Human Monoclonal Antibodies to the Human Immunodeficiency Virus Type I" (HIV-1) Transmembrane Glycoprotein gp41 Enhance HIV-1 Infection *in Vitro*," *Proc. Natl. Acad. Sci. USA*, 87:3185; Robinson, W. E., M. K. Gorny, J.-Y. Xu, W. M. Mitchel and S. Zolla-Pazner. 1991. "Two Immunodominant Domains of gp41 Bind Antibodies Which Enhance Human Immunodeficiency Virus Type 1 Infection *in Vitro*," *J. Virol.*, 65:4169.

94 Porterfield, J. S. 1988. "Aberrant Responses to Infectious Agents: Immune Enhancement of Viral Infectivity," in *Technological Advances in Vaccine Development*, p. 539.

95 Goudsmit, J., J. de Jong, A. do Ronde, M. Tersmette and P. Nara. 1990. "Antigenic Variation of HIV-1 and Its Role in the Pathogenesis of AIDS" (abstr. L025), *UCLA Symposia on Molecular and Cellular Biology. HIV and AIDS: Pathogenesis, Therapy and Vaccine*, S.14D:90.

96 Meloen, R. H., R. M. Liskamp and J. Goudsmit. 1989. "Specificity and Function of the Individual Amino Acids of an Important Determinant of HIV-1 that Induces Neutralising Activity," *J. Gen. Virol.*, 70:1505.

97 Holley, L. H., J. Goudsmit and M. Karplus. 1991. "Prediction of Optimal Peptide Mixtures to Induce Broadly Neutralizing Antibodies to Human Immunodeficiency Virus Type 1," *Proc. Natl. Acad. Sci. USA*, 88:6800.

98 Devash, Y., T. J. Matthews, J. E. Drummond, K. Javaherian, D. J. Waters, L. O.

Arthur, W. A. Blattner and J. R. Rusche. 1990. "C-Terminal Fragments of gp120 and Synthetic Peptides from Five HTLV-III Strains: Prevalence of Antibodies to the HTLV-III-MN Isolate in Infected Individuals," *AIDS Res. Human Retrovir.*, 6:307.

99 Goudsmit, J., C. L. Kuiken and P. L. Nara. 1989. "Linear Versus Conformational Variation of V3 Neutralization Domains of HIV-1 during Experimental and Natural Infection," *AIDS*, 3(suppl. 1):S119.

100 Tersmette, M., R. E. Y. deGoede, F. de Wolf, J. Goudsmit, J. G. Huisman and F. Miedema. 1989. "Evolution of the Biological Phenotype of Sequential Human Immunodeficiency Virus (HIV) Isolates in Seroconverting Homosexual Men" (abstr. M.C.0.8), *V International Conference on AIDS*.

101 Levy, J. A. 1989. "Human Immunodeficiency Viruses and the Pathogenesis of AIDS," *JAMA*, 261:2997.

102 Fauci, A. S. 1988. "The Human Immunodeficiency Virus: Infectivity and Mechanisms of Pathogenesis," *Science*, 239:617.

103 Haseltine, W. A. 1988. "Replication and Pathogenesis of the AIDS Virus," *AIDS*, 1:217.

104 Hoffmann, G. W., T. A. Kion and M. D. Grant. 1991. "An Idiotypic Network Model of Aids Immunopathogenesis," *PNAS USA*, 88:3060.

105 Orentas, R. J., J. E. K. Hildreth, E. Obah, M. Polydefkis, G. E. Smith, M. L. Clements and R. F. Siliciano. 1990. "Induction of CD4⁺ Human Cytolytic T Cells Specific for HIV-Infected Cells by a gp160 Subunit Vaccine," *Science*, 248:1234.

106 Siliciano, R. F., T. Lawton, C. Knall, R. W. Karr, P. Berman, T. Gregory and E. L. Reinherz. 1988. "Analysis of Host-Virus Interactions in AIDS with Anti-gp120 T Cell Clones: Effect of HIV Sequence Variation and a Mechanism for CD4⁺ Cell Depletion," *Cell*, 54:561.

107 Bolognesi, D. P. 1989. "HIV Antibodies and Vaccine Design," *AIDS*, 3:S111.

108 Goudsmit, J. 1988. "Immunodominant B-Cell Epitopes of the HIV-1 Envelope Recognized by Infected and Immunized Hosts," *AIDS*, 2:S41.

109 Cease, K. B. 1990. "Peptide Component Vaccine Engineering: Targeting the AIDS Virus," *Int. Rev. Immunol.*, 7:85.

110 Back, N. K. T., C. Thiriart, L. Van Der Hoek, C. Bruck and J. Goudsmit. 1989. "Human Antibodies to HIV-1 gp160 Inhibit Attachment to CD4" (abstr. Th.C.P.34), *Vth International Conference on AIDS*.

111 Dowbenko, D., G. Nakamura, C. Fennie, C. Shimasaki, L. Riddle, R. Harris, T. Gregory and L. Lasky. 1988. "Epitope Mapping of the Human Immunodeficiency Virus Type 1 gp120 with Monoclonal Antibodies," *J. Virol.*, 52:4703.

112 Linsley, P. S., J. A. Ledbetter, E. Kinney-Thomas and S. L. Hu. 1988. "Effects of Anti-gp120 Monoclonal Antibodies on CD4 Receptor Binding by the Envelope Protein of Human Immunodeficiency Virus Type 1," *J. Virol.*, 62:3695.

113 Back, N. K., C. Thiriart, A. Delers, C. Ramautarsing, C. Bruck and J. Goudsmit. 1990. "Association of Antibodies Blocking HIV-1 gp160-sCD4 Attachment with Virus Neutralizing Activity in Human Sera," *J. Med. Virol.*, 31:200.

114 Steimer, K. S., C. J. Scandella, P. V. Skiles and N. L. Haigwood. 1991. "Neutralization of Divergent HIV-1 Isolates by Conformation-Dependent Human Antibodies to gp120," *Science*, 254:105.

115 Ho, D. D., J. A. McKeating, X. L. Li, T. Moudgil, E. S. Daar, N.-C. Sun and J. E. Robinson. 1991. "Conformational Epitope on gp120 Important in CD4 Bind-

ing and Human Immunodeficiency Virus Type-1 Neutralization Identified by a Human Monoclonal Antibody," *J. Virol.*, 65:489.

116 Weiner, D. B., W. V. Williams, M. J. Merva, K. Huebner, J. A. Berzofsky and M. I. Greene. 1990. "HIV Infectivity: Analysis of Viral Envelope Determinants and Target Cell Requirements for Infectivity by HIV-1," *Vaccines*, 90:339.

117 Kieber-Emmons, T., A. Whalley, W. M. Williams, T. Ryskamp, W. J. W. Morrow, I. Schmid, J. V. Giorgi, J. F. Krowka, W. V. Williams, M. J. Merva and D. B. Weiner. 1990. "Biological Characteristics of an HIV-1 Envelope-Derived Synthetic Peptide," *Vaccines*, 90:1.

118 Ugen, K. E., B. Perussia, M. Kamoun, M. Merva, W. V. Williams, P. Nara, T. Kieber-Emmons and D. B. Weiner. 1991. "Inhibition of HIV-1 Cellular Infection by Immunologic Reagents," *Vaccines*, 91:115.

119 Tyler, D. S., S. D. Stanley, S. Zolla-Pazner, M. K. Gorny, P. P. Shadduck, A. J. Langlois, T. J. Matthews, D. P. Bolognesi, T. J. Palker and K. J. Weinhold. 1990. "Identification of Sites within gp41 that Serve as Targets for Antibody-Dependent Cellular Cytotoxicity by Using Human Monoclonal Antibodies," *J. Immunol.*, 145:3276.

120 Bixler, G. S., Jr. and M. Z. Atassi. 1984. "T Cell Recognition of Lysozyme. III. Recognition of the 'Surface-Stimulation' Synthetic Antigenic Sites," *J. Immunogenet.*, 11:245.

121 Francis, M. J., C. M. Fry, D. J. Rowlands, F. Brown, J. L. Bittle, R. A. Houghten and R. A. Lerner. 1985. "Immunological Priming with Synthetic Peptides of Foot-and-Mouth Disease Virus," *J. Gen. Virol.*, 66:2347.

122 Gallaher, W. R., J. M. Ball, R. F. Garry, M. C. Griffen and R. C. Montelaro. 1989. "A General Model for the Transmembrane Proteins of HIV and Other Retroviruses," *AIDS Res. Human Retrovir.*, 5:431.

123 Wang, J. J. G., S. Steel, R. Wisniewolski and C. Y. Wang. 1986. "Detection of Antibodies to Human T-Lymphotropic Virus Type III by Using a Synthetic Peptide of 21 Amino Acid Residues Corresponding to a Highly Antigenic Segment of gp41 Envelope Protein," *Proc. Natl. Acad. Sci. USA*, 83:6159.

124 Klasse, P. J., R. Pipkorn and J. Blomberg. 1988. "Presence of Antibodies to a Putatively Immunosuppressive Part of Human Immunodeficiency Virus (HIV) Envelope Glycoprotein gp41 Is Strongly Associated with Health among HIV-Positive Subjects," *Proc. Natl. Acad. Sci. USA*, 85:5225.

125 Lange, J., A. Vahine, J. Dekker, F. De Wolf and J. Goudsmit. 1989. "Antibodies to an HIV-1 Synthetic Peptide with Partial Homology to MULV p15 Do Not Protect against AIDS," *AIDS*, 3:402.

126 Robert-Guroff, M., M. S. J. Reitz, W. G. Robey and R. C. Gallo. 1986. "*In vitro* Generation of an HTLV-III Variant by Neutralizing Antibody," *J. Immunol.*, 137:3306.

127 Reitz, M. S. J., C. Wilson, C. Naugle, R. C. Gallo and M. Robert-Guroff. 1988. "Generation of a Neutralization-Resistant Variant of HIV-1 Is due to Selection for a Point Mutation in the Envelope Gene," *Cell*, 54:57.

128 Wilson, C., M. S. J. Reitz, K. Aldrich, P. J. Klasse, J. Blomberg, R. C. Gallo and M. Robert-Guroff. 1990. "The Site of an Immune-Selected Point Mutation in the Transmembrane Protein of Human Immunodeficiency Virus Type 1 Does Not Constitute the Neutralization Epitope," *J. Virol.*, 64:3240.

129 Qureshi, N. M., D. H. Coy, R. F. Garry and L. A. Henderson. 1990. "Character-

ization of Putative Cellular Receptor for HIV-1 Transmembrane Glycoprotein Using Synthetic Peptides," *AIDS*, 4:553.

130 Golding, H., F. A. Robey, F. T. Gates, III, W. Linder, P. R. Beining, T. Hoffman and B. Golding. 1988. "Identification of Homologous Regions in Human Immunodeficiency Virus 1 gp41 and Human MHC Class II β 1 Domain," *J. Exp. Med.*, 167:914.

131 Golding, H., G. M. Shearer, K. Hillman, P. Lucas, J. Manischewitz, R. A. Zajac, M. Clerici, R. E. Gress, R. N. Boswell and B. Golding. 1989. "Common Epitope in Human Immunodeficiency Virus (HIV) 1-GP41 and HLA Class II Elicits Immunosuppressive Autoantibodies Capable of Contributing to Immune Dysfunction in HIV I-Infected Individuals," *J. Clin. Invest.*

132 Young, J. A. T. 1988. "HIV and HLA Similarity," *Nature*, 333:215.

133 Garrett, T. P. G., M. A. Saper, P. J. Bjorkman, J. L. Strominger and D. C. Wiley. 1989. "Specificity Pockets for the Side Chains of Peptide Antigens in HLA-Aw68," *Nature*, 342:692.

134 Frelinger, J. A., F. M. Gotch, H. Zweerink, E. Wain and A. J. McMichael. 1990. "Evidence of Widespread Binding of HLA Class I Molecules to Peptides," *J. Exp. Med.*, 172:827.

135 Choppin, J., F. Martinon, E. Gomard, E. Bahraoui, F. Connan, M. Bouillot and J.-P. Lévy. 1990. "Analysis of Physical Interactions between Peptides and HLA Molecules and Application to the Detection of Human Immunodeficiency Virus 1 Antigenic Peptides," *J. Exp. Med.*, 172:889.

136 Takahashi, H., J. Cohen, A. Hosmalin, K. B. Cease, R. Houghten, J. L. Cornette, C. DeLisi, B. Moss, R. N. Germain and J. A. Berzofsky. 1988. "An Immunodominant Epitope of the HIV Envelope Glycoprotein gp160 Recognized by Class I Major Histocompatibility Molecule-Restricted Murine Cytotoxic T Lymphocytes," *Proc. Natl. Acad. Sci. USA*, 85:3105.

137 Takahashi, H., J. Cohen, A. Hasmalin, K. B. Cease, R. A. Houghten, J. L. Cornette, C. DeLisi, S. Merli, R. N. Germain, B. Moss and J. A. Berzofsky. 1989. "Limited Epitope Repertoire Recognized with Class I MHC Molecules by Murine Cytotoxic T Lymphocytes on the HIV gp160 Envelope Glycoprotein," *Vaccines*, 89:109.

138 Aichele, P., H. Hengartner, R. M. Zinkernagel and M. Schulz. 1990. "Antiviral Cytotoxic T Cell Response Induced by *in vivo* Priming with a Free Synthetic Peptide," *J. Exp. Med.*, 171:1815.

139 DeLisi, C. and J. A. Berzofsky. 1985. "T-Cell Antigenic Structures Tend to Be Amphipathic Structures," *Proc. Natl. Acad. Sci. USA*, 82:7048.

140 Berzofsky, J. A., K. B. Cease, J. L. Cornette, J. L. Spouge, H. Margalit, I. J. Berkower, M. F. Good, L. H. Miller and C. DeLisi. 1987. "Protein Antigenic Structures Recognized by T Cells: Potential Applications to Vaccine Design," *Immunol. Rev.*, 98:9.

141 Cease, K. B., H. Margalit, J. L. Cornette, S. D. Putney, W. G. Robey, C. Ouyand, H. Z. Streicher, P. J. Fischinger, R. C. Gallo, C. DeLisi and J. A. Berzofsky. 1987. "Helper T-Cell Antigenic Site Identification in the Acquired Immunodeficiency Syndrome Virus gp120 Envelope Protein and Induction of Immunity in Mice to the Native Protein Using a 16-Residue Synthetic Peptide," *Proc. Natl. Acad. Sci. USA*, 84:4249.

142 Rothbard, J. B. 1986. "Peptides and the Cellular Immune Response," *Ann. Inst. Pasteur Virol.*, 137E:518.

143 Whitton, J. L., H. Lewicki, J. R. Gebhard, A. Tishon, P. J. Southern and M. B. A. Oldstone. 1988. "Virus Epitopes that Induce Cytotoxic T Lymphocytes Can Be Recognized as Short Peptides and Are Selected by Class I Molecules," *Vaccines*, 88:215.

144 Claverie, J. M., P. Kourilsky, P. Langlade-Demoyen, A. Chalufour-Prochnicka, G. Dadaglio, F. Tekaia, F. Plata and L. Bougueleret. 1988. "T-Immunogenic Peptides Are Constituted of Rare Sequence Patterns. Use in the Identification of T Epitopes in the HIV Gag Protein," *Eur. J. Immunol.*, 18:1547.

145 Bouillot, M., J. Choppin, F. Cornille, F. Martinon, T. Papo, E. Gomard, M. C. Fournie-Zaluski and J.-P. Lévy. 1989. "Physical Association between MCH Class I Molecules and Immunogenic Peptides," *Nature*, 339:473.

146 Choppin, J., F. Martinon, F. Connan, E. Gomard and J.-P. Lévy. 1991. "HLA-Binding Regions of HIV-1 Proteins. I. Detection of Seven HLA Binding Regions in the HIV-1 Nef Protein," *J. Immunol.*, 147:569.

147 Choppin, J., F. Martinon, F. Connan, M. Pauchard, E. Gomard and J.-P. Lévy. 1991. "HLA-Binding Regions of HIV-1 Proteins. II. A Systematic Study of Viral Proteins," *J. Immunol.*, 147:575.

148 Cox, J. H., J. W. Yewdell, L. C. Eisenlohr, P. R. Johnson and J. R. Bennick. 1990. "Antigen Presentation Requires Transport of MHC Class I Molecules from the Endoplasmic Reticulum," *Science*, 247:715.

149 Moore, M. W., F. R. Carbone and M. J. Bevan. 1988. "Introduction of Soluble Protein into the Class I Pathway of Antigen Processing and Presentation," *Cell*, 54:777.

150 Hosaka, Y., F. Sasao, K. Yamanaka, J. R. Bennink and J. W. Yewdel. 1988. "Recognition of Noninfectious Influenza Virus by Class I–Restricted Murine Cytotoxic T Lymphocytes," *J. Immunol.*, 140:606.

151 Yewdell, J. W., J. R. Bennink and Y. Hosada. 1988. "Cells Process Exogenous Proteins for Recognition by Cytotoxic T Lymphocytes," *Science*, 239:637.

152 Staerz, U. D., H. Karasuyama and A. M. Garner. 1987. "Cytotoxic T Lymphocytes against a Soluble Protein," *Nature*, 329:449.

153 Jin, Y., J. W. Sih and I. Berkower. 1988. "Human T Cell Response to the Surface Antigen of Hepatitis B Virus (HBsAg). Endosomal and Nonendosomal Processing Pathways Are Accessible to Both Endogenous and Exogenous Antigen," *J. Exp. Med.*, 168:293.

154 Barnaba, V., A. Franco, A. Alberti, C. Balsano, R. Benvenuto and F. Balsano. 1989. "Recognition of Hepatitis B Virus Envelope Proteins by Liver-Infiltrating T Lymphocytes in Chronic HBV Infection," *J. Immunol.*, 143:2650.

155 Ishioka, G. Y., J. I. Krieger, S. Colon, C. Miles, H. M. Grey, and R. W. Chestnut. 1990. "Class I MHC-Restricted, Peptide-Specific Cytotoxic T Lymphocytes Generated by Peptide Priming *in Vivo*," *Vaccines*, 90:7.

156 Barnaba, V., A. Franco, A. Alberti, R. Benvenuto and F. Balsano. 1990. "Selective Killing of Hepatitis B Envelope Antigen-Specific B Cells by Class I-Restricted, Exogenous Antigen-Specific T Lymphocytes," *Nature*, 345:258.

157 Carbone, F. R. and M. J. Bevan. 1989. "Induction of Ovalbumin-Specific Cytotoxic T Cells by *in vivo* Peptide Immunization," *J. Exp. Med.*, 169:603.

158 Bevan, M. J. 1976. "Cross-Priming for a Secondary Cytotoxic Response to Minor H Antigens with H-2 Congenic Cells Which Do Not Cross-React in the Cytotoxic Assay," *J. Exp. Med.*, 143:1283.

159 Carbone, F. R., M. W. Moore, J. M. Sheil and M. J. Bevan. 1988. "Induction of Cytotoxic T Lymphocytes by Primary *in vitro* Stimulation with Peptides," *J. Exp. Med.*, 167:1767.

160 Deres, K., H. Schild, K.-H. Wiesmüller, G. Jung and H.-G. Rammensee. 1989. "*In vivo* Priming of Virus-Specific Cytotoxic T Lymphocytes with Synthetic Lipopeptide Vaccine," *Nature*, 342:561.

161 Morein, B., B. Sundquist, S. Höglund, K. Dalsgaard and A. Osterhaus. 1984. "ISCOM, a Novel Structure for Antigenic Presentation of Membrane Proteins from Enveloped Viruses," *Nature*, 308:457.

162 Morein, B., K. Lövgren, S. Höglund and B. Sundquist. 1987. "The ISCOM: An Immunostimulating Complex," *Immunol. Today*, 8:333.

163 Morein, B. 1988. "The ISCOM Antigen-Presenting System," *Nature*, 332:287.

164 Lövgren, K., J. Lindmark, R. Pipkorn and B. Morein. 1987. "Antigenic Presentation of Small Molecules and Peptides Conjuated to a Preformed ISCOM as Carrier," *J. Immunol. Meth.*, 98:137.

165 Berezin, V. E., V. M. Zaides, E. S. Isaeva, A. F. Artamonov and V. M. Zhdanov. 1988. "Controlled Organization of Multimolecular Complexes of Enveloped Virus Glycoproteins: Study of Immunogenicity," *Vaccine*, 6:450.

166 Harding, C. V., D. S. Collins, J. W. Slot, H. J. Geuze and E. R. Unanue. 1991. "Lipsome-Encapsulated Antigens Are Process in Lysosomes, Recycled, and Presented to T Cells," *Cell*, 64:393.

167 Lövgren, K. and B. Morein. 1988. "The Requirement of Lipids for the Formation of Immunostimulating Complexes (ISCOMs)," *Biotechnol. Appl. Biochem.*, 10:161.

168 Takahashi, H., T. Takeshita, B. Morein, S. Putney, R. N. Germain and J. A. Berzofsky. 1990. "Induction of CD8+ Cytotoxic T Cells by Immunization with Purified HIV-1 Envelope Protein in ISCOMs," Nature, 344:873.

169 Watari, E., B. Dietzschold, G. Szokan and E. Heber-Katz. 1987. "A Synthetic Peptide Induces Long-Term Protection from Lethal Infection with Herpes Simplex Virus 2," *J. Exp. Med.*, 165:459.

170 Byrne, J. A. and M. B. Oldstone. 1984. "Biology of Cloned Cytotoxic T Lymphocytes Specific for Lymphocytic Choriomeningitis Virus: Clearance of Virus *in Vivo*," *J. Virol.*, 51:682.

171 Lukacher, A. E., V. L. Braciale and T. J. Braciale. 1984. "*In vivo* Effector Function of Influenza Virus-Specific Cytotoxic T Lymphocyte Clones Is Highly Specific," *JEM*, 160:814.

172 Reddehase, M. J., W. Mutter, K. Münch, H.-J. Bühring and U. H. Koszinowski. 1987. "CD8-Positive T Lymphocytes Specific for Murine Cytomegalovirus Immediate-Early Antigens Mediate Protective Immunity," *J. Virol.*, 61:3102.

173 Cannon, M. J., E. J. Stott, G. Taylor and B. A. Askonas. 1987. "Clearance of Persistent Respiratory Syncytial Virus Infections in Immunodeficient Mice Following Transfer of Primed T Cells," *Immunology*, 62:133.

174 Moskophidis, D., S. P. Cobbold, H. Waldmann and F. Lehmann-Grube. 1987. "Mechanisms of Recovery from Acute Virus Infection: Treatment of Lymphocytic Choriomeningitis Virus-Infected Mice with Monoclonal Antibodies Reveals that Lyt-2+ T Lymphocytes Mediate Clearance of Virus and Regulate the Antiviral Antibody Response," *J. Virol.*, 61:1867.

175 Hom, R. C., R. W. Finberg, S. Mullaney and R. M. Ruprecht. 1991. "Protective

Cellular Retroviral Immunity Requires both CD4⁺ and CD8⁺ Immune T Cells," *J. Virol.* , 65:220.

176 Mawle, A. C., M. R. Ridgeway, M.-P. Kieny and A. R. Lifson. 1990. "HIV-1-Specific CTL Responses in Long-Term Asymptomatic Seropositive Individuals" (abstr. #L529), *UCLA Symposia on Molecular and Cellular Biology, HIV and AIDS: Pathogenesis, Therapy and Vaccine*, S.14D:173.

177 Salahuddin, S. Z., R. M. Rose, J. E. Groopman, P. D. Markham and R. C. Gallo. 1986. "Human T-Lymphotropic Virus Type III Infection of Human Alveolar Lung Macrophages," *Blood*, 68:281.

178 Autran, B., C. M. Mayaud, M. Raphael, F. Plata, M. Denis, A. Bourguin, J. M. Guillon, P. Debre and G. Akoun. 1988. "Evidence for a Cytotoxic T-Lymphocyte Alveolitis in Human Immunodeficiency Virus–Infected Patients," *AIDS*, 2:179.

179 Plata, F. A., B. L. P. Martins, S. Wain-Hobson, M. Raphael, C. Mayaud, M. Denis, J.-M. Guillon and P. Debré. 1987. "AIDS Virus–Specific Cytotoxic T Lymphocytes in Lung Disorders," *Nature*, 328:348.

180 Lanzavecchia, A., E. Roosnek, T. Gregory, P. Berman and S. Abrignani. 1988. "T Cells Can Present Antigens Such as HIV gp120 Targeted to Their Own Surface Molecules," *Nature*, 334:530.

181 Mills, K. H. G., D. F. Nixon and A. J. McMichael. 1989. "T-Cell Strategies in AIDS Vaccines: MHC-Restricted T-Cell Responses to HIV Proteins," *AIDS*, 3:S101.

182 Walker, B. D. and F. Plata. 1990. "Editorial Review. Cytotoxic T Lymphocytes against HIV," *AIDS*, 4:177.

183 Nixon, D. F., A. R. M. Townsend, J. G. Elvin, C. R. Rizza, J. Gallwey and A. J. McMichael. 1988. "HIV-1 Gag-Specific Cytotoxic T Lymphocytes Defined with Recombinant Vaccinia Virus and Synthetic Peptides," *Nature*, 336:484.

184 Walker, B. D., S. Chakrabarti, B. Moss, T. J. Paradis, T. Flynn, A. G. Durno, R. S. Blumberg, J. C. Kaplan, M. S. Hirsch and R. T. Schooley. 1987. "HIV-Specific Cytotoxic T Lymphocytes in Seropositive Individuals," *Nature*, 3328:345.

185 Riviere, Y., F. Tanneau-Salvadori, A. Regnault, O. Lopez, P. Sansonetti, B. Guy, M.-P. Kieny, J.-J. Fournel and L. Montagnier. 1989. "Human Immunodeficiency Virus-Specific Cytotoxic Responses of Seropositive Individuals: Distinct Types of Effector Cells Mediate Killing of Targets Expressing Gag and Env Proteins," *J. Virol.*, 63:2270.

186 Achour, A., O. Picard, D. Zagury, P. S. Sarin, R. C. Gallo, P. H. Naylor and A. L. Goldstein. 1990. "HGP-30, a Synthetic Analogue of Human Immunodeficiency Virus (HIV) p17, Is a Target for Cytotoxic Lymphocytes in HIV-Infected Individuals," *Proc. Natl. Acad. Sci. USA*, 87:7045.

187 Walker, B. D., C. Flexner, T. J. Paradis, T. C. Fuller, M. S. Hirsch, R. T. Schooley and B. Moss. 1988. "HIC-1 Reverse Transcriptase is a Target for Cytotoxic T Lymphocytes in Infected Individuals," *Science*, 240:64.

188 Koenig, K., T. R. Fuerst, L. V. Wood, R. M. Woods, J. A. Suzich, G. M. Jones, V. F. De la Cruz, R. T. Davey, Jr., S. Venkatesan, B. Moss, W. E. Biddison and A. S. Fauci. 1990. "Mapping the Fine Specificity of a Cytolytic T Cell Response to HIV-1 Nef Protein," *J. Immunol.*, 145:127.

189 Cullmann, B., E. Gomard, M.-P. Kiény, B. Guy, F. Dreyfus, A.-D. Saimot, D. Sereni, D. Sicard and J.-P. Lévy. 1991. "Six Epitopes Reacting with Human Cyto-

toxic CD8⁺ T cells in the Central Region of the HIV-1 Nef Protein," *J. Immunol.*, 146:1560.

190 Culmann, B. E., E. Gomard, M. P. Kiény, B. Guy, F. Dreyfus, A. G. Saimot, D. Sereni and J. P. Lévy. 1989. "An Antigenic Peptide of the HIV-1 Nef Protein Recognized by Cytotoxic T Lymphocytes of Seropositive Individuals in Association with Different HLA-B Molecules," *Eur. J. Immunol.*, 19:2383.

191 Tanneau, F., P. Sansonett, M. P. Kiény, O. Lopez, L. Montagnier and Y. Riviere. 1989. "Analysis of the Structural and Non-Structural Proteins of HIV-1 Recognized by Primary Cytotoxic T Lymphocytes," *V International Conference on AIDS*, abstract W.C.O.44.

192 Takahashi, H., R. Houghten, S. D. Putney, D. H. Margulies, B. Moss, R. N. Germain and J. A. Berzofsky. 1989. "Structural Requirements for Class I MHC Molecule–Mediated Antigen Presentation and Cytotoxic T Cell Recognition of an Immunodominant Determinant of the Human Immunodeficiency Virus Envelope Protein," *J. Exp. Med.*, 1770:2023.

193 Barnes, D. M. 1987. "Solo Actions of AIDS Virus Coat," *Science*, 237:971.

194 Ruegg, C. L., C. R. Monell and M. Strand. 1989. "Inhibition of Lymphoproliferation by a Synthetic Peptide with Sequence Identity to gp41 of Human Immunodeficiency Virus Type 1," *J. Virol.*, 63:3257.

195 Ruegg, C. L., C. R. Monell and M. Strand. 1989. "Identification, Using Synthetic Peptides, of the Minimum Amino Acid Sequence from the Retroviral Transmembrane Protein p15E Required for Inhibition of Lymphoproliferation and Its Similarity to gp21 of Human T-Lymphotropic Virus Types I and II," *J. Virol.*, 63:3250.

196 Ruegg, C. L., J. E. Clements and M. Strand. 1990. "Inhibition of Lymphoproliferation and Protein Kinase C by Synthetic Peptides with Sequence Identity to the Transmembrane and Q Proteins of Visna Virus," *J. Virol.*, 64:2175.

197 Cianciolo, G. J., H. Bogerd and R. Synderman. 1988. "Human Retrovirus-Related Synthetic Peptides Inhibit T Lymphocyte Proliferation," *Immunol. Lett.*, 19:7.

198 Cianciolo, G. J., T. D. Copeland, S. Oroszlan and R. Snyderman. 1985. "Inhibition of Lymphocyte Proliferation by a Synthetic Peptide Homologous to Retroviral Envelope Proteins," *Science*, 230:453.

199 Kleinerman, E. S., L. B. Lachman, R. D. Knowllees, R. Snyderman and G. J. Cianciolo. 1987. "A Synthetic Peptide Homologous to the Envelope Proteins of Retroviruses Inhibits Monocyte-Mediated Killing by Inactivating Interleukin 1," *J. Immunol.*, 1139:2329.

200 Wahl, S. M., J. B. Allen, S. Gartner, J. M. Orenstein, M. Popovic, D. E. Chenoweth, L. O. Arthur, W. L. Farrar and L. M. Wahl. 1989. "HIV-1 and Its Envelope Glycoprotein Down-Regulate Chemotactic Ligand Receptors and Chemotactic Function of Peripheral Blood Monocytes," *J. Immunol.*, 1442:3553.

201 Brenneman, D. E., G. L. Westbrook, S. P. Fitzgerald, D. L. Ennist, K. L. Elkins, M. R. Ruff and C. B. Pert. 1988. "Neuronal Cell Killing by the Envelope Protein of HIV and Its Prevention by Vasoactive Intestinal Peptide," *Nature*, 335:639.

202 Greve, J. M., G. Davis, A. M. Meyer, C. P. Forte, S. Connolly Yost, C. W. Marlor, M. E. Kamarck and A. McClelland. 1989. "The Major Human Rhinovirus Receptor is ICAM-1," *Cell*, 56:839.

203 Staunton, D. E., V. J. Merluzzi, R. Rothlein, R. Barton, S. D. Marlin and T. A.

Springer. 1989. "A Cell Adhesion Molecule, ICAM-1, Is the Major Surface Receptor for Rhinoviruses," *Cell*, 56:849.

204 Mendelsohn, C. L., E. Wimmer and V. R. Racaniello. 1989. "Cellular Receptor for Poliovirus: Molecular Cloning, Nucleotide Sequence, and Expression of a New Member of the Immunoglobulin Superfamily," *Cell*, 56:855.

205 Kowalski, M., J. Potz and L. Basinipour, et al. 1987. "Functional Regions of the Envelope Glycoprotein of Human Immunodeficiency Virus Type 1," *Science*, 237:1351.

206 Cordonnier, A., L. Montagnier and M. Emerman. 1989. "Single Amino Acid Changes in the HIV Envelope Affect Viral Tropism and Receptor Binding," *Nature*, 340:571.

207 Cordonnier, A., Y. Rivière, L. Montagnier and M. Emerman. 1989. "Effects of Mutations in Hyperconserved Regions of the Extracellular Glycoprotein of Human Immunodeficiency Virus Type 1 on Receptor Binding," *J. Virol.*, 63:4464.

208 Clapham, P. R., J. N. Weber, D. Whitby, K. McIntosh, A. G. Gagleish, P. J. Maddon, K. C. Deen, R. W. Sweet and R. A. Weiss. 1989. "Soluble CD4 Blocks the Infectivity of Diverse Strains of HIV and SIV for T-Cells and Monocytes but Not for Brain and Muscle Cells," *Nature*, 337:368.

209 Fisher, R. A., J. M. Bertonis, W. Meier, V. A. Johnson, D. S. Costopoulos, T. Liu, R. Tizard, B. Walker, M. S. Hirsch, R. T. Schooley and R. A. Flavell. 1988. "HIV Infection Is Blocked *in vitro* by Recombinant Soluble CD4," *Nature*, 331:76.

210 Hussey, R. E., N. E. Richardson, M. Kowalski, N. R. Brown, H.-C. Chang, R. F. Siliciano, T. Dorfman, B. Walker, J. Sodroski and E. R. Reinherz. 1988. "A Soluble CD4 Protein Selectively Inhibits HIV Replication and Syncytium Formation," *Nature*, 331:78.

211 Deen, K. C., J. S. McDougal, R. Inacker, G. Folena-Wasserman, J. Arthos, J. Rosenberg, P. J. Maddon, R. Axel and R. W. Sweet. 1988. "A Soluble Form of CD4 (T4) Protein Inhibits AIDS Virus Infection," *Nature*, 331:82.

212 Traunecker, A., W. Lüke and K. Karjalainen. 1988. "Soluble CD4 Molecules Neutralise Human Immunodeficiency Virus Type 1," *Nature*, 331:84.

213 Sekigawa, I., S. M. Chamow, J. E. Groopman and R. A. Byrn. 1990. "CD4 Immunoadhesin, but Not Recombinant Soluble CD4, Blocks Syncytium Formation by Human Immunodeficiency Virus Type 2–Infected Lymphoid Cells," *J. Virol.*, 64:5194.

214 Lifson, J. D., K. M. Hwang, P. L. Nara, B. Fraser, M. Padgett, N. M. Dunlop and L. E. Eiden. 1988. "Synthetic CD4 Peptide Derivatives that Inhibit HIV Infection and Cytopathicity," *Science*, 241:712.

215 Nara, P. L., K. M. Hwang, D. M. Rausch, J. D. Lifson and L. E. Eiden. 1989. "CD4 Antigen–Based Antireceptor Peptides Inhibit Infectivity of Human Immunodeficiency Virus *in vitro* at Multiple Stages of the Viral Life Cycle," *PNAS*, 86:7139.

216 Hayashi, Y., K. Ikuta, N. Fujii, K. Ezawa and S. Kato. 1989. "Inhibition of HIV-1 Replication and Syncytium Formation by Synthetic CD4 Peptides," *Arch. Virol.*, 105:129.

217 Jameson, B. A., P. E. Rao, L. I. Kong, B. H. Hahn, G. M. Shaw, L. E. Hood and S. B. Kent. 1988. "Location and Chemical Synthesis of a Binding Site for HIV-1 on the CD4 Protein," *Science*, 240:1335.

218 Finberg, R. W., D. C. Diamond, D. B. Mitchell, Y. Rosenstein, G. Soman, T. C.

Norman, S. L. Schreiber and S. J. Burakoff. 1990. "Prevention of HIV-1 Infection and Preservation of CD4 Function by the Binding of CPFs to gp120," *Science*, 249:287.

219 Daar, E. S., X. L. Li, T. Moudgil and D. D. Ho. 1990. "High Concentrations of Recombinant Soluble CD4 Are Required to Neutralize Primary Human Immunodeficiency Virus Type 1 Isolates," *Proc. Natl. Acad. Sci. USA*, 87:6574.

220 Rossmann, M. G., E. Arnold, J. W. Erickson, E. A. Frankenberger, J. P. Griffith, H.-J. Hecht, J. E. Johnson, G. Kamer, M. Luo, A. G. Mosser, R. R. Rueckert, B. Sherry and G. Vriend. 1985. "Structure of a Human Common Cold Virus and Functional Relationship to Other Picornoviruses," *Nature*, 317:145.

221 Rossmann, M. G. 1988. "Antiviral Agents Targeted to Interact with Viral Capsid Proteins and a Possible Application to Human Immunodeficiency Virus," *Proc. Natl. Acad. Sci. USA*, 85:4625.

222 Rossmann, M. G. 1989. "The Structure of Antiviral Agents that Inhibit Uncoating When Complexed with Viral Capsids," *Antiviral Res.*, 11:3.

223 Chapman, M. S., I. Minor and M. G. Rossmann. 1991. "Human Rhinovirus 14 Complexed with Antiviral Compound R 61837," *J. Mol. Biol.*, 217:455.

224 Bergelson, J. M., M. P. Shepley, B. M. C. Chan, M. E. Hemler and R. W. Finberg. 1992. "Identification of the Integrin VLA-2 as a Receptor for Echovirus 1," *Science*, 255:1718.

225 Leonard, C. K., M. W. Spellman, L. Riddle, R. J. Harris, J. N. Thomas and T. J. Gregory. 1990. "Assignment of Intrachain Disulfide Bonds and Characterization of Potential Glycosylation Sites of the Type 1 Recombinant Human Immunodeficiency Virus Envelope Glycoprotein (gp 120) Expressed in Chinese Hamster Ovary Cells," *Jour. Biol. Chem.*, 265:10373–10382.

Peptides as Molecular Probes of Immune Responses

ELLEN HEBER-KATZ[1]
HILDEGUND C. J. ERTL[1]

INTRODUCTION

PEPTIDES have been used in immunology as defined synthetic antigens which have the potential to be made in large quantities and with the hope of producing safe vaccines without the worry of infections. Peptides have been shown to be useful as probes in measuring antigen-specific responses in both the B cell and the T cell arm of the immune response. In this review, we will cover studies in two very different systems, the T cell response to an internal protein of rabies virus and the T cell response to a surface glycoprotein of herpes simplex virus (HSV), which have yielded very different results and lead us to believe that it is difficult to draw major conclusions about the use of peptides in immune responses and vaccines in general. Rather it appears that each system is unique and that further studies with peptides must be done on an individual basis. Thus, one will have to take into account the individual peptide, the individual protein, and each individual virus.

DEFINITION OF IMMUNODOMINANCE

The hallmark of an immune response to a complex antigen is the striking ability to generate a diversity of specific molecules, known as antibodies. These are produced by cells that are just as diverse. However, it was noticed that when inbred animals were immunized with antigens of re-

[1]The Wistar Institute, 3601 Spruce Street, Philadelphia, PA 19104, U.S.A.

stricted structural heterogeneity, there was a segregation of antigen-specific responses. Thus, it was found that animals of a given histocompatibility or MHC genotype could respond to restricted antigen and animals of a second MHC genotype could not. This was seen both at the level of antibodies or B cells and at the level of delayed-type hypersensitivity (DTH) or T cells, known to be responsible for helping B cells to make antibody.

A set of clever experiments were able to dissect the problem revealing that the inability to respond lay with the T cells and not with the B cells. Thus, if one could bypass the nonresponder T cells and provide nonspecific help, then the B cells would be free to respond to any antigen. Not so for the T cells. With the discovery that T cells needed to see antigen in the context of MHC it became clear that certain MHC molecules were permissive for the presentation of antigens and others were not. This implied that T cells were directly involved in the recognition of MHC structures. Thus, T cells were attributed with the important role of regulating the immune response.

To bring this to the present, it is now known that T cells respond to protein antigens in association with MHC molecules. These antigens are recognized as peptides which have been processed from whole protein molecules by antigen-presenting cells. One level of selection of a stimulatory peptide is the ability of a particular peptide or antigenic determinant to interact with different MHC molecules. Thus, it becomes clear how the MHC determines T cell fine specificity. When animals are immunized with a whole protein molecule the T cell response that follows can be shown to be specific for only one or a very limited number of determinants, a phenomenon known as immunodominance.

METHODS OF DEFINING IMMUNODOMINANT T CELL EPITOPES

Numerous epitopes have been identified for murine as well as human T cells. The initial work was done with well-defined proteins such as cytochrome c [1], lysozyme [2], or myoglobin [3]. In viral systems, the response to several pathogens such as influenza A virus [4,5], hepatitis B virus (HBV) [6,7], and human immunodeficiency virus (HIV) [8,9] has been investigated as well as those studies done in rabies virus and HSV in our own laboratories which will be described in Tables 10.1 and 10.2.

Most of the experiments designed to define epitopes used either cells derived from virus-immune animals or humans that were subsequently restimulated *in vitro* with a number of synthetic peptides of 10–20 amino acids in length that were delineated from the viral protein of interest, in many cases a viral surface antigen such as the hemagglutinin of influenza A virus [6] or gp160 or 120 of HIV [8]. In other cases, T cell epitopes were

TABLE 10.1. Class II Restricted Responses to Peptides.

Virus	Antigen	Peptide	Restricting Element Species	Reference
Influenza A	HA	307-318	human	Lamb et al. [5]
		126-138	mouse [IA^d]	Eisenlohr et al. [46]
		302-313	mouse [IE^d]	
		111-119	mouse [H-2^d]	
	Matrix	17-31	human [HLA-DR1]	Rothbard and Taylor [47]
HIV	gp120	428-442	mouse, human	Cease et al. [8] and Bersowsky et al. [48]
		112-124	mouse, human	
		426-450	nonhuman primates	Krohn et al. [49]
		410-429	human [HLA-DR1]	Lusso et al. [50]
HBV	HBsAg	212-226, 269-283	mouse [H-2^q]	Milich et al. [7]
	S region	284-311, 314-328	mouse [H-2^k]	
		193-202	human [Dpw4]	Celis et al. [6]
		212-226, 284-311	human	Milich et al. [7]

(continued)

TABLE 10.1. (continued).

Virus	Antigen	Peptide	Restricting Element Species	Reference
HBV	pre S	12-21, 53-73, 94-117	mouse [H-2^{s,f}]	Milich et al. [51]
	nucleocapsid	120-131	mouse [H-2^s]	Milich et al. [52-54]
		129-140	mouse [H-2^b]	
		100-110	mouse [H-2^f]	
		100-120	mouse [H-2^q]	
		85-100	mouse [H-2^b]	
Rabies	nucleoprotein	404-418	mouse [H-2^k]	Ertl et al. [12]
		21-35, 394-408	mouse [H-2^b]	
		11-25, 281-294	mouse [IA^q]	Celis et al. [55]
		201-215, 121-135	human [HLA-DR7]	Celis et al. [56]
		11-25	human [HLA-DQw3]	
	glycoprotein	292-323	mouse [IE^d]	
		283-323	human [HLA-DR7]	Celis et al. [55]
HSV	gIp2	1-16	mouse [IA^k]	Heber-Katz and Dietzschold [57]
		8-23	mouse [IE^k]	

TABLE 10.2. Class I Restricted Responses to Peptides.

Virus	Antigen	Peptide	Restricting Element	Reference
Influnza A	NP	147-161	mouse [H-2K^d]	Taylor et al. [58]
		50-63	mouse [H-2K^k]	Bastin et al. [59]
		365-380	mouse [H-2D^b]	Townsend et al. [60]
		339-347	human [HLA-B37]	Townsend et al. [60]
		335-349	human [HLA-B37, A1, B13]	McMichael et al. [61]
	matrix	56-68	human [HLA-A2]	Gotch et al. [62]
HIV	gp160	308-322, 315-329	mouse [H-2^d]	Takahashi et al. [9]
LCMV	gp2	272-293	mouse [H-2^b]	Whitton et al. [63]

identified by the use of virus-specific T cell clones or hybridomas. Both of
these methods address the question of the antigenicity of peptides. Both
methods yield in general comparable results and both have advantages and
disadvantages.

In the rabies virus system, we compared both methods and obtained the
following results. Our studies concentrated on identifying T helper (Th)
cell epitopes of the viral nucleoprotein (N protein). Animals immunized
with either N protein, presented in the form of ribonucleoprotein (RNP),
a complex that consists of the viral genome, the N protein, a nominal
phosphoprotein (NS protein), and a few copies of a viral polymerase [10]
or with N protein purified from insect cells infected with a baculo N protein recombinant virus [11], were shown to be protected against a subsequent potentially lethal challenge with rabies virus. In addition, lymphokine secreting T cells of mice that were injected with inactivated rabies
virus, in our experiments of the Evelyn Rokitniki Abelseth (ERA) strain,
responded if tested on purified viral proteins better to the N protein than
to any of the other viral proteins [12].

In order to identify Th cell epitopes of this internal viral protein, we
stimulated lymphocytes derived from popliteal and para-aortal lymph
nodes of ERA virus–immune mice with 40 synthetic peptides of an average length of 15 amino acids that overlapped at each end for five amino
acids with the adjacent peptide and that covered nearly the entire sequence
of the ERA N protein. Initially, proliferation was tested two or three days
later with a [³H]thymidine pulse. The results we obtained using this
method were disappointing; the background proliferation of lymphocytes
cultured in absence of antigen was unacceptably high and in addition proliferation in response to antigens known to be recognized was generally at
most two fold above control data. We then developed a lymphokine release
assay which at least in our system was shown to be more sensitive. Again,
lymph node lymphocytes from virus-immune mice were cultured in presence or absence of antigen. After 20–24 hrs parts of the supernatants were
removed and transferred onto a lymphokine dependent T cell line such as
the HT-2 cell line. Proliferation versus cell death of this cell line could
either be assessed visually after 48 hrs or be measured by [³H]thymidine
incorporation. Using this method we were able to identify one epitope in
H-2^k mice expressed by peptide 31D (residues 404-418), and two epitopes
in H-2^b mice expressed by peptides 3D (21-35) and 30D (394-408) [12].
Using this type of mixed population has the advantage that a number of
mouse strains could be tested easily. Furthermore, this method facilitates
the recognition of dominant epitopes as it is presumably too insensitive to
detect minor epitopes.

Epitopes of cytolytic T (Tc) cells can be identified in a similar way by
priming lymphocytes *in vivo* with antigen, in our system live rabies virus,

followed by an *in vitro* stimulation with inactivated virus. Epitope-specific effector cells can then be determined in a ^{51}Cr-release assay by lysis of H-2 compatible target cells pretreated with different peptides.

The second method, i.e., generation of T cell clones and/or hybridomas directed against virus, followed by selection of T cells that respond to a given protein (in our case the N protein) has several advantages. Once the clones are established a multitude of experiments designed to further define the epitope can be performed rapidly. These include using peptide analogous of the antigen, determining MHC binding specificity by using stimulator or target cells from different congenic mice, or by conducting peptide inhibition experiments. Furthermore the differences between negative and positive responses are much more pronounced with T cell clones as compared to primary cultures. Potential disadvantages are that culture conditions might select for T cell clones to minor rather than major epitopes. For the ERA N protein as far as the 31D epitope was concerned the primary response showed good correlation with the results obtained with T cell clones. Only peptide 31D elicited a response from ERA–N protein immune H-2^k mice. Accordingly more than 95% of the T cell clones derived from H-2^k mice specific for the N protein responded to peptide 31D thus confirming its immunodominance [12]. Another disadvantage is that the generation and maintenance of T cell clones is expansive and labor intensive and not always successful. As an alternative one can generate T cell hybridomas by fusion of either primary T cells or already established and characterized T cell clones with a myeloma cell line such as BW. This approach can generally not be used for class I restricted Tc cells as they loose their lytic activity upon fusion. In our experience with Th cells to peptide 31D the specificity of these hybridomas was identical to that of the parental T cell clones [13]. While T cell hybridomas have the advantage to be easier to maintain (as they do not require stimulator cells or exogenous lymphokines) and can be grown up to large quantities, they have the disadvantage of generally losing specificity more rapidly than T cell clones, which requires frequent subcloning.

Peptides can be tested on Th cell clones either for induction of proliferation or for stimulation of lymphokine release. T cell hybridomas that grow constituetively can only be tested for release of lymphokines in response to antigen. Both methods, i.e., proliferation and release of lymphokines have basically the same sensitivity and give comparable results. For an initial screening of different peptides the lymphokine release assay might be superior as proliferation is inhibited in the presence of excessive amounts of peptides. For example peptide 31D showed optimal stimulation if present at 0.2 μM. Another peptide that we identified to carry a dominant epitope of the nominal phosphoprotein (NS protein) stimulated best if used at 0.04 μM concentration and was inhibitory at 0.2 μM concentrations if tested in a proliferation assay. This shows that antigenic concentrations vary tremendously from peptide to peptide not only depending on the length of the peptide but presumably also on the structure which might determine the affinity for the MHC molecule. Testing peptides for induction of lymphokine release might thus be advantageous.

Most epitopes to date have been defined by the use of overlapping, synthetic peptides. Although some investigators used a limited number of peptides relying on one of the currently available predictions for T cell epitopes, these predictions are somewhat unreliable and using them might lead to missing important epitopes. Synthesizing overlapping peptides that cover the entire length of a large virus is a prohibitively time consuming and expensive endeavor.

An alternative approach in identifying epitopes of viral proteins was used in the murine cytomegalovirus system to define epitopes of Tc cells [14]. We have subsequently used the same approach to define Tc as well as Th epitopes of the rabies virus NS protein (J. Larson et al., manuscript in preparation). In principle, initially the gene that encodes the antigen of interest is cloned. A set of serial carboxy-terminal truncations of the cDNA are generated that encode proteins that are serially shortened by 20–50 amino acids. These truncated genes are expressed under an early promoter in a host virus such as vaccinia virus. The recombinant viruses are tested for expression of the inserted gene by Southern and Northern blot. Subsequently, the expression of full length or truncated foreign proteins is determined by Western blot. The recombinant virus can be used to either prime lymphocytes *in vivo* that are then tested *in vitro* for a response to the parental virus. Alternately virus-immune T cells can be tested for an *in vitro* response to the recombinant virus either by using the recombinant virus as antigen in a proliferation or lymphokine release assay to identify Th cells or by infecting target cells with the recombinant virus to test for Tc cell activity. Using this method a putative epitope can be narrowed down to a stretch of 20–50 amino acids. Synthetic peptides delineated from this area of the protein can then be used to further define the epitope.

Immunogenicity of a Th cell epitope can be tested directly by injecting mice with the synthetic peptide in adjuvants such as CFA and subsequently restimulating lymphocytes with the viral antigen or the peptide. In our experience all peptides that were antigentic *in vitro* for virus-induced T cells, were able to induce T cells that secreted lymphokines to the virus and to the homologous peptide *in vivo*. As an additional asay for Th cells mice can be primed with peptides and then be boosted several weeks later with a low dose of inactivated virus. For example in the case of rabies virus we were able to show that 31D in H-2^k mice and 3D in H-2^b mice induced T cells that upon booster immunization with inactivated rabies virus caused an accelerated and enhanced B cell response to the viral glycoprotein [12].

It is currently not possible to test the immunogenicity of peptides that carry Tc cell epitopes by simply immunizing mice with peptides as this approach generally does not cause stimulation of Tc effector cells.

T CELL EPITOPES OF VIRAL ANTIGENS: IMMUNODOMINANCE VERSUS DIVERSITY

Herpes Simplex Viral System

In the herpes simplex viral (HSV) system, the focus has been on the glycoprotein D (gD). This molecule is 393 amino acids long and has a molecular weight of 59,000 Da [15-17]. gD is expressed both on the viral envelope and also on the surface of infected cells [18]. It is known to be a target of antibody neutralization and there have been described seven major B cell antigenic determinants [17]. Our studies on the T cell response to the gD was initially begun by the examination of N-terminal peptides of this protein. Immunization with the 23 amino acid peptide was found to stimulate T cells in the B10.A (H-2^a) strain of mouse. Furthermore, there were two determinants in this region, one found in residues 1-16 and one found in residues 8-23 [19]. To determine the potential protective effect of these peptides against an HSV infection, we immunized BALB/c (H-2^d) mice, animals which are highly susceptible to lethal HSV infections, with a peptide construct. We found that the 1-23 peptide could protect and that this protection was T cell–mediated [20] (see the next section). We thus concluded that this must be an important T cell determinant that is probably immunodominant.

Recombinant gD was obtained from Rae Lynn Burke at Chiron Corp. [21] and studies of immunodominance revealed that this N-terminal peptide was not an immunodominant peptide in any of the mouse strains examined. As shown in most systems [22], immunization with this protein in complete Freund's adjuvant (CFA) yielded T cells from draining lymph nodes which were reactive to only one synthetic peptide determinant. In H-2^d mice, peptide number 13, residues 241-260, was stimulatory, as previously reported [23]. On the other hand, in H-2^k mice peptide number 26, residues 211-230, was stimulatory. In both H-2^b and H-2^f mice, at least six different peptides were stimulatory. This supported the idea of immunodominance and Ir gene control and specific association of given peptides with the MHC genotype of the mouse (at least for H-2^d and H-2^k mice).

Given the fact, however, that the 1-23 peptide could protect animals from disease and that in this case the immunogen was not gD in CFA but rather infectious virus, we attempted to dissect the T cell response to the gD molecule after priming with infectious HSV. Seven days after injection of 10^6 PFU of HSV-1, draining lymph nodes were removed and tested for responses to HSV, gD, and the complete panel of synthetic peptides. We found that in BALB/c mice, T cells responsive to gD could respond to peptide number 13, as was seen after immunization with gD in CFA, but now we also saw responses to the majority of the peptides used. Thus, the phenomenon of immunodominance seemed to disappear. Furthermore, culturing these cells with gD did not result in a dominant peptide number 13 response. Cloning T cells with specific peptides from HSV-infected mice yielded T cells which could cross-react with gD, peptide, and HSV showing that the peptide responses were not due to aberrant cross-reactions but represented true diversity in the gD response. Further evidence of diversity was shown with the finding of BALB/c T cell lines to these many different peptide determinants displayed both I-A and I-E restricted responses [24]. This finding indicates that there is probably more than one determinant in each of the 20 amino acid long synthetic peptides examined. Preliminary data from other mouse strains injected with infectious virus also show responsiveness to a diversity of peptide determinants. At present then, it appears that 80% of the glycoprotein D molecule is immunogenic for T cells. Why there is such a difference between the response to gD in the form of a protein injected as an emulsion or as a protein expressed as a result of an infection is unclear. However, most studies with class II restricted T cells indicate that exogenous routes of antigen processing occur and it is in this case that immunodominance is seen. However, it is possible that other routes of antigen processing occur for endogenously produced antigen which may lead to the diversity to determinants seen [25–29]. These findings have implications in terms of selection of determinants that are used to elicit antiviral T cell responses and the relevance of immunodominance when defined by proteins which have been injected in CFA as opposed to a natural infection.

It is interesting that in humans, the same lack of immunodominance may be occurring when priming is a result of an HSV infection. Thus, examination of a panel of infected individuals showed a response to the 1-23 peptides irrespective of the MHC haplotype of the individual [30].

Rabies Viral System

In contrast in the herpes virus system, the murine T cell response to the rabies virus N protein focuses on only a limited or restricted number of determinants in 2/3 haplotypes tested. Mice immunized with rabies virus of the H-2^k (or H-2^a) haplotype responded to only one peptide (i.e., peptide 31D) while H-2^b mice responded to peptides 3D and 30D but failed to respond to 31D [12]. Lack of responsiveness to peptide 31D was unlikely to be caused by tolerance due to mimicry of a self antigen as (H-2^k × H-2^b)

F_1 mice responded to all three peptides. Mice that carried the H-2^d haplotype responded weakly to a number of peptides (including 3D and 31D) none of which was clearly immunodominant [12]. As far as what has been tested for H-2^b and H-2^k mice, neither the route of inoculation (i.e., into the footpad or intraperitoneally) nor the ability of the virus to multiply changes the epitope pattern for Th cells.

We have presented two viral systems yielding results at two ends of the spectrum: one in which there is strict immunodominance and one in which there is none. The latter system might be explained by the fact that HSV in this system is not limiting since virus replicates in cells at the site of injection and probably in the antigen-presenting cell. On the other hand, rabies virus only multiplies in neuronal cells that are in general not accessible to the peripheral immune system. This suggests that immunodominance at the T cell level may be a function of the availability of antigenic peptide fragments.

THE ROLE OF PEPTIDE STRUCTURE IN T CELL RESPONSES

One of the first antigens to be carefully dissected in terms of helper T cell responsiveness to peptide determinants was cytochrome *c*, where it was noted that a helical structure seemed to be preferred [31]. Support for this idea was extended to the myoglobin system [32]. If indeed such a structural correlation could be found for predicting T cell determinants, it would be easy to see how useful this would be.

Using a data base of 23 known Th cell epitopes H. Margalit et al. [33] postulated that antigenic sites on proteins are helical in structure with one side predominantly polar and the opposite side mainly apolar. The authors suggest that the strong correlation between immunodominant T cell epitopes and regions able to form peptides that fold into amphipathic helixes indicates that this structure might facilitate binding to MHC via the hydrophobic part of the molecule, with subsequent recognition by the TcR of the hydrophilic part. From the limited number of T cell epitopes the authors compared, ~75% contained an amphipathic helix while the other sites were not predicted by the algorithm. None of the immunodominant regions of the rabies N protein we identified [12] had a tendency to form an amphipathic helix and would have certainly been missed if we had selected peptides on the basis of the above described prediction.

Rothbard and Taylor [34], analyzing a similar set of data, proposed that T cell epitopes in contrast to B cell epitopes seem to be clustered in areas that are poorly exposed on the surface of a protein, which they suggest protects them from enzymatic cleavage. Furthermore 29 out of 30 peptides analyzed had a charged residue or a glycine followed by two hydrophobic residues that in 22 cases were followed by a charged or polar residue. If the fourth amino acid in this pattern was hydrophobic, a charged polar amino acid was commonly found in the fifth position. Although this prediction is more general our peptides in the rabies virus N protein system would not have been predicted by this pattern either [12].

Another general observation is that T cell epitopes seem to be clustered in variable regions of viral proteins. This was observed with HIV [8] or in the case of the rabies N protein [12] where two out of three immunodominant T cell epitopes were identified in regions of this otherwise fairly conserved molecule that showed amino acid exchanges between the two rabies virus N proteins (i.e., that of the Pasteur virus (PV) and the ERA virus strains) that have been sequenced to date.

HSV

In our studies with the HSV peptides, we found support for immunogenic determinants which were not only helical structures but also nonhelical structures [35]. Within the first 23 amino acids of the gD, we found that the two identified T cell determinants differed structurally. Using a set of peptides with the sequence of HSV-1 and HSV-2, which differed by two residues, and a hybrid of those two molecules, we compared the structure and function of those peptides which were 23 amino acids long [1-23(1), 1-23(2), and 1-23(H)], peptides from the N-terminus [1-16(1) and 1-16(2)], and peptides from the C-terminus [8-23(1) and 8-23(2)]. Using circular dichroism to measure helicity in the helix-promoting solvent TFE, it was found that the 1-16(1) and 1-16(2) peptides as well as the 1-23(1) peptide were helical, whereas the 8-23(1) and 8-23(2) peptides as well as the 1-23(2) and 1-23(H) peptides were non-helical (See Table 10.1). Functional analysis showed that the T cells induced by the 1-23(1) peptide which is helical induced a response to the peptides that were strictly helical, thus to the 1-23(1), 1-16(1), and 1-16(2) peptides. Furthermore, such a response was restricted to the I-A molecule. On the other hand, the 1-23(H) peptide, which was nonhelical, induced a T cell response to the peptides which were nonhelical, the 1-23(H), 1-23(2), 8-23(1), and 8-23(2) peptides. In this case, the T cell response was found to be only I-E restricted. The association of these different structures has been seen in other studies [36].

From these studies, we were also able to provide the first evidence that residues distant from the actual antigenic determinant could affect both structure and responsiveness, though other studies have confirmed this [37]. Using such T cell populations specific for the nonhelical determinant, 8-23(1), we found that the addition of the 1-7 residues resulting in the 1-23(1) sequence resulted in a change from a nonhelical to a helical structure and nonresponsiveness to the 8-23 encompassed in that structure.

Also, T cell populations reactive to the helical 1-16 peptides were now found to be nonreactive in the 1-23(H) molecule which had been made nonhelical by the addition of the 17-23(2) sequence added at the end (see Table 10.3).

RABIES VIRUS

In the rabies virus system the response to peptide 31D was investigated with a panel of Th cell clones in order to define minimal structural requirements for this peptide to retain antigenicity [13]. The initial 31D (AVY TRIMMNGGRLKR) peptide was a 15 amino acid long peptide corresponding to residues 404-418 of the N protein. This peptide stimulated T cell clones if used at concentrations ranging from 10^{-7} to 10^{-8} M. Extending the sequence by an additional 17 amino acids increased the antigenicity of the peptide that was shown to be positive at 10^{-9} M concentrations thus suggesting that the antigenic potency of a peptide might be up to a point directly correlated with the length of a peptide. Accordingly two 10 amino acid long peptides delineated from the N- or C-terminus of peptide 31D (AVYTRIMMNG and IMMNGGRLKR), which were both shown to stimulate 31D specific T cells, had to be used at concentrations of 10^{-6} and 10^{-5} M, respectively. As those two 10 amino acid long peptides only have the IMMNG sequence in common, a 5 amino acid peptide that contains this sequence was synthetized and shown to induce a response if added at concentrations of 10^{-3} M. At these concentrations a 4 amino acid peptide of the MMNG sequence was positive as was a tripeptide that contained MNG. Another trimer, i.e., MMN was only weakly positive and single

TABLE 10.3. Relationship of the Helix Contents of Synthetic Peptides of the First 23 Amino Acid Residues of HSV gD and Their Function.

Peptide	Helix Content (%)*	1-23(1) Response†	1-23(H) Response‡
1. 1-23(1)**	17	+	−
2. 1-23(2)	<5	−	+
3. 1-23(H)	5	−	+
4. 1-16(1)	17	+	−
5. 1-16(2)	15	+	−
6. 8-23(1)	<10	−	+
7. 8-23(2)	<5	−	+

* Helix content determined in TFE derived from the spectra by the method of Greenfield and Fasman [38].
** The sequences of the HSV-1 and HSV-2 and a hybrid of the two gD molecules.
† The response of T cells from animals primed with the helical 1-23(1) peptide.
‡ The response of T cells from animals primed with the nonhelical 1-23(H) peptide.

amino acids such as M or N did not elicit a response at any of the concentrations tested.

In the next set of experiments, we investigated the specificity of the response. T cell clones that recognized peptide 31D responded to most rabies virus strains we tested. They did not respond to the PV strain that is known to have one amino acid exchange within the sequence that is represented by peptide 31D where in position 410 the methionine of the ERA strain was replaced by an isoleucine in the PV strain. A 15 amino acid peptide that corresponded to the 31D sequence of the PV N protein (AVYTRIIMNG GRLKR) was not being recognized by 31D specific T cells although an excess of this peptide inhibited the response of T cells to peptide 31D indicating that lack of responsiveness was caused by lack of recognition by the TcR rather than inappropriate binding of the peptide to MHC. A 5 amino acid long peptide corresponding to the middle part of the PV peptide, i.e., IIMNG was recognized by T cells to the same extent as the original IMMNG peptide. A number of 4 and 5 amino acid long peptides was subsequently analyzed and most of them such as QIINM, a sequence found in gp 120 of HIV, MMDG, MMQG or GNMM induced responses of 31D specific T cell clones. Two other peptide analogues, i.e., IMVNG and MVNG had a markedly reduced antigenicity for some T cell clones or were negative for others. Unrelated peptides such as KEKE or KSPV did not induce a response either. The response to small peptides was specific in as much as T cell clones that recognized different epitopes either of rabies virus or of an unrelated protein failed to respond to these small peptides. Both the response to virus or larger peptides as well as the response to smaller peptides was restricted to IE^k and could be inhibited by unrelated peptides known to bind to IE^k. Our data clearly demonstrate two points. First the antigenic potency of a peptide is directly correlated with the length of a peptide, i.e., longer peptides of >30 amino acids stimulate at 10^{-9} M while a 10^6 times higher concentration is needed of 3–5 amino acid long peptides to achieve similar activation of T cells as measured by proliferation or lymphokine release. Second, the specificity of the response is directly correlated with the length of a peptide. Longer peptides are exclusively specific and the change of one crucial amino acid, such as a methionine to isoleucine, can abolish antigenicity. Smaller peptides show a high degree of flexibility and the same amino acid exchange has no effect on antigenicity. The higher degree of non-specificity could not be explained by the higher concentration of peptide needed to elicit a response, as the 15 amino acid long peptide delineated from the N protein of the PV strain failed to induce a response even if added in mg amounts.

It is hard to explain how 3–5 amino acid long peptides that do not even have to be conserved can induce a specific response. Structurally the antigenic peptides had a tendency for a β-turn; peptide analogues that were designed to have a weakened β-turn potential by, for example replacing the methionine in position three of the pentapeptide by a valine, lost antigenicity suggesting that a β-turn played a role either in binding of the peptide to MHC or for recognition by the TcR.

PROTECTION FROM VIRAL INFECTIONS BY PEPTIDE VACCINES

The ability of stimulate an immune response using a synthetic replica of a pathogen and especially a small part of that pathogen suddenly becomes very interesting when thinking about the possibility of a vaccine. Such small synthetic molecules are not only easy to produce in large quantities but they cannot replicate and thus are considered to have little if any detrimental effects. The only issue is efficacy and as stated above, a given peptide is thought to associate with only one or a few MHC haplotypes and therefore would not be good as a general tool. However, that may not always be the case.

HSV

In the HSV system, as discussed previously, we were able to achieve a protective response from a lethal HSV infection in the susceptible BALB/c strain of mouse using the 1-23 peptides [20]. This was not accomplished by the injection of free peptide in saline but rather required a particular construct involving the peptide coupled to a fatty acid and then incorporated into a liposome. Previously studies had indicated that both the use of fatty acid side chains and the use of liposomes could enhance antigenicity by measuring antibody responses against particular viral proteins [39,40]. The two lipids however had not been used together. The use of our peptide-lipid construct yielded several interesting results. First, there was no detectable antibody produced. This might seem surprising since the liposome and fatty acid side chain alone enhanced antibody production. However, there have been previous reports indicating that lipids in fact enhance DTH responses (attributed to T cells) over antibody responses [41,42]. Second, the protection could be adoptively transferred with T cells and this protective activity could be eliminated by anti-CD8 antibody. This was the first report that peptide could induce a CD8-positive T cell, a cell generally considered to be important in an antiviral response. Third, the protective response induced was long lasting. Thus, one injection of the construct yielded protection of susceptible BALB/c mice after eight months. Finally, the peptide used was not the immunodominant peptide of the T cell response to glycoprotein D. Thus, it might be possible to use many peptides previously thought not to be significant.

RABIES

All of the N protein peptides that stimulated rabies virus specific Th cells *in vitro* were shown to induce a rabies virus specific Th cell response *in vivo*. For example the 31D peptide induced T cells that upon *in vitro* resimulation with whole virus, viral RNP, the N protein or peptide 31D release lymphokines, mainly IL-2. Peptides that failed to stimulate ERA virus primed T cells did not apparently induce a virus specific or even peptide specific T cell response *in vivo*. Even the small peptides such as IMMNG, MMNG or MNG induced virus specific T cells *in vivo* while control peptides such as IMVNG or MVNG did not.

Mice that were primed with immunogenic peptides developed upon booster immunization with whole virus an accelerated and enhanced neutralizing antibody response presumably by N protein specific Th cells providing help to glycoprotein specific B cells via a bystander effect [12].

Nevertheless mice that were immunized with peptide failed to be protected against a subsequent lethal challenge with rabies virus [12] thus demonstrating that neither Th cells nor an accelerated virus neutralizing antibody response upon challenge sufficed for protection. In order to test whether mice could be protected by peptide vaccines at all we synthetized longer peptides that in addition to a T cell epitope (in this case 31D) contained the sequence of a linear B cell epitope either of the viral N protein (such as contained in peptide V10c) or of the viral glycoprotein (such as defined by peptide G-24). Immunization with either peptide lead to induction of rabies virus N protein specific Th cells as well as of antibodies either to the N or the G protein. Mice immunized with these peptides *were* protected against a subsequent challenge with rabies virus [43,44].

A peptide-lipid construct similar to that described above for HSV was used with another rabies peptide (N-V12b) derived from the N protein to immunize mice. A decrease in the mortality rate of an intramuscular challenge of rabies virus was seen [45].

CONCLUSION

We have presented here what appears to be conflicting data relating to the studies of peptides as molecular probes of T cell responses. In the rabies system there is clear immunodominance and Ir gene control whereas in the herpes system there is no dominance and what appears to be no Ir gene control. In terms of protection and vaccination, in the herpes system there is clear support for such an approach while in the rabies system support for the use of peptides is less clear. A major point of this review actually shows that one cannot generalize and that any given system is unique and therefore analysis of peptides as molecular probes must be carried out in each case studied.

ACKNOWLEDGEMENTS

We would like to thank Bernhard Dietzschold, Laszlo Otvos, Jr., Jovi Larson, Keizo Yamashita, and Eiji Watari for all their work and advice. This work was supported by grants from the NIH (AI 22528F and AI27435).

REFERENCES

1 Solinger, A. M., M. E. Ultee, E. Margoliash and R. H. Schwartz. 1979. *J. Exp. Med.*, 150:830.

2 Katz, M. E., R. M. Maizels, I. Wicker, A. Miller and E. E. Sercarz. 1982. *Eur. J. Immunol.*, 12:535.

3 Berkower, I., G. K. Buckenmeyer, F. R. N. Gurd and J. A. Berzofsky. 1982. *Proc. Nat. Acad. Sci. USA*, 79:4723.

4 Hackett, C. J., J. L. Hurwitz, B. Dietzschold and W. Gerhard. 1985. *J. Immunol.*, 135:1391.

5 Lamb, J. R., D. D. Eckkels, P. Lake, J. N. Woody and N. Green. 1982. *Nature*, 300:66.

6 Celis, E., D. Ou and L. Otvos, Jr. 1985. *J. Immunol.*, 140:1808.

7 Milich, D. R., D. L. Peterson, G. G. Leroux-Roels, R. A. Lerner and F. V. Chisari. 1985. *J. Immunol.*, 134:4203.

8 Cease, K., H. Mardalit, J. Cornette, S. Putney, W. Robey, C. Wuyang, H. Streicher, P. Fischinger, R. Gallo, C. Delisi and J. A. Bersofsky. 1987. *Proc. Natl. Acad. Sci. USA*, 184:4249.

9 Takahashi, H., J. Cohen, A. Hosmalin, K. B. Cease, R. Houghten, J. L. Cornette, C. DeLisi, B. Moss, R. N. Germain and J. A. Berzofsky. 1988. *Proc. Natl. Acad. Sci. USA*, 85:3105.

10 See Reference 49.

11 Fu, Z.-F., B. Dietzschold, C. I. Schumacher, W. N. Wunner, H. C. J. Ertl and H. Koprowski. *Proc. Nat. Acad. Sci. USA*, in press.

12 Ertl, H. C. J., B. Dietzschold, M. Gore, L. Otvos, Jr., J. K. Larson, W. Wunner and H. Koprowski. 1989. *J. Virol.*, 63:2885.

13 Ertl, H. C. J., B. Dietzschold and L. Otvos, Jr. *Eur. J. Immunol.*, in press.

14 Del Val, M., H. Volkmer, J. B. Rothbard, S. Jonjic, M. Messerle, J. Shickedanz, M. J. Reddehase and U. H. Koszinowski. 1988. *J. Virol.*, 62:3965.

15 Balachandran, N., D. Harnish, W. E. Rawls and S. Bachetti. 1982. *J. Virol.*, 44:344.

16 Eisenberg, R. J., D. Long, L. Pereira, B. Hamper, M. Zweig and G. H. Cohen. 1982. *J. Virol.* 41:478.

17 Watson, R. J. 1983. *Gene*, 158:303.

18 Spear, P. G. 1984. In *Herpes Viruses, Vol. 3*, B. Roizman, ed., New York: Plenum, p. 315.

19 Heber-Katz, E., S. Valentine, B. Dietzschold and C. Burns-Purzycki. 1988. *J. Exp. Med.*, 167:275.

20 Watari, E., B. Dietzschold, G. Szokan and E. Heber-Katz. 1987. *J. Exp. Med.*, 165:451.

21 Sanchez-Pescador, L., R. L. Burke, G. Ott and G. Van Nest. 1988. *J. Immunol.*, 141:1720.

22 Berzofsky, J. 1987. In *The Antigens*, M. Sela, ed., New York: Academic Press, pp. 1–146.

23 Chestnut, R., P. Berman and S. Grammer. 1987. *12th International Herpesvirus Workshop*, p. 191.

24 Yamashita, K. and E. Heber-Katz. 1989. *J. Exp. Med.*, 170:997.

25 Adorini, L., E. Appella, G. Doria and Z. A. Nagy. 1988. *J. Exp. Med.*, 168:2091.

26 Eisenlohr, L. C. and C. J. Hackett. 1989. *J. Exp. Med.*, 169:921.

27 Mills, K. H., J. J. Skehel and D. B. Thomas. 1986. *J. Exp. Med.*, 163:1477.

28 Atassi, M. A. and J. Kurisaki. 1984. *Immunol. Commun.*, 13:539.

29 Brachiale, T. J., M. T. Sweetser, L. A. Morrison, D. J. Kittlesen and V. L. Brachiale. 1989. *Proc. Natl. Acad. Sci. USA*, 86:277.

30 DeFreitas, E. C., B. Dietzschold and H. Koprowski. 1985. *PNAS*, 82:3425.

31 Pincus, M., F. Gerewitz, R. H. Schwartz and H. Scheraga. 1983. *PNAS*, 80:3297.

32 Berkower, I., L. Matis, F. R. N. Gurd, D. Longo and J. A. Berzofsky. 1984. *J. Immunol.*, 132:1370.

33 Margalit, H., J. L. Spouge, J. L. Cornette, K. B. Cease, C. DeLisi and J. A. Berzofsky. 1987. *J. Immunol.*, 138:2213.

34 Rothbard, J. B. and W. R. Taylor. 1988. *EMBO J.*, 7:93.

35 Heber-Katz, E., M. Hollosi, B. Dietzschold, F. Hudenc and G. Fasman. 1985. *J. Immunol.*, 135:1385.

36 Sette, A., S. Buus, S. Colon, C. Miles and H. M. Grey. 1989. *J. Immunol.*, 142:35.

37 Gammon, G., N. Shastri, J. Cogswell, S. Wilbur, S. Sadegh-Nasseri, U. Kryzych, A. Miller and E. Sercarz. 1987. *Immun. Rev.*, 98:53.

38 Greenfield, N. and G. D. Fasman. 1969. *Biochemistry*, 8:4108.

39 Hopp, T. P. 1984. *Mol. Immunol.*, 21:13.

40 Thibodeau, L., F. Naud and A. Baudreault. 1981. In *Genetic Variation Among Influenza Viruses*, D. P. Nayak, ed., New York: Academic Press, p. 587.

41 Coon, J. and R. J. Hunter. 1973. *J. Immunol.*, 110:183.

42 Dailey, M. O. and R. J. Hunter. 1974. *Can. J. Immunol.*, 25:267.

43 Dietzschold, B., M. Gore, I. J. T. M. Claassen, F. G. C. M. Uytdehaag, B. Dietzschold, W. H. Wunner, A. D. M. E. Osterhaus and H. J. Koprowski. 1989. *Gen. Virol.*, 70:291.

44 Dietzschold, B. and H. C. J. Ertl. 1991. *CRC Critical Rev. in Immunol.*, 10:427.

45 Dietzschold, B., H. Wang, C. E. Rupprecht, E. Celis, M. Tollis, H. Ertl, E. Heber-Katz and H. Koprowski. 1987. *PNAS*, 87:9165.

46 Eisenlohr, L. C., W. Gerhard and C. J. Hackett. 1988. *J. Immunol.*, 141:2581.

47 Rothbard, J. B., R. I. Lechler, K. Howland, V. Bal, D. D. Eckels, R. Sekaly, E. O. Long, W. R. Taylor and J. R. Lamb. 1988. *Cell*, 52:515.

48 Berzofsky, J. A., A. Bensussan, K. B. Cease, J. F. Bourge, R. Cheynier, Z. Lurhuma, J. J. Salaun, R. C. Gallo, G. M. Shearer and D. Zagury. 1988. *Nature*, 334:706.

49 Krohn, K. J. E., P. Lusso, R. C. Gallo, A. Ranki, L. O. Arthur, B. Moss and S. Putney. 1988. In *Vaccines 88*, H. Ginsberg, F. Brown, R. A. Lerner and R. M. Chanock, eds., NY: Cold Spring Harbor Lab. CSH, p. 357.

50 Lusso, P. A., A. Ranki, R. C. Gallo, K. J. E. Krohn, P. D. Markham and S. S. Kueberuwa. 1988. In *Vaccines 88*, H. Ginsberg, F. Brown, R. A. Lerner and R. M. Chanock, eds., NY: Cold Spring Harbor Lab. CSH, p. 361.

51 Milich, D. R., A. McLachlan, A. Moriarty and G. B. Thornton. 1987. *J. Immunol.*, 138:4457.

52 Milich, D. R., J. L. Hughes, A. McLachlan, G. B. Thornton and A. Moriarty. 1988. *Proc. Natl. Acad. Sci. USA*, 85:1610.

53 Milich, D. R. and A. McLachlan. 1986. *Science*, 234:1398.

54 Milich, D. R., A. McLachlan, A. Moriarty and G. B. Thornton. 1987. *J. Immunol.*, 139:1223.

55 Celis, E., D. Ou, B. Dietzschold, L. Otvos, Jr. and H. Koprowski. 1989. *Hybridoma*, 3:263.

56 Celis, E., R. W. Karr, B. Dietzschold, W. H. Wunner and H. Koprowski. 1988. *J. Immunol.*, 141:2721.

57 Heber-Katz, E. and B. Dietzschold. 1988. *Current Topics in Microbiol. and Immunol.*, 130:51.

58 Taylor, P. M., J. Davey, K. Howland, J. B. Rothbard and B. A. Askona. 1987. *Immunogenetics*, 26:267.

59 Bastin, J., J. Rothbard, J. Davey, I. Jones and A. Townsend. 1987. *J. Exp. Med.*, 165:1508.

60 Townsend, A. R. M., J. Rothbard, F. M. Gotch, G. Behadur, D. Wraith and G. G. Brownlee. 1986. *Cell*, 39:1.

61 McMichael, A. J., F. M. Gotch and J. Rothbard. 1986. *J. Exp. Med.*, 164:1397.

62 Gotch, F. M., A. J. McMichael, G. L. Smith and B. Moss. 1986. *J. Exp. Med.*, 165:408.

63 Whitton, J. L., H. Lewicki, J. R. Gebherd, A. Tishon, P. J. Southern and M. B. A. Oldstone. 1988. In *Vaccines 88*, H. Ginsberg, F. Brown, R. A. Lerner and R. M. Chanock, eds., NY: Cold Spring Harbor Lab. CSH, p. 215.

CHAPTER 11

The Design of MHC Binding Peptides

ALESSANDRO SETTE[1]
ALAN G. LAMONT[1]
HOWARD M. GREY[1]

INTRODUCTION

MORE than five years ago, it was shown that class II MHC molecules act as cellular receptors for peptidic antigens [1-4]. Since then, data have been accumulating which define, in various experimental systems, the structural requirements for MHC interaction of different model peptides [5-10]. Based on the reported association between certain autoimmune diseases and certain MHC types [11], it is hoped that high affinity MHC binding peptides acting as MHC blockers could prove a useful tool in fighting autoimmune diseases. In the present report, we wish to summarize some of the recent data bearing relevance to the design of such MHC binding peptides.

The design of MHC binding antagonists could be, for ease of discussion, arbitrarily subdivided into three different stages. In the first stage, after identification of an active peptide molecule, the crucial structural features that endow that particular sequence with its MHC binding capacity are defined. Some rational (or empirical) strategies can then be applied to enhance binding affinities and/or modulate the specificity of interaction (stage two). Stage three will entail further modification of the peptide molecule to enhance *in vivo* activity. These types of modification will be targeted, for example, at improving stability and bioavailability, and at the same time reduce renal clearance, liver uptake, and toxicity.

[1]Cytel, 3525 John Hopkins Court, San Diego, CA 92121, U.S.A.

STRUCTURAL FEATURES OF HIGH AFFINITY MHC BINDERS

Peptide-MHC interactions have been analyzed in detail in various model systems. Allen, Unanue, and colleagues have analyzed the structural requirements for the interaction between an HEL-derived peptide (HEL 46-61) and purified IA^k molecules [5]. We have experimentally addressed the same question for the IA^d/OVA 323-339 interaction [6], and another HEL-derived peptide (HEL 107-116) with IE^d [7]. More recently, a similar analysis has been presented for the human class II molecule, DR1, and the hemagglutinin-derived peptide Ha 307-319 [8]. Similar experimental questions have also been addressed by Schwartz and co-workers using cytochrome c-derived peptides [9].

In these studies, crucial binding regions on the peptide molecule have been defined by truncation analysis (i.e., by synthesizing and testing for class II binding a panel of analogs sequentially truncated from either the C- or N-terminal of the peptide) Without exception, the crucial core regions defined are relatively short with an average size of about six amino acids.

To further analyze within such core binding regions the relative role of different amino acid residues, each position has been varied by introducing different single amino acid substitutions. The resulting analogs have been tested for their capacity to bind MHC, activate T cells, or induce an immune response. In all cases, only a few (one to three of the peptide amino acid side chains) were shown to be crucial for MHC interactions. Furthermore, the interaction between class II molecules and their peptide ligands is very permissive. Class II molecules typically accept a large number (~ 70–80%) of different single amino acid substitutions of the peptide molecule without noticeable effects. On the other hand, T cell interactions appear to be very specific, in that they accept only a few (10–20%) of the single amino acid substitutions tested. The extreme permissiveness of peptide–class II interactions allows for rather extreme modifications of the peptide molecules without losing the binding capacity. Conversely, even minor modifications can dramatically affect T cell recognition.

In a complementary approach [12–14], sequence analysis methods have been used in our attempt to define common structural traits shared by the majority of good binding peptides but infrequent in nonbinding peptides. Indeed, the great permissiveness of this interaction allows class II molecules to bind through the same binding site a large number of unrelated peptides, thus providing a sufficiently large repertoire of MHC-binding antigens available for T cell recognition. Recognition of vast numbers of unrelated peptides is accomplished by recognition of structurally broad "motifs." In the case of IA^d and IE^d molecules [6,7,14] for which binding motifs have been defined, the structural motifs appear to be rather different from one another. Thus, while in the case of IA^d interaction the most crucial residues of the peptide molecule were hydrophobic, in the case of IE^d, positive charge appears to play the major role.

Finally, the data obtained have some bearing on the long-debated issue of what conformation is required for binding to MHC. In the literature, conflicting reports have invoked different conformations, mainly α-helices, as crucial for these interactions. If a helical conformation were to be required, the residues involved in interaction with either the T cell receptor or the MHC molecule would be expected to segregate on different faces of the helix. In the case of IA^k/HEL 46-61, a segregation compatible with recognition of an α-helical conformation has, in fact, been observed [5]. An involvement of α-helical regions in class II peptide binding has also been invoked on the basis of indirect studies [10]. However, in the case of IE^d/HEL 107-116, there is no apparent segregation between residues crucial for Ia and T cell recognition, and all the crucial class II residues also appear to be involved in T cell recognition [7]. Similar data were obtained in the case of IA^d/OVA 323-337 [6] and IE^k/p cyt$_c$ 88-103 [9]. These data suggest that, at least in these instances, the peptide may be recognized in a planar conformation, sandwiched between the T cell receptor and the Ia molecule [6].

STRUCTURAL MODIFICATIONS OF MHC BINDING PEPTIDES

Following the analysis described in the previous paragraphs, modification of the peptide structure can be attempted. Most commonly, the desired goals will be increases in binding affinities and changes in the peptide binding specificity, such that cross-reactivity with other MHC molecules will either be increased or decreased. Higher binding single amino acid substituted or truncated analogs can sometimes be identified. Similarly, we have been able to significantly alter the specificity pattern of several epitopes, either by truncation or single amino acid substitutions. For example, removal of the last three N-terminal residues from a Myoglobin-derived peptide (MyoY 106-118) increased its IE^d binding capacity >50-fold, while the IA^d binding capacity remained essentially unchanged [15]. Another example of specificity modulation is shown in Table 11.1, where different analogs derived from the peptide, OVA 324-334 (good IA^d binder, weak IA^k binder) and Ha 132-142 (good IA^d and IA^k binders) were tested for their IA^d and IA^k binding capacities [15]. Preliminary data showed that the weak reactivity of the OVA peptide with IA^k centered around residues 327-332, i.e., the same region of the OVA peptide identified as the core region crucial for IA^d binding. If the same region of the Ha peptide was responsible for the interaction with both IA^d and IA^k, then "grafting" the Ha core region 135-140 within OVA-derived flanking re-

TABLE 11.1. IA Binding Capacity of OVA 324-334 and Ha 132-142 Chimeric Peptides.

Peptide	Amino Acid Position in the Peptide Sequence											Relative Binding Capacity to:	
	1	2	3	4	5	6	7	8	9	10	11	IA^k	IA^d
Ha 134-142	T	N	G	V	T	A	A	S	S	H	E	1.00	1.00
OVA 324-334	S	Q	A	V	H	A	A	H	A	E	–	0.04	0.53
OVA/Ha 5, 8, 9	S	Q	A	V	T	A	A	S	S	E	–	0.53	1.00
OVA/Ha 5	S	Q	A	V	T	A	A	H	A	E	–	0.58	0.89
OVA/Ha 8	S	Q	A	V	H	A	A	S	A	E	–	0.05	1.14
OVA/Ha 9	S	Q	A	V	H	A	A	H	S	E	–	0.05	0.80
OVA/Ha 5, 8	S	Q	A	V	T	A	A	S	A	E	–	0.21	1.00
OVA/Ha 5, 9	S	Q	A	V	T	A	A	H	S	E	–	0.51	2.00
OVA/Ha 8, 9	S	Q	A	V	H	A	A	S	S	E	–	0.07	1.00

AC → S substitution was introduced at position 140 to avoid cysteine-related problems in the synthesis and purification of the peptide series. The introduction of this substitution did not affect the capacity of Ha 130-142 to bind IA^d or IA^k (data not shown). The amount of each peptide necessary to inhibit by 50% the binding of ^{125}I-labeled OVA Y323-339 to IA^d or of ^{125}I-labeled HEL Y46-61 to IA^k was measured by a gel filtration method (4) and normalized to the highest binder (Ha 132-142) of the peptide series. The data represent the average of two to five experiments. The 50% inhibition doses of the Ha 132-142 before normalization were 55 μM for IA^d and 24 μM for IA^k. The dash indicates a relative binding capacity ≤0.01.

gions should yield a chimeric peptide capable of binding strongly to both IA^d and IA^k. The data presented in the third line of Table 11.1 show that this was indeed the case. Inasmuch as the OVA and Ha sequences differ in their core region by only three amino acids, we synthesized the six possible "chimeric" core regions derived, in part, from the Ha sequence. These peptides were then tested for IA^d and IA^k binding, to determine which residues of the Ha sequence were critical for its IA^k binding capacity. These results are also shown in Table 11.1. Although all the peptides were essentially equivalent in IA^d binding capacity, they differed markedly in their capacity to interact with IA^k. Peptides carrying the Ha-derived threonine residue (T) in position five were good IA^k binders, whereas peptides carrying the histidine residue derived from the OVA sequence in that same position bound only weakly to IA^k. Thus, these data suggest that IA^d and IA^k recognize very similar structures on the peptide, but differ in their fine specificity, as illustrated by the finding that an H in position five is compatible with strong IA^d binding, but markedly limits the capacity of the same peptide to bind IA^k.

More elaborate types of modification are those attempting to influence peptide conformation, in the hope of significant increases in binding affinities resulting from selective stabilization of the particular conformation assumed by the peptide when bound to the MHC. In recent years, much debate has been devoted to the conformational requirements for antigen molecules to bind MHC molecules and activate T cells. As already mentioned, different groups, mostly on the basis of indirect functional or biochemical data, have argued for or against regular secondary structures (mainly α-helix) as the main conformational requirement.

We and others [10,16–18] analyzed the effect of dipole modification on peptide binding capacities. Recent studies [19] indicated that modification of the dipole moment of peptide molecules has a pronounced effect on their propensity to form α-helices. More precisely, negative charges at the N-terminus and positive charges at the C-terminus tend to stabilize helix structures, while positive charges at the N-terminus or negative charges at the C-terminus tend to destabilize helical structures. It was indeed shown [5] that an increased dipole analog of the IA^k binding peptide HEL 52-61 was significantly more effective than the parental molecule in activating HEL-specific T cell hybridomas.

To test the effect of introducing modifications that alter the stabilization of α-helices on the capacity of OVA 323-336 to bind IA^d, analogs with various dipole modifications were synthesized and tested for their IA^d binding capacity. We were unable to detect any improvement of the MHC binding capacity following these modifications [17]. In fact, a relatively weak inverse correlation between α-helix propensity and binding capacity was apparent. These data do not, therefore, support the notion that MHC molecules recognize α-helical structures. Interestingly, when the same peptide molecules were tested for their capacity to activate two IA^d-restricted T cell hybridomas, it was found that amidation and acetylation of the peptide 322-336 led to increased biologic activity for one, but not the other hybridoma. Similar findings have recently been reported by Allen and co-workers, who observed a > 100-fold increase in antigenicity without a substantial change in affinity of interaction with MHC′ with dipole-modified analogs [16].

In another series of experiments, we have analyzed whether we could modulate binding affinity and specificity by addition of nonnatural amino acid sequences to the crucial IA^d binding core region of OVA 323-339. A similar approach has been followed by Paterson and colleagues, in the analysis of the interaction between IE^k and p cyt_c-derived peptides [20,21]. We extended the IA^d binding core region (OVA 327-332) defined within the peptide OVA 323-339 at both the N- and C-termini with three to four amino acid residues [17]. These additions were designed so that the peptides could be predicted to assume particular secondary structures, thus allowing an examination of whether a correlation existed between binding affinity for Ia molecules and peptide conformation. Although no such correlation was observed [17], the core extension approach generated peptides with a wide range of binding affinities, including several peptides with a higher affinity than the native OVA peptide for IA^d.

In the experiments shown in Table 11.2, a panel of 10 core-extended peptides was tested for its ability to bind purified IA^d, IA^k, and IE^d molecules *in vitro*. All the peptides except one (DE) retained the ability to bind IA^d. Four of these (YT, AK, AM, and NV) bound with a two- to 10-fold greater affinity than the parent OVA 323-336 sequence, while for two (MH and KM), the affinity for IA^d remained approximately equivalent. The remaining three peptides (TN, ES, and VI) bound 10- to 100-fold less efficiently than the parental peptide. While most of the peptides shared a relatively low IA^k binding capacity (0.01–0.06), similar to that of the OVA 323-336 peptide, two core-extended peptides (AM and AK) displayed increased IA^k reactivities. Similarly, the majority of peptides were negative for IE^d binding, as was the parental OVA 323-336 molecule. The exceptions displaying good IE^d binding capacity were the AK and KM peptides. Thus, these data indicate that the core extension approach can be used not only to increase the affinity of peptide binding for a particular MHC molecule, but also to generate analogs with different class II MHC binding specificities than the native peptide sequence.

We have subsequently developed an approach that, like the core-extension approach, is capable of yielding peptides with increased MHC binding capacities [22]. The experiments leading to definition of such an approach were prompted by the observation that within a large collection

TABLE 11.2. Capacity of Core-Extended Peptides
to Bind MHC Class II Molecules.

Peptide			Relative Binding Capacity to:		
			IA^d	IE^d	IA^k
ISQA	VHAAHA	EINE	1.00	—	0.02
YTYT	-------------	YTYT	10.00	0.01	0.01
AKAK	-------------	AKAK	4.55	0.24	0.35
AMAM	-------------	AMAM	6.30	—	0.11
NVNV	-------------	NVNV	2.78	—	0.02
MHMH	-------------	MHMH	1.76	—	0.06
KMKM	-------------	KMKM	0.64	2.66	0.04
TNTN	-------------	TNTN	0.07	—	0.06
ESES	-------------	ESES	0.07	—	0.06
VIVI	-------------	VIVI	0.01	—	0.06
DEDE	-------------	DEDE	—	0.01	0.02

The amount of each peptide required to inhibit by 50% the binding of ^{125}I-labeled OVA Y323-339 to IA^d, ^{125}I-labeled repressor Y12-26 to IE^d, or ^{125}I-labeled HEL Y46-61 to IA^k was measured by a gel filtration method [4]. Figures for relative binding were obtained by dividing the values obtained for the control peptide (OVA 323-336 for IA^d, λ-repressor 12-26 for IE^d, and HEL 46-61 for IA^k) by those for the core-extended peptides. The figures represent the mean of two to three experiments, and a dash indicates a relative binding capacity of <0.01. The 50% inhibitory concentrations before normalization were: OVA 323-336, 19 μM; λ-repressor 12-26, 1 μM; HEL 46-61, 1 μM.

of tested peptides for IE^d binding capacity, the naturally occurring opioid peptide, Dynorphin, stood out as being the best. The sequence of this peptide (Table 11.3) was noteworthy, in that it possessed three overlapping IE^d binding motifs containing three basic residues. To evaluate whether multiple MHC binding determinants occurring in the same peptide molecule

TABLE 11.3. IA^d Binding Capacity of Reiterative Motif Peptides.

Peptide	Peptide Sequence	Relative Binding Capacity to:	
		IA^d	IE^d
Dynorphin 1-13	YGGFLRRIRPKLK	—	13.6
OVA 323-339	ISQAVHAAHAEINEAGR	1.00	—
ROI	VHAAHAVHAAHAVHA	27.7	—
HEL 105-120	MNAWVAWRNRCKGTDV	—	0.48
RHI	AWRNRAKAWRNRAKAWRNRAK	0.04	17.0
λ rep 12-26	LEDARRLKAIYEKKK	0.10	1.00
RLI	ARRLKARRLKARRLK	—	3.9

Relative binding figures were obtained as described in Table 11.2. The figures represent the mean of two to three experiments, and a dash indicates a relative binding capacity of <0.01. The 50% inhibitory concentrations before normalization were: OVA 323-336, 2.1 μM; λ-repressor 12-26, 2.4 μM.

could act in a cooperative manner, we synthesized three "reiterative motif" peptides derived by repeating two or three times the MHC binding core region (as defined by truncation analysis) of three naturally occurring peptide sequences. Thus, the three good MHC binding peptide sequences previously analyzed in detail [1,3,11] and selected as core region donors were: OVA 323-339, IA^d binder, core region = VHAAHA; λ rep 12-26, IE^d (and IA^d) binder, IE^d, core region = (A)RRLK; HEL 105-120, IE^d binder, core region = AWRNRCK. The reiterative motif peptide analogs that were synthesized are shown in Table 11.1 (ROI, RLI, RHI). When these peptides were tested for IA^d binding in an inhibition assay, it was found that ROI bound IA^d molecules very strongly, 27-fold better than the original OVA peptide. The specificity of the interaction was retained, in that no IE^d binding capacity was demonstrable. Similarly, RHI showed a dramatic increase in IE^d binding capacity (compared to HEL 105-120) and remained IA^d-negative. Finally, RLI showed increased IE^d binding capacity, albeit more modest than the other two, and also scored negative for IA^d binding. The loss of IA^d binding of the RLI peptide probably reflects the fact that the IA^d binding core region of the parental peptide (DARRLKAI) is only partially overlapping with its IE^d core binding region. Thus, these data demonstrate that multiple MHC binding core regions can, in some way, act cooperatively, thereby resulting in an enhanced Ia binding capacity. The phenomenon appears to be somewhat generalizable, in that the strategy was successful with three different determinants and two different class II isotypes so far analyzed.

In an attempt to gain some insight into the molecular basis of the cooperative effect observed, we synthesized another series of reiterative analogs in which two core regions were linked by a three-residue spacer derived from the natural sequence of the original OVA, HEL, or λ rep peptides. As controls, peptides were synthesized in which two core regions were contiguous to one another, and the tri-peptide spacer was added at the C-terminus of the peptide. We reasoned that if reiterative analogs acted by binding to and cross-linking two class II molecules to one another, the insertion of the tri-peptide would either not affect the binding or would facilitate it by making the two core regions more accessible for binding to multiple MHC molecules. Alternatively, if the cooperative effect was due to some other mechanism, such as the cooperative stabilization of peptide secondary structures favorable to class II binding, insertion of the tri-peptide spacer might be detrimental to the binding capacity of the reiterative analogs. The results of these experiments are shown in Table 11.4. In the case of the OVA-derived analogs, the peptide in which the tri-peptide spacer was inserted between the two core regions (ROII) did not bind appreciably better than the original OVA 323-339 peptide, whereas when the two core regions were synthesized contiguously and the spacer placed at the C-terminus (ROIII), a very marked increased binding capacity was

TABLE 11.4. Class II Binding of Reiterative Analogs.

Peptide	Peptide Sequence	Relative Binding Capacity to:	
		IA^d	IE^d
OVA 323-339	ISQA<u>VHAAHA</u>EINEAGR	1.00	—
ROII	VHAAHAEINVHAAHA	1.62	—
ROIII	VHAAHAVHAAHAEIN	24.8	—
ROIV	AHAAHAAHAAHAAHAA	34.0	—
HEL 105	MNAWN<u>AWRNRC</u>KGTDV	ND	0.48
RHII	AWRNRAKGTDAWRNRAK	ND	0.07
RHIII	AWRNRAKAWRNRAKGTD	ND	15.1

observed. Again, specificity was retained, since all these peptides were negative for IE^d binding. Similarly, in the case of the HEL reiterative motif analogs, the peptides with contiguous core regions (RHIII) bound 200-fold better than the one in which the tri-peptide spacer was inserted between the two core regions (RHII).

Inspection of the sequence of the ROI analog (Table 11.3) reveals that only three different amino acids are present in that sequence (valine, alanine, and histidine). Moreover, it was known [4] that a Val → Ala substitution at position 323 did not deleteriously affect the binding of the OVA peptide to IA^d. For this reason, we synthesized and tested for IA^d binding the analog ROIV (Table 11.4), which, in fact, differs from ROI only because of the replacement of valine residues by alanine. This simple peptide, consisting of only two amino acids, binds very strongly to IA^d. The binding appears to be specific, in that no IE^d binding was detectable. To study the binding capacity of this peptide more directly, a tyrosine residue was included at the N-terminal end of the peptide, that was then radiolabeled. This radiolabeled reiterative peptide (ROIV) bound much more efficiently to IA^d than ^{125}I-radiolabeled OVA 323-339. Furthermore, both the OVA 323-339 and the ROIV peptide appeared to compete for the same binding site, in that the binding of either one of them to purified IA^d molecules was inhibitable, in a dose-dependent fashion, by excess unlabeled OVA 323-336 or ROIV. Availability of this radiolabeled probe also enabled us to analyze ROIV-IA^d complexes by size exclusion TSK 3000 HPLC chromatography. The apparent sizes of IA^d-OVA 323-339 complexes and IA^d-ROIV complexes were found to coincide exactly. Thus, there was no evidence that reiterative motif analogs, at least in the case of ROIV and IA^d, act by cross-linking MHC molecules.

Based on the experimental results described in the previous sections, it would be predicted that naturally-occurring reiterative motif structures in proteins would also be associated with cooperatively enhanced binding capacity. This type of phenomenon could play some role in selecting immunodominant regions in protein antigens. It is tempting for us to interpret, in this light, some data obtained with a set of 11 residue peptides (overlapping by 10) spanning through residues 307-339 of OVA. These peptides were tested for their capacity to bind purified IA^d molecules. Positive binding capacity was detected in all 18 peptides contained within residues 310-337. Since many of these undeca peptides are non-overlapping, it must be concluded that more than one IA^d binding site exists in the OVA 310-337 region. In fact, three broad peaks of activity were detected in this analysis, and suggest that at least three IA^d binding sites situated very close to each other in this immunodominant peptide region may exist.

In conclusion, having eliminated the possibility that the duplicated core binding regions enhanced activity by cross-linking individual MHC molecules to one another, we are left with no clear mechanism by which reiterated motifs lead to increased binding affinity. It is possible that the effect is mediated by the capacity of these core regions to form some particular secondary conformation, and that by repeating the core regions, this conformation is stabilized to a greater extent than it would be with unrelated peptide flanking regions. Alternatively, the enhanced binding activity of the reiterated core regions may reflect distinct subsites of interaction with similar specificities within the MHC-peptide binding site. Thus, repeating the binding regions would enable a single peptide to bind to two independent subsites, thereby increasing the affinity of the interaction.

The detection of naturally-occurring clustered class II binding sites suggests a possible role of "reiterative motif" structures *in vivo* in the generation of immunodominant regions. Naturally-occurring clustered class II binding sites have been detected, as discussed above, in the case of the OVA 323-339 sequence and the opioid peptide, Dynorphin. In addition, other cases of naturally-occurring immunogenic and/or immunodominant regions containing more than one class II binding site have been described. Examples are the Ha 121-146 region (two apparent IA^k sites [15]), the HEL 105-129 region (two apparent IE^d sites [14]), the p cyt 81-104 region (two apparent IE^k sites [23]), and the Nase 1-40 region (at least two independent IE^k sites [24]). Interestingly, immunological properties of "head-to-tail" synthetically joined determinants have also been described independently by Ria et al. [25]. In their case, however, a hybrid peptide was obtained by joining core regions derived from two different T cell antigens. It was found that one determinant could dramatically alter the properties of the other contiguous one. Further studies on the immunogenicity of peptides containing multiple contiguous binding regions should allow for an evaluation of the biologic importance of this phenomenon.

PEPTIDE MODIFICATIONS AND BIOLOGICAL ACTIVITY

The ultimate goal of designing peptides with improved MHC binding characteristics is, as already mentioned, their usage *in vivo* as modulators of autoimmune diseases. Indeed, MHC blockade has been demonstrated in *in vitro* systems by inhibiting presentation of peptide antigens to specific T cells, using an excess of another competing peptide [5,8–13,26–30]. Recently, the system of antigenic competition between peptides has been extended to preventing the induction of an immune response *in vivo* [31]. In this case, a T cell proliferative response to a hen egg lysozyme peptide (HEL 46-61) in association with IA^k was prevented by an excess of a mouse lysozyme peptide 46-62, which was capable of binding to the same restriction element with a similar affinity. In the experiments described below, we have used "core-extended" peptides to evaluate whether this approach could be used to generate peptide molecules capable of acting *in vivo* as inhibitors of the induction of T cell proliferative responses, and to examine the conditions under which an *in vitro* test for inhibition of antigen presentation could predict the *in vivo* activity of a peptide inhibitor.

For this purpose, the core-extended peptides AK and YT were compared with the native OVA 323-339 peptide for their ability to inhibit the induction of a T cell proliferative response to *Staph. nuclease* res. 61-80 (Nase 61-80), previously shown to elicit a vigorous IA^d-restricted T cell response after immunization [24]. Animals were immunized with an antigen/CFA emulsion containing 6 nmoles Nase 61-80, together with a five- or 20-fold excess of inhibitor peptide. Control animals received Nase 61-80 alone. The lymph node proliferative responses to the Nase peptide were assessed nine to 11 days later.

With the AK-extended peptide, some inhibition of the response was observed at five-fold excess, and inhibition was virtually complete at a 20-fold excess [Figure 11.1(a)]. In contrast, the YT peptide, despite having as high or higher relative binding affinity than AK, was noninhibitory when used at a five-fold excess, and was only partially inhibitory at a 20-fold excess of inhibitor [Figure 11.1(b)]. A control peptide with no affinity for IA^d, DE was unable to cause any inhibition [32]. When OVA 323-339 was used to inhibit, there was a partial reduction in response in the 20-fold excess group, but this was only observed at the highest challenge dose of antigen (19 μM) [Figure 11.1(c)]. Thus, our results show that core-extended peptides can effectively compete with a nominal peptide antigen for the induction of an immune response *in vivo*. However, the poor inhibitory capacity of certain peptides with good MHC binding capacity (YT and OVA 323-339) indicates that competition *in vivo* is not determined solely by binding affinity for Ia molecules.

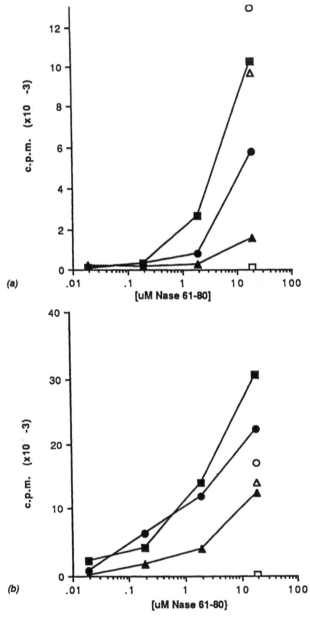

(a)

[uM Nase 61-80]

(b)

[uM Nase 61-80]

Figure 11.1 *In vivo* competition by core-extended peptides. Mice were immunized with a CFA emulsion containing 6 nmoles Nase 61-80, either alone (square symbol) or in conjunction with a five-fold (circular symbol) or 20-fold (triangular symbol) molar excess of inhibitor peptide. Draining lymph nodes were removed 9–11 days later to test for proliferative responses *in vitro* to Nase 61-80 (■, ●, ▲), or to the inhibitor peptide (19 µm: □, ○, △). Competition was assessed for the AK (a) and YT (b) core-extended peptides, and compared to the parental OVA 323-339 peptide (c). The background responses (unstimulated control) ranged from 50–650 cpm, and were subtracted from the stimulated response values before plotting. The figures shown are one representative experiment from three performed for each peptide.

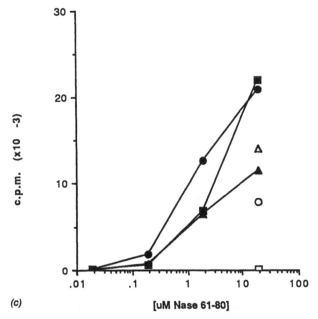

(c)

Figure 11.1 (continued) *In vivo* competition by core-extended peptides. Mice were immunized with a CFA emulsion containing 6 nmoles Nase 61-80, either alone (square symbol) or in conjunction with a five-fold (circular symbol) or 20-fold (triangular symbol) molar excess of inhibitor peptide. Draining lymph nodes were removed 9–11 days later to test for proliferative responses *in vitro* to Nase 61-80 (■, ●, ▲), or to the inhibitor peptide (19 μm: □, ○, △). Competition was assessed for the AK (a) and YT (b) core-extended peptides, and compared to the parental OVA 323-339 peptide (c). The background responses (unstimulated control) ranged from 50–650 cpm, and were subtracted from the stimulated response values before plotting. The figures shown are one representative experiment from three performed for each peptide.

One possibility was that the YT peptide was more rapidly degraded than the other peptides. Therefore, in an attempt to more closely mimic the *in vivo* fate of antigen in an *in vitro* assay, the pulse period was prolonged to 20 hours. A panel of 10 core-extended peptides tested previously were examined in this system, and in addition, the nonstimulatory truncation of OVA 323-339 (OVA 323-336) was included in these assays (Table 11.5). In contrast to the data obtained with a short pulse period, only three of the seven peptides with similar or greater binding affinity than OVA 323-339 (AK, NV, and KM) gave ID_{50} values of > 10 μM, while the remaining four (YT, AM, MH, and OVA 323-336) showed significantly reduced or even abolished capacity to act as inhibitors of antigen presentation. All other peptides were inactive in this assay. However, when a protease inhibitor cocktail was included during the pulse period, a similar pattern to that observed with the short pulse period was obtained, in that the ability to inhibit was restored to the YT, AM, and to a lesser extent, MH peptides. Also, the inhibitory activity of OVA 323-336 was similar to the other high affinity IA^d binding peptides. Thus, by extending the pulse period to 20 hours, an excellent correlation between the *in vitro* capacity of peptides to inhibit antigen presentation and their ability to inhibit *in vivo* was obtained. Furthermore, direct evidence was obtained for the role of proteolysis in influencing the efficacy of peptides as inhibitors, since the inclusion of protease inhibitors during the assay differentially enhanced the inhibitory capacity of some of the peptides.

To further analyze the susceptibility of the YT and AK peptides to degradation, we examined their stability in 1% FCS containing medium, either in the presence or absence of fixed APC, by HPLC analysis of the peptides at various incubation times. In good agreement with the cellular data, the AK peptide was found to be remarkably stable, with less than 20% being degraded in 24 hours. In contrast, the YT peptide was extremely susceptible to degradation, with a half-life of less than eight hours. Finally, and most interestingly, substitution of the N- and C-terminal residues of the YT peptide with D-amino acids greatly increased its stability. The pattern observed was, in fact, very similar to that of the AK peptide with T 1/2 of >24 hours.

From the above experiment, it was determined that the rapid degradation of the YT peptide could be greatly reduced by substitution of the N- and C-terminal residues with D-amino acid isomers. Therefore, we next examined how such substitutions affected the interaction of the YT peptide with IA^d, both in the direct binding assay and in the inhibition of antigen presentation assay. From the data in Table 11.6, it is clear that D-amino acid substitutions in the AK peptide had little effect on either the affinity of binding to IA^d (4.6 versus 6.2) or the ID_{50} (7 μM versus 12 μM). In contrast, with the YT peptide, although the substitutions did not affect binding affinity (5.5 versus 4.1) they greatly increased the ability of the peptide to inhibit activation of the T cell hybridoma in the cellular assay (ID_{50}: 7 μM versus 68 μM) when the APC were pulsed for 20 hours in the absence of protease inhibitors. Thus, enhancing the stability of the YT peptide with N- and C-terminal D-amino acid substitutions greatly increased its capacity to function as an inhibitor of antigen presentation.

CONCLUSIONS

Development of a direct binding assay to detect peptide-MHC interactions has opened the way to attempts to modify the structure of MHC-binding peptides, in order to increase binding constants and stability and

TABLE 11.5. Degradation of Core-Extended Peptides Undermine Their Ability to Inhibit Antigen Presentation *in vitro*.

Protease Inhibitors: Peptide	Dose Required for 50% Inhibition of Response (μM)	
	−	+
YT	41.4	3.6
AK	6.9	1.2
AM	65.5	1.5
NV	7.5	1.7
MH	66.3	15.1
KM	6.9	2.3
TN	>90	ND
ES	>90	ND
VI	>90	>90
DE	>90	>90
OVA 323-336	>90	4.7

Stimulator and inhibitor peptides were added to A20 cells in the presence or absence of protease inhibitors, and the cells were incubated for 20 hrs before washing and adding to T cells. Incubation was continued for 18–20 hrs, at which time a sample of supernatant was removed for determination of IL-2 concentration. The figures represent the concentration of inhibitor peptide required to reduce IL-2 secretion of the T cell hybridoma by 50%, and are the mean of two to four independent determinations. ND, not determined.

to modulate binding specificity. Some of the approaches aimed at accomplishing this task have been reviewed herein. In general, it was found that it is possible to alter binding constants and specificity of MHC-binding peptides using several different methods. It was also found that in order for a peptide to exhibit *in vivo* activity, not only high binding capacity, but also resistance to proteolytic degradation was required.

TABLE 11.6. Binding Affinity and Inhibitory Capacity of Core-Extended Peptides Containing N- and C-terminal D aa Substitutions.

Peptide	Relative Binding Affinity	Dose Required for 50% Inhibition (μM)
YT	4.1	68
D aa YT	5.5	7
AK	6.2	12
D aa AK	4.6	7

The amount of each peptide required to inhibit by 50% the binding of ^{125}I-labeled OVA Y323-339 to IA^d was measured by gel filtration and normalized as before. The figures for inhibition in the cellular assay represent the amount of peptide required to reduce IL-2 secretion of the T cell by 50% in the 20 hr inhibition assay in the absence of protease inhibitors. The data represent the means from two to three experiments.

REFERENCES

1 Babbitt, B. P., P. M. Allen, G. Matsueda, E. Haber and E. R. Unanue. 1985. *Nature*, 317:359.

2 Buus, S., S. Colon, C. Smith, J. H. Freed, C. Miles and H. M. Grey. 1986. *Proc. Natl. Acad. Sci. USA*, 83:3968.

3 Allen, P. M., B. Babbitt and E. Unanue. 1987. *Immunol. Rev.*, 98:172.

4 Buus, S., A. Sette and H. M. Grey. 1987. *Immunol. Rev.*, 98:115.

5 Allen, P. M., G. R. Matsueda, R. J. Evans, J. B. Dunbar, Jr., G. R. Marshall and E. Unanue. 1987. *Nature*, 327:713.

6 Sette, A., S. Buus, S. Colon, J. A. Smith, C. Miles and H. M. Grey. 1987. *Nature*, 328:395.

7 Sette, A., L. Adorini, S. Buus, E. Appella, S. M. Colon, C. Miles, G. Doria, Z. A. Nagy, S. Tanaka and H. M. Grey. 1989. *J. Immunol.*, 143:3289.

8 Jardetzky, T. S., J. C. Gorga, R. Busch, J. Rothbard, J. L. Strominger and D. C. Wiley. 1990. *EMBO J.*, 9:1797.

9 Fox, B. S., C. Chen, E. Fraga, C. A. French, B. Singh and R. H. Schwartz. 1987. *J. Immunol.*, 139:1578.

10 Rothbard, J. B., R. I. Lechler, K. Howland, V. Bal, D. D. Eckels, R. Sekaly, E. O. Long, W. R. Taylor and J. R. Lamb. 1988. *Cell*, 52:515.

11 Todd, J. A., H. Acha-Orbea, J. I. Bell, N. Chao, Z. Fronek, C. O. Jacob, M. McDermott, A. A. Sinha, L. Timmerman, L. Steinman and H. O. McDevitt. 1988. *Science*, 240:1003.

12 Rothbard, J. and W. Taylor. 1988. *EMBO J.*, 7:93.

13 Sette, A., S. Buus, S. Colon, C. Miles and H. M. Gray. 1988. *J. Immunol.*, 141:45.

14 Sette, A., S. Buus, E. Appella, J. A. Smith, R. Chestnut, C. Miles, S. M. Colon and H. M. Grey. 1989. *Proc. Natl. Acad. Sci. USA*, 86:3296.

15 Sette, A., S. Buus, S. Colon, C. Miles and H. M. Grey. 1989. *J. Immunol.*, 142:35.

16 Allen, P., G. R. Matsueda, S. Adams, J. Freeman, R. W. Roof, L. Lambert and E. R. Unanue. 1989. *Int. Immunol.*, 1:141.

17 Sette, A., A. Lamont, S. Buus, S. M. Colon, C. Miles and H. M. Grey. 1989. *J. Immunol.*, 143:1268.

18 Rothbard, J. B., R. Busch, K. Howland, V. Bal, C. Fenton, W. R. Taylor and J. R. Lamb. 1989. *Int. Immunol.*, 1:479.

19 Shoemaker, K. R., P. S. Kim, E. J. York, J. M. Stewart and R. L. Baldwin. 1987. *Nature*, 326:563.

20 Bhayani, H., F. R. Carbone and Y. Paterson. 1988. *J. Immunol.*, 141:377.

21 Collawn, J. F., H. Bhayani and Y. Paterson. 1989. *Molec. Immunol.*, 26:1069.

22 Sette, A., J. Sidney, M. Albertson, C. Miles, S. M. Colon, T. Pedrazzini, A. G. Lamont and H. M. Grey. 1990. *J. Immunol.*, 145:1809.

23 Carbone, F. R., U. D. Staerz and Y. Paterson. 1987. *Eur. J. Immunol.*, 17:897.

24 Schaeffer, E. B., A. Sette, D. L. Johnson, M. C. Bekoff, J. A. Smith, H. M. Grey and S. Buus. 1989. *Proc. Natl. Acad. Sci. USA*, 86:4649.

25 Ria, F., B. M. C. Chan, M. T. Scherer, J. A. Smith and M. L. Gefter. 1990. *Nature*, 343:381.

26 Buus, S., A. Sette, S. M. Colon, C. Miles and H. M. Grey. 1987. *Science*, 235:1353.

27 Guillet, J., M. Lai, T. Briner, J. Smith and M. Gefter. 1986. *Nature*, 324:260.

28 Babbitt, B. P., P. M. Allen, G. Matsueda, E. Haber and E. R. Unanue. 1986. *Proc. Natl. Acad. Sci. USA*, 83:4509.

29 Buus, S. and O. Werdelin. 1986. *J. Immunol.*, 136:459.

30 Lakey, E. K., E. Margoliash, G. Flouret and S. K. Pierce. 1986. *Eur. J. Immunol.*, 16:721.

31 Adorini, L., S. Muller, F. Cardinaux, P. V. Lehmann, F. Falcioni and Z. A. Nagy. 1988. *Nature*, 334:623.

32 Lamont, A. G., M. F. Powell, S. M. Colón, C. Miles, H. M. Grey and A. Sette. 1990. *J. Immunol.*, 144:2493.

CHAPTER 12

Biology and Chemistry of Extracellular Matrix Cell Attachment Peptides

FRANK A. ROBEY[1]

INTRODUCTION

CELL attachment, chemotaxis, differentiation and metastasis: these are words that describe related biological phenomena involving components of extracellular matrix. Extracellular matrix is a general term used to describe a mass of diverse, specialized molecular components, mostly organic, which reside on the outside of cells and tissues and which are thought to have specific molecular properties and binding specificities. Each component of an extracellular matrix is considered to be multifunctional, e.g., some components may have specific cellular receptors and a distant binding site(s) to an unrelated component. Although the biological function of a particular extracellular matrix is determined by its molecular constituents and the interactions of these constituents, in general and in an overall sense, extracellular matrix is the material responsible for the organization and support of cells and tissues throughout the body.

Knowledge of the biology and chemistry of extracellular matrices has increased immensely from information derived using molecular biology and, using these techniques, the amino acid sequences of many of the extracellular matrix proteins have been determined. For several years now, we have been able to use this information to reconstruct parts of the active regions of these large proteins using synthetic peptides derived from the parent proteins.

[1]Peptide and Immunochemistry Unit, Laboratory of Cellular Development and Oncology, National Institute of Dental Research, National Institutes of Health, Bethesda, MD 20892, U.S.A.

It is not the intention of this chapter to review the literature about extracellular matrix proteins *per se*; much of this has been accomplished in several review articles [1–10]. There are three primary goals of this chapter: first, to describe concisely some of the biologically active peptides derived from extracellular matrix proteins, most notably, fibronectin and laminin, along with a brief history of the discovery of these peptides; second, to present ways in which these peptides are being used and/or modified and third, to summarize the current thinking about the peptides derived from the extracellular matrix with respect to their research and/or possible therapeutic uses.

COMPONENTS AND PEPTIDES FROM EXTRACELLULAR MATRICES

FIBRONECTIN

The purification of fibronectin from plasma was first described in 1970 by Mosesson and Umfleet [11]. Since that time, fibronectin has been the most studied of all extracellular matrix proteins possibly because a plasma form exists, which is now readily purified [12], in addition to the extracellular matrix form. Its ability to interact with cells to promote cell attachment [13] is the most celebrated activity of fibronectin *in vitro*. Rapid advances in functional studies on fibronectin have provided explanations relating to detailed issues of cell attachment, migration, and specificity.

Fibronectin is regarded as being a general cell attachment protein; most cell types except erythrocytes will adhere to fibronectin immobilized to certain surfaces by interacting specifically with fibronectin.

Fibronectin is a disulfide-linked dimer with a molecular mass of about 550 k. The structure of fibronectin varies depending on the cell type producing the protein. In addition to being a glycoprotein, various sites on fibronectin may be phosphorylated, sulfated, and acetylated; the significance of these modifications is not fully understood. It is believed that glycosylation can modify the functional properties of fibronectin [10].

The fibronectin molecule has several domains which are specific for various ligands. The binding sites include those for fibrin, heparin, collagen, DNA, cells, amyloid P component, and fibrin(ogen). The collagen binding activity of fibronectin has been developed for the affinity purification of plasma-derived fibronectin; gelatin (collagen) containing support matrices are commercially available and are used to specifically bind fibronectin in plasma; elution of fibronectin is accomplished with urea or citrate [12].

Active Peptides from Fibronectin

In 1984, two reports appeared in the literature which described the ability of small fragments derived from fibronectin to inhibit cell binding to immobilized fibronectin and to support the attachment of cells to plastic [14,15]. The approach taken by the groups doing this work involved finding proteolytic fragments of the parent protein that have the inhibitory activity. By determining the structure of the fragments, the groups were able to construct the active fragments, all of which contained the sequence Arg-Gly-Asp-Ser (RGDS).

The discovery of RGDS and related derivatives established the use of small peptides to study much larger proteins derived from extracellular matrix. For fibronectin, other peptides have been discovered that have similar activities, some of which, like the RGDS-containing peptide, may be involved in cell attachment *in vivo*. In 1987, Humphries et al. showed that a region of fibronectin not containing RGDS had the ability to inhibit the spreading of B16-F10 melanoma cells on fibronectin whereas the same peptide had no effect on the spreading of baby hamster kidney cells on fibronectin [16].

Recently, McCarthy et al. [17] reported an RGD-independent cell adhesion fragment from the heparin binding region of fibronectin. This peptide, Tyr-Glu-Lys-Pro-Gly-Ser-Pro-Pro-Arg-Glu-Val-Val-Pro-Arg-Pro-Arg-Pro-Gly-Val (YEKPGSPPREVVPRPRPGV), was reported to bind to heparin and to cells. In addition, a peptide that bound cells independent of any interaction with heparin was identified [17].

Other attachment factors in the form of peptides derived from fibronectin have been discovered and others will follow in the very near future; the cell attachment activity of fibronectin for various cell types is intricately regulated by various features within the fibronectin molecule.

OTHER RGD-CONTAINING PROTEINS

Since the original discovery of RGDS, several other proteins capable of mediating cell adhesion onto biological or artificial surfaces have been isolated from either body fluids or extracellular matrices. Some of the cell adhesion proteins containing Arg-Gly-Asp (RGD), the core of cell attachment sites, include bone sialoprotein [18], fibrinogen [19], osteopontin [20], thrombospondin [21], and vitronectin [22]. See the review article by Rouslahti [10] for additional information.

Most recently, a region of the tat protein from HIV-1, the causative agent of AIDS was discovered to contain RGD [23]. This is particularly interesting in light of the finding by Ensoli et al. [24] that the tat protein is released from HIV-1-infected cells *in vitro* and may stimulate the growth of Karposi's sarcoma lesions in patients suffering from AIDS.

As is quite obvious, the true contribution of the RGD-containing regions of these proteins and many other proteins in their overall biological function is a very active topic of research. However, the RGD sequence can be found in over 120 other proteins that have no known adhesive properties; vague arguments related to conformation have been used to account for this.

Integrins are a class of cellular receptors which bind RGD-containing proteins [25]. Since the microenvironment of the RGD residues appears to be unique to each protein, each integrin is believed to have an optimal microenvironment of its own to cater to the designated protein. In this respect, the word "optimal" is emphasized because it has been shown that the RGD sequence in different proteins can take on different conformations [10] and this implies different cellular specificities. As with peptides derived from extracellular matrix proteins, the topic and import of integrins is fast-growing.

LAMININ

Laminin is the most abundant glycoprotein in basement membranes and is both a structural and biologically active component. Laminin was first isolated from the mouse Engelbreth-Holm-Swarm (EHS) tumor in 1979 by P. G. Robey [26]. As with fibronectin [2,3,6,10], several review articles have been written describing the various structure-function aspects of laminin [7-9].

The variety of biological functions displayed by laminin include cell attachment, induction of mitogenesis, chemotaxis, binding to heparin sulfate proteoglycans, collagen IV, osteonectin, and nidogen/entactin, and growth and differentiation of various cell types [7-9]. Laminin has the ability to promote neurite outgrowth. As with fibronectin, primary fragments of laminin are being studied to locate regions in the parent molecule having these and other biological activities.

Laminin is a four-armed flexible protein with a molecular mass of about 850 k. There are three short arms and a single long arm. The three polypeptide chains that make up the entire laminin molecule have been named the A chain (molecular weight, 400 kDa), the B1 chain (molecular weight approximately 200 kDa), and the B2 chain (molecular weight approximately 200 kDa). The complete primary structures of each of the three chains have been determined [27-29].

It is important to note that murine EHS-derived laminin is the most readily purified form of laminin and, therefore, the most studied.

Although human placenta-derived laminin has been found to be similar to EHS laminin [30] there may be considerable variations between laminin from other species. Laminins from several other species have been isolated and studied to a lesser degree than the EHS-derived laminin.

There is much to be assimilated about laminin but it is believed that, as in other species, laminin participates in self association as a part of a complex polymer network of the basement membrane. Thus, for understanding these interactions as well as the way(s) by which laminin binds cells, many research teams have taken to the study of synthetic peptides derived from active laminin fragments.

RGD-Containing Region of Laminin

Laminin is one of many proteins with an RGD sequence of amino acids that is implicated as a major cell attachment point for laminin to integrin-like receptors on cells. However, laminin binding to an integrin-like receptor on some cells was not inhibited by peptides containing the RGD sequence [31]. It is believed by some that, in intact basement membrane, the RGD region in the laminin structures are perhaps buried and, therefore, laminin may be unable to bind cells through its RGD-containing region [32]. On the other hand, it has been shown that the binding of bovine aortic endothelial cells to laminin is inhibited by soluble RGD-containing peptides [33]. Thus, with respect to laminin, there is still much to be clarified about the role, if any, played by the RGD-containing region.

Active Peptides from Laminin

The first unique synthetic peptide derived from laminin to be shown to have some biological activity was Cys-Asp-Pro-Gly-Tyr-Ile-Gly-Ser-Arg (CDPGYIGSR). The peptide was discovered by making antibodies to synthetic peptides derived from various regions along the B1 chain of laminin and observing which antibodies inhibited HT1080 cell attachment to laminin [34]. By making various peptides surrounding the epitope which blocked cell attachment, the peptide, Tyr-Ile-Gly-Ser-Arg (YIGSR), was unveiled [35,50].

Human melanoma cells (MeWo) express a novel integrin receptor for laminin [36]. Binding of the receptor to laminin was found to be independent of RGD- or YIGSR-like sequences but required divalent cations. In addition, an association was deduced between the 67-kDa elastin receptor and the 67-kDa tumor cell laminin receptor [37]. In this work, a peptide from elastin, Val-Gly-Val-Ala-Pro-Gly (VGVAPG) and a similar peptide from laminin, Leu-Gly-Thr-Ile-Pro-Gly (LGTIPG) were found to be capable of eluting the receptor from elastin and laminin affinity columns. YIGSR was relatively inactive in eluting this receptor from a laminin affinity column.

Charonis et al. [38] described a 20–amino acid peptide from the B1 chain of laminin with heparin-binding and cell adhesion–promoting activity. The peptide, Arg-Tyr-Val-Val-Leu-Pro-Arg-Pro-Val-Cys-Phe-Glu-Lys-Gly-Met-Asn-Tyr-Thr-Val-Arg (RYVVLPRPVCFEKGMNYTVR), promotes cell adhesion of murine melanoma cells, fibrosarcoma, glioma, pheochromocytoma, and aortic endothelial cells. This finding suggests that cell surface-associated heparin-like molecules may act as receptors for certain laminin domains.

An additional peptide believed to act synergistically with YIGSR, and located proximal to YIGSR in the B1 chain, is Pro-Asp-Ser-Gly-Arg (PDSGR). This pentapeptide, similar to YIGSR, has the ability to stimulate cell events such as adhesion and chemotaxis. PDSGR also blocks metastasis but with less potency that YIGSR [39]. The physiological significance of this is still a subject of conjecture.

A peptide found in the long A chain of laminin has been identified and found to mediate cell attachment, migration, and neurite outgrowth [40,55]. This hydrophobic peptide, Ile-Lys-Val-Ala-Val (IKVAV), was unique at the time because, unlike other laminin-derived peptides, it had the ability to promote neurite outgrowth or cell spreading. In addition, IK-VAV is able to stimulate axonal-like processes of cerebral neurons and PC12 cells [40].

A peptide from the B2 chain of laminin has been found to stimulate neurite outgrowth [40]. The peptide, Arg-Asn-Ile-Ala-Glu-Ile-Ile-Lys-Asp-Ala (RNIAEIIKDA), is the first and only peptide from the B2 chain of laminin to be reported as having biological activity. Others are expected to follow.

TYPE 4 COLLAGEN

Type 4 collagen is a highly studied form of collagen found in basement membranes, a form of extracellular matrix. A summary of the properties of type 4 collagen can be found in Reference [9]. A recent observation by Chelberg et al. provided evidence that type 4 collagen is broken down into at least one active peptide, Gly-Val-Lys-Gly-Asp-Lys-Gly-Asn-Pro-Gly-Trp-Pro-Gly-Ala-Pro (GVKGDKGNPGWPGAP), with much of the *in vitro* biological activity found in the parent protein [42]. This peptide requires the three proline residues for its activity and represents a cell-specific adhesion, spreading, and motility domain of type 4 collagen.

CONJUGATES AND USES OF PEPTIDES FROM
EXTRACELLULAR MATRIX

RGDS-PROTEIN CONJUGATES

In the first paper that described RGDS, that by Pierschbacher and Ruoslahti [14], a description of experiments is given by the authors who used both a cell attachment assay and an inhibition assay to unveil the active RGDS. Without going into specifics, it was found that newborn rat kidney (NRK) cells would adhere to RGDS immobilized to Sepharose via a 6-carbon spacer. Similarly, by conjugating the small peptide to rabbit immunoglobulin and binding this conjugate to plastic, they were able to demonstrate cell attachment. Finally, using high concentrations of soluble forms of the small peptide, the authors were able to inhibit the binding of cells to fibronectin. The significance of their approach to these assays will be discussed later. The affinity constant of 6×10^{-4} M is quite weak compared to many physiological activities and, therefore, there was some doubt as to the true physiological significance of their discovery. However, the finding that other peptides at similar concentrations were inactive clearly strengthened their argument.

In the work described by Yamada and Kennedy [15], slightly different assays were used to reach the same conclusion: RGDS was a major site on fibronectin to interact with cells. These authors used the phenomenon of fibronectin-mediated cell spreading and the inhibition of the observed spreading by the various peptides for their assay. The baby hamster kidney (BHK) cells used in this assay bound but did not spread when added to collagen-coated plastic dishes. The addition of fibronectin with the cells resulted in the spreading phenomenon which was observed with phase-contrast microscopy. The affinity of the small peptide was slightly larger than that reported by Pierschbacher and Ruoslahti [14], but this could readily be attributed to a different assay system and cell type used by these researchers.

From a chemical viewpoint, the most impressive aspects of both studies were that a major function of a very large protein could be localized to a small peptide, four amino acids in length, and the design of very creative experiments to show binding of a very small, highly charged molecule. A peptide such as RGDS would be expected to contain very little hydrophobic character and the prediction is that RGDS binds poorly to plastic. Therefore, a conjugate to RGDS to rabbit IgG was made in Pierschbacher and Ruoslahti [14] and this was used to coat the plastic to demonstrate cell attachment. Thus, the active conjugate given in Pierschbacher and Ruoslahti [14] used Gly-Arg-Gly-Asp-Ser-Cys, GRGDS(C), where the amino terminus included glycine and the highly reactive cysteine was added to the carboxy terminus to react with a heterobifunctional cross-linker to make the conjugate.

CYCLIC RGDS

To demonstrate the concept regarding conformational restrictions of certain RGD-containing substances, Pierschbacher and Ruoslahti [43] used a cyclized form of RGDS to show potent inhibition of cell binding to vitronectin with little inhibition of cells adhering to fibronectin. Whereas RGDS was equally potent in blocking the activity of fibronectin and vitronectin, only the cyclized form was capable of discriminating between the two proteins.

TRUNCATED PROTEIN A CONTAINING RGDS

Using molecular biological techniques, RGDS has been introduced into a truncated form of protein A, a staphylococcal immunoglobulin–binding protein [44]. The mutated protein was able to bind IgG and, in addition, could mediate binding and spreading of cells to an inert surface. Thus, the cell adhesive and immunoglobulin binding activities of this single protein appeared to function coordinately. The approach taken in Maeda et al. [44] is only representative of whole new groups of "designer proteins" which are now being produced with dual functions in mind.

POLYMERIC RGD

Polymers of the peptide RGD have been synthesized using diphenyl-phosphorylazide to cross-link monomers of RGD. The polymers have been used extensively to study inhibition of metastases by certain RGD receptor–containing metastatic cells (*vide infra*), [45,46]. The diphenyl-phosphorylazide method of polymerizing peptides is described elsewhere [47].

AN RGD-GLASS CONJUGATE

A method has been developed by Massia and Hubbell to covalently immobilize small peptides that are active in cell adhesion in order to promote the adhesion and spreading of cells to glass surfaces [48]. Small synthetic peptides will have a tendency to desorb or become degraded by proteases when noncovalently adsorbed to surfaces and thus, the hope is that covalent immobilization of cell attachment peptides might overcome these problems. Adhesion of cells to impermeable glass might be a useful alternative to the adhesion of cells to penetrable surfaces such as polyacryl-amide gels onto which RGD peptides have been covalently linked [49].

VARIOUS FORMS OF YIGSR

For the use of YIGSR, it was found that the amide form of the C-terminus was more active than the free carboxyl form [50]. The amide was made initially because of the possibility that the positive charge from the arginine could interact with the negative charge of its own carboxyl group. If the total positive charge on the arginine of YIGSR is necessary for the peptide's biological activity, an adjacent negatively charged carboxyl group could be detrimental (G. R. Martin and F. A. Robey, unpublished observation). In retrospect, it seems rational to make most peptides from larger proteins in the amide form at the C-terminus instead of in the free carboxylic acid form; the additional negative charge could greatly influence the behavior of the peptide in terms of hydrophilic character and conformation. The exception of course would be for those peptides that naturally exist as the C-termini of their parent proteins.

Various forms of YIGSR have been synthesized in this laboratory in an effort to improve the observed biological activities. The only synthetic form to have appreciable activity was the cyclic YIGSR which was synthesized by first adding a bromoacetyl moiety to the N-terminus and a cysteine residue at the C-terminus. By placing this into a buffered aqueous solution at pH 7–8, the free sulfhydryl reacted with the bromoactyl to give the cyclic YIGSR [39,51]. Interestingly, this method was used in an attempt to make polymers of the YIGSR but the cyclic version formed quantitatively (F. A. Robey, unpublished data). Attempts to find cell attachment activity in YIGSR conjugated to bovine serum albumin with HT1080 cells (H. K. Kleinman and F. A. Robey, unpublished data) were not successful even though there was a considerable amount of YIGSR conjugated to the albumin [52]. For these experiments, YIGSR was conjugated to albumin through its amino terminal region [52].

Unlike RGD-containing peptides, YIGSR is not as ubiquitous as initially expected in terms of its cell attachment activity; YIGSR is unique to laminin and the original thinking was that YIGSR would be one of laminin's most active components, similar to the dominant role played by RGD-containing peptides in fibronectin. However, YIGSR does not support the attachment of many cell types nor compete with laminin in supporting the attachment of several cell types. In some instances, YIGSR may be responsible for the spreading phenomenon seen when cells bind to laminin but not the initial binding [33]. YIGSR was found to inhibit the migration of neutral crest cells along basement membrane substrata [53]. YIGSR has the ability to abolish completely the migratory activity of cardiac mesenchymal cells within three dimensional gels of laminin [54]. Thus, certain cells appear to have a YIGSR-specific receptor which may function differently depending on the cell type.

Much of the concern for YIGSR may be explained in its inability to bind strongly to surfaces. The recent report showing cell attachment activity on glass plates to which YIGSR was convalently attached proves that YIGSR is active in supporting the activity of human foreskin fibroblasts. However, cells spread at much slower rates on the YIGSR-containing surface than on the RGDS-derivatized glass surface [48]. It is clear that much is left to be learned about YIGSR, its analogues, and its receptors before general statements concerning its activity and physiological relevance can be made. Unlike RGD-containing proteins, YIGSR appears to be unique to laminin and for this reason alone, the applications of its use may be governed by the limited role(s) played *in vivo* by laminin itself.

EXPERIMENTAL METASTASIS

The perils of cancer reside in the proficiency of cancer cells to metastasize to various parts of the body. To do this, malignant cells must transverse the extracellular matrix to depart from the primary tumor and to relocate. To prevent this, a thorough understanding of the ways by which cells bind to, move on, and penetrate through extracellular matrix is of importance. With this knowledge, cell-specific targeting agents could be rationally designed and used to prevent the spread of cancer.

The complex, multistep process of metastasis involves malignant cell surface components and the use of these components by malignant cells as substrata to migrate and to traverse endothelial basement membranes. Tumor cells pass through basement membrane during both entrance and departure from the circulation. Attachment is thought to be the initial step in metastasis and type 4 collagen, laminin, and fibronectin—components of basement membranes and extracellular matrix—are thought to be major mediators in the metastatic process by binding cell surface components [56–62].

The ability to promote cell migration via cell adhesion led investigators to consider invasion and metastases as possible events in which fibronectin and other extracellular matrix proteins might play a role [57]. Specific interactions between tumor cells and host cells and components are fundamental to the metastatic process. Among these interactions, cell attachment and detachment are considered to be of significance.

Studies conducted by Humphries et al. [63] using B16-F10 cells, a murine melanoma cell line, clearly showed that GRGDS inhibited lung colonization presumably through its ability to interfere with cellular processes. The conclusion that GRGDS interfered with *in vivo* cell attachment and migration and therefore, metastases, is yet to be definitively validated but, based on enormous amounts of supportive *in vitro* data, such a conclusion is warranted.

In 1984, it was reported that laminin strongly stimulated metastasis formation when metastatic murine melanoma cells were preincubated with whole laminin followed by tail vein injection [58]. Recently, a publication reported an amino acid sequence from the laminin A chain that stimulates metastasis [64]. The peptide, composed of 19 amino acids (Cys-Ser-Arg-Ala-Arg-Lys-Gln-Ala-Ala-Ser-Ile-Lys-Val-Ala-Val-Ser-Ala-Asp-Arg)   also increased collagenase 4 activity, a key enzyme in the breakdown of basement membranes. These results indicate that understanding the relationship of laminin to the metastatic process is of paramount importance.

Following the studies on metastases with RGD-containing peptides, researchers have studied the ability of laminin's YIGSR to inhibit the metastasis of B16-F10 melanoma cells in mice [65]. YIGSR was found to block the formation of lung tumor colonies in mice when co-injected with tumor cells. The YIGSR was varied in concentration from 50 μg/mouse to 1 mg/mouse. Only the highest concentration was considered to be highly successful in blocking metastases. Cyclic YIGSR is even more potent than the noncyclized YIGSR [39]. As with RGD-containing peptides, polymers of YIGSR have been synthesized and found to inhibit the metastastic formation of malignant tumor cells in the lung more effectively than the pentapeptide [66].

As for laminin, fragments appear to have the ability to either stimulate or suppress metastases. YIGSR is one active component of laminin and the amide [50], polymeric [45,66], and cyclized [39,51] forms of YIGSR are all more potent than the linear YIGSR in blocking experimental metastases.

The results compound the issue of targeting the binding of metastatic cells to specific peptides in laminin but they reinforce the notion that laminin plays a major role in metastasis. As mentioned in the introduction to this chapter, a vast amount of work is being done at the present time to unravel these important issues.

Type 4 collagen, a major component of basement membrane also contains a peptide sequence which is capable of inhibiting experimental metastases. This is the same peptide reported by Chelberg et al., containing three proline residues which inhibits the binding of cells to type 4 collagen [42].

FUTURE APPLICATIONS OF PEPTIDES DERIVED FROM EXTRACELLULAR MATRIX PROTEINS

Studying biologically active peptides derived from extracellular matrix proteins is a very useful means to delineate the complex array of the extracellular matrix and the cell surface binding components. The net result at present is a greater understanding of how living organisms are arranged and manage to function biologically. Knowledge of extracellular matrix peptides has reached a point at which the peptides could be developed for uses aimed not so much at research but at diagnosis and therapy for vastly disparate groups of diseases.

It is quite possible that peptides derived from extracellular matrix proteins could have clinical uses. In 1990, no extracellular matrix peptide has been approved but, for some, preclinical investigations under the auspices of the appropriate regulatory agencies are being conducted. These include toxicology studies in small animals to study the general safety and tolerance levels of the peptides and/or their derivatives. Because the peptides are quite small, limitations on manufacturing kilogram amounts should be surpassed readily. Quality control of the synthetic peptides will require the use of mass spectrometry in addition to the commonly used techniques for characterizing peptides, i.e., high performance liquid chromatography and amino acid analysis.

From a regulatory point of view, safety and efficacy are the criteria upon which approval of a drug substance is based. Therefore, the challenge to those developing the peptide-containing material lies not in the mass production of a peptide but in demonstrating consistency in modifying or conjugating the active peptide in the final form in which it will be used clinically.

As metastases inhibitors, peptides derived from type 4 collagen, laminin and fibronectin have proved to be efficacious. Whether these findings ever translate into something actually clinically useful will depend largely on the results of toxicity tests; because the peptides are so small, their circulating half-life in serum may be very short, on the order of minutes. Therefore, use of these small peptides (perhaps prophylactically following surgical removal of a primary tumor) could require perfusion of the patient over a period of several days with large amounts and therein lies the importance of the toxicology (safety) studies.

Wound healing is a very promising application for these synthetic peptides. The specific areas are quite varied and extend from soft tissue to bone. Inert matrices that carry extracellular matrix peptides could be used to bind new cells at a site of tissue damage and enhance the repair by providing substrata upon which new cells can attach and proliferate.

Artificial organs and blood vessels may be improved with the use of peptides derived from extracellular matrix because the substrata of inert substance could carry the biologically active peptide and allow neighboring tissue to bind specifically to the inert material. This will be especially useful in the artificial limb and dental implant areas. The tough, inert materials used to replace bones and teeth today are poor substrates for bone cell adsorption and growth. Thus, the implanted materials take several months to take hold *in vivo*.

Platelet aggregation is inhibited by RGD-containing peptides [19]. Today, thrombolytic therapy is a major approach for the treatment of myocardial infarcts and many approaches to preventing *in vivo* arterial thrombus formation in the vasculature target platelets. Perhaps the RGD-containing peptides could be developed to either dissociate platelets in the thrombus or used to prevent clot formation before it develops in an artery or vein. Considering the high prevalence of cardiac disease throughout the world, uses of RGD for treatment of heart disease will certainly be studied very closely.

New methods of conjugation chemistry are needed to attach these extracellular matrix peptides to biocompatible, inert materials, some of which have yet to be discovered. The combined peptide-biomaterial must have only the desired activities and not elicit undesirable side effects such as being immunogenic in the host.

Uses of the adhesion peptides has progressed away from extracellular matrix and into the immune system where the foundations developed by studying extracellular matrix are finding additional clear-cut uses as research tools. Understanding the science governing recognition, adhesion, and interactions of immune cells with targets is a fundamental challenge of immunologists. This understanding will enhance our knowledge of how the immune system functions but it will also allow new ways to manipulate the immune system by targeting.

Great strides are being made at the present time in the area of immune recognition in part because of our understanding about cell recognition, adhesion, chemotaxis, and proliferation coming from extracellular matrix studies. The same can be said about understanding the organization and workings of the nervous system, one of biomedical research's last frontiers.

REFERENCES

1 Piez, K. A., ed. 1985. *Extracellular Matrix Biochemistry.* New York, NY: Elsevier.

2 Bernfield, M., ed. 1989. *Extracellular Matrix, Current Opinion in Cell Biology,* 1:953.

3 Mosher, D. F. 1989. *Fibronectin.* New York, NY: Academic Press.

4 Mayne, R. and R. E. Burgeson. 1987. *Structure and Function of Collagen Types.* Orlando, FL: Academic Press.

5 Mecham, R. P. and T. N. Wight. 1987. *Biology of Proteoglycans.* Orlando, FL: Academic Press.

6 Yamada, K. M. 1989. "Fibronectins: Structure, Functions and Receptors," *Cur. Op. in Cell Biol.*, 1:956–963.

7 Martin, G. R. and R. Timpl. 1987. "Laminin and Other Basement Membrane Components," *Ann. Rev. Cell Biol.*, 3:57–85.

8 Beck, K., I. Hunter and J. Engel. 1990. "Structure and Function of Laminin: Anatomy of a Multidomain Glycoprotein," *FASEB J.*, 4:148–160.

9 Yurchenco, P. D. and J. C. Schnittny. 1990. "Molecular Architecture of Basement Membranes," *FASEB J.*, 4:157–1590.

10 Ruoslahti, E. 1988. "Fibronectin and Its Receptors," *Ann. Rev. Biochem.*, 57:375–413.

11 Mosesson, M. W. and R. A. Umfleet. 1970. "The Cold-Insoluble Globulin of Human Plasma. I. Purification, Primary Characterization, and Relationship to Fibrinogen and Other Cold Insoluble Fractions Components," *J. Biol. Chem.*, 245(21):5728–5736.

12 Miekka, S. I., K. C. Ingham and D. Menache. 1982. "Rapid Methods for Isolation of Human Plasma Fibronectin," *Thromb. Res.*, 27:1–14.

13 Klebe, R. J. 1984. "Isolation of a Collagen-Dependent Cell Attachment Factor," *Nature*, 250:248–251.

14 Pierschbacher, M. D. and E. Ruoslahti. 1984. "Cell Attachment Activity of Fibronectin Can Be Duplicated by Small Synthetic Fragments of the Molecule," *Nature*, 309:30–33.

15 Yamada, K. M. and D. W. Kennedy. 1984. "Dualistic Nature of Adhesive Protein Function: Fibronectin and Its Biologically Active Peptide Fragments Can Autoinhibit Fibronectin Function," *J. Cell. Biol.*, 99:29–36.

16 Humphries, M. J., A. Komoriya, S. K. Akiyama, K. Olden and K. M. Yamada. 1987. "Identification of Two Distinct Regions of the Type III Connecting Segment of Human Plasma Fibronectin That Promote Cell Type-Specific Adhesion," *J. Biol. Chem.*, 262:6886–6892.

17 McCarthy, J. B., A. P. N. Skubitz, Q. Zhao, X. Yi, D. J. Mickelson, D. J. Klein and L. T. Furcht. 1990. "RGD-Independent Cell Adhesion to the Carboxy-Terminal Heparin-Binding Fragment of Fibronectin Involves Heparin-Dependent and -Independent Activities," *J. Cell. Biol.*, 110:777–787.

18 Fisher, L. W., O. W. McBride, J. D. Termine and M. F. Young. 1990. "Human Bone Sialoprotein. Deduced Protein Sequence and Chromosomal Localization," *J. Biol. Chem.*, 265:2347–2351.

19 Gartner, T. K. and J. S. Bennett. 1985. "The Tetrapeptide Analogue of the Cell Attachment Site of Fibrinogen Inhibits Platelet Aggregation and Fibrinogen Binding to Activated Platelets," *J. Biol. Chem.*, 260:11891–11894.

20 Oldberg, A., A. Franzen and D. Heinegard. 1986. "Cloning and Sequence Analysis of Rat Bone Sialoprotein (Osteopontin) cDNA Reveals an Arg-Gly-Asp Cell-Binding Sequence," *Proc. Nat. Acad. Sci. USA*, 83:8819–8823.

21 Lawler, J. and R. O. Hynes. 1986. "The Structure of Human Thrombospondin: An Adhesive Glycoprotein with Multiple Calcium-Binding Sites and Homologies with Several Different Proteins," *J. Cell. Biol.*, 103:1635–1648.

22 Suzuki, S., Å. Oldberg, E. Hayman, M. D. Pierschbacher and E. Ruoslahti. 1985. "Complete Amino Acid Sequence of Human Vitronectin Deduced from cDNA. Similarity of Cell Attachment Sites in Vitronectin and Fibronectin," *EMBO J.*, 4:2519–2524.

23 Brake, D. A., C. Debouck and G. Biesecker. 1990. "Identification for an Arg-Gly-Asp (RGD) Cell Adhesion Site in Human Immunodeficiency Virus Type 1 Transactivation Protein, Tat," *J. Cell. Biol.*, 111:1275–1281.

24 Ensoli, B., G. Barillari, S. Z. Salahuddin, R. C. Gallo and F. Wong-Stall. 1990. "Tat Protein of HIV-1 Stimulates Growth of Cells Derived from Karposi's Sarcoma Lesions of AIDS Patients," *Nature*, 345:84–86.

25 Hynes, R. O. 1987. "Integrins: A Family of Cell Surface Receptors," *Cell*, 48:549–554.

26 Timpl, R., H. Rohde, P. G. Robey, S. I. Rennard, J. M. Foidart and G. R. Martin. 1979. "Laminin—A Glycoprotein from Basement Membranes," *J. Biol. Chem.*, 254:9932–9933.

27 Sasaki, M., S. Kato, K. Kohno, G. R. Martin and Y. Yamada. 1987. "Sequence of the cDNA Encoding the Laminin B1 Chain Reveals a Multidomain Protein Containing Cysteine-Rich Repeats," *Proc. Nat. Acad. Sci. USA*, 84:935–939.

28 Sasaki, M. and Y. Yamada. 1987. "The Laminin B2 Chain Has a Multidomain Structure Homologous to the B1 Chain," *J. Biol. Chem.*, 262:17111–17117.

29 Sasaki, M., H. K. Kleinman, H. Huber, R. Deutzmann and Y. Yamada. 1988. "Laminin, a Multidomain Protein: the A Chain Has a Unique Globular Domain and Homology with the Basement Membrane Proteoglycan and the Laminin B Chains," *J. Biol. Chem.*, 263:16536–16544.

30 Ohno, M., A. Martinez-Hernandez, N. Ohno and N. A. Kefalides. 1985. "Comparative Study of Laminin Found in Normal Placental Membrane with Laminin of Neoplastic Origin," in *Basement Membranes*, S. Shibata, ed., Amsterdam: Elsevier Science Publ. (Japan: Mishima) pp. 3–11.

31 Gehlsen, K. R., L. Dillner, E. Engvall and E. Ruoslahti. 1988. "The Laminin Receptor Is a Member of the Integrin Family of Cell Adhesion Receptors," *Science*, 241:1228–1229.

32 Schnittny, J. C., R. Timpl and J. Engel. 1988. "High Resolution Immunoelectron Microscopic Localization of Functional Domains of Laminin, Nidogen, and Heparin Sulfate Proteoglycan in Epithelial Basement Membrane of Mouse Cornea Reveals Different Topological Orientations," *J. Cell. Biol.*, 107:1599–1610.

33 Basson, C. T., W. J. Knowles, L. Bell, S. M. Albelda, V. Castronovo, L. A. Liotta and J. A. Madri. 1990. "Spatiotemporal Segregation of Endothelial Cell Integrin Extracellular Matrix-Binding Proteins during Adhesion Events," *J. Cell. Biol.*, 110:789–801.

34 Graf, J., Y. Iwamoto, M. Sasaki, G. R. Martin, H. K. Kleinman, F. A. Robey and Y. Yamada. 1987. "Identification of an Amino Acid Sequence in Laminin Mediating Cell Attachment, Chemotaxis and Receptor Binding," *Cell*, 48:989–996.

35 Iwamoto, Y., J. Graf, M. Sasaki, H. K. Kleinman, D. R. Greatorex, G. R. Martin, F. A. Robey and Y. Yamada. 1988. "Synthetic Pentapeptide from the B1 Chain of Laminin Promotes B16F10 Melanoma Cell Migration," *J. Cell. Phys.*, 134:287–291.

36 Kramer, R. H., K. A. McDonald and M. P. Vu. 1989. "Human Melanoma Cells Express a Novel Integrin Receptor for Laminin," *J. Biol. Chem.*, 264:15642–15649.

37 Mecham, R. P., A. Hinek, G. L. Griffin, R. M. Senior and L. A. Liotta. 1989. "The Elastin Receptor Shows Structural and Functional Similarities to the 67-kDa Tumor Cell Laminin Receptor," *J. Biol. Chem.*, 264:16652–16657.

38 Charonis, A. S., A. P. N. Skubitz, G. G. Koliakos, L. A. Reger, J. Dege, A. M. Vogel, R. Wohlhueter and L. T. Furcht. 1988. "A Novel Synthetic Peptide from the B1 Chain of Laminin with Heparin-Binding and Cell Adhesion–Promoting Activities," *J. Cell. Biol.*, 107:1253–1260.

39 Kleinman, H. K., J. Graf, Y. Iwamoto, M. Sasaki, C. S. Schasteen, Y. Yamada, G. R. Martin and F. A. Robey. 1989. "Identification of a Second Active Site in Laminin for Promotion of Cell Adhesion and Migration and Inhibition of *in vivo* Melanoma Lung Colonization," *Arch. Biochem. Biophys.*, 272:39–45.

40 Sephel, G. C., K.-I. Tashiro, M. Sasaki, D. Greatorex, G. R. Martin, Y. Yamada and H. K. Kleinman. 1989. "Laminin A Chain Synthetic Peptide Which Supports Neurite Outgrowth," *Biochem. Biophys. Res. Comm.*, 162:821–829.

41 Liesi, P., A. Närvänen, J. Soos, H. Sariola and G. Snounou. 1989. "Identification of a Neurite Outgrowth-Promoting Domain of Laminin Using Synthetic Peptides," *FEBS Lett.*, 244:141–148.

42 Chelberg, M. K., J. B. McCarthy, A. P. N. Skubitz, L. T. Furcht and E. C. Tsilibary. 1990. "Characterization of a Synthetic Peptide from Type IV Collagen That Promotes Melanoma Cell Adhesion, Spreading and Motility," *J. Cell. Biol.*, 111:262–270.

43 Pierschbacher, M. D. and E. Ruoslahti. 1987. "Influence of Stereochemistry of the Sequence Arg-Gly-Asp-Xaa on Binding Specificity in Cell Adhesion," *J. Biol. Chem.*, 262:17294–17298.

44 Maeda, T., R. Oyama, K. Ichihara-Tanaka, F. Kimizuka, I. Kato, K. Titani and S. Kiyotoshi. 1989. "A Novel Cell Adhesive Protein Engineered by Insertion of the Arg-Gly-Asp-Ser Tetrapeptide," *J. Biol. Chem.*, 264:15165–15168.

45 Saiki, I., J. Iida, J. Murata, R. Ogawa, N. Nishi, K. Sugimura, T. Seiichi and I. Azuma. 1989. "Inhibition of Metastasis of Murine Malignant Melanoma by Synthetic Polymeric Peptides Containing Core Sequences of Cell-Adhesive Molecules," *Can. Res.*, 49:3815–3822.

46 Saiki, I., J. Murata, J. Iida, N. Nishi, K. Sugimura and I. Azuma. 1989. "The Inhibition of Murine Lung Metastasis by Synthetic Polypeptides [Poly(Arg-Gly-Asp) and Poly(Tyr-Ile-Gly-Ser-Arg)] with a Core Sequence of Cell Adhesion Molecules," *Br. J. Cancer*, 59:194–197.

47 Nishi, N., B. Nakajima, N. Hasebe and J. Noguchi. 1980. "Polymerization of Amino Acid or Peptides with Diphenylphosphoryl Azide (DPPA)," *Int. J. Biol. Macromol.*, 2:53.

48 Massia, S. P. and J. A. Hubbell. 1990. "Covalent Surface Immobilization of Arg-Gly-Asp- and Tyr-Ile-Gly-Ser-Arg-Containing Peptides to Obtain Well-Defined Cell Adhesive Substrates," *Analyt. Biochem.*, 187:292–301.

49 Bradley, B. K. and R. L. Schnaar. 1988. "Binding RGD Peptides to Polyacrylamide Gels," *Analyt. Biochem.*, 172:270–278.

50 Graf, J. , R. C. Ogle, F. A. Robey, M. Sasaki, G. R. Martin, Y. Yamada and H. K. Kleinman. 1987. "A Pentapeptide from the B1 Laminin Chain Mediates Cell Adhesion and Binds the 67,000 Laminin Receptor," *Biochem.*, 26:6896–6900.

51 Robey, F. A. and R. L. Fields. 1989. "Automated Synthesis of N-Bromoacetyl-Modified Peptides for the Preparation of Synthetic Peptide Polymers, Peptide-Protein Conjugates and Cyclic Peptides," *Analyt. Biochem.*, 177:373–377.

52 Kolodny, N. and F. A. Robey. 1990. "Conjugation of Synthetic Peptides to Proteins: Quantitation from S-Carboxymethylcysteine Released Upon Acid Hydrolysis," *Analyt. Biochem.*, 187:136–140.

53 Bilozur, M. E. and E. D. Hay. 1988. "Neural Crest Migration in 3D Extracellular Matrix Utilizes Laminin, Fibronectin or Collagen," *Dev. Biol.*, 125:19–33.

54 Davis, L. A., R. C. Ogle and C. D. Little. 1989. "Embryonic Heart Mesenchymal Cell Migration in Laminin," *Dev. Biol.*, 133:37–43.

55 Tashiro, K., G. C. Sephel, B. Weeks, M. Sasaki, G. R. Martin, H. K. Kleinman and Y. Yamada. 1989. "A Synthetic Peptide Containing the IKVAV Sequence from the A Chain of Laminin Mediates Cell Attachment, Migration and Neurite Outgrowth," *J. Biol. Chem.*, 264:16174–16182.

56 Liotta, L. A., J. Kleinerman, P. Catanzara and D. Rynbrandt. 1977. "Degradation of Basement Membrane by Murine Tumor Cells," *J. Natl. Cancer Inst.*, 58: 1427–1439.

57 Liotta, L. A., C. N. Rao and S. H. Barsky. 1983. "Tumor Invasion and the Extracellular Matrix," *Lab. Invest.*, 49:636–649.

58 Barsky, S. H., C. N. Rao, J. E. Williams and L. A. Liotta. 1984. "Laminin Molecular Domains Which Alter Metastases in a Murine Model," *J. Clin. Invest.*, 74:843–848.

59 Rao, C. N., I. M. Margulies, T. S. Tralka, V. P. Terranova, J. A. Madri and L. A. Liotta. 1982. "Isolation of a Subunit of Laminin and Its Role in Molecular Structure and Tumor Cell Attachment," *J. Biol. Chem.*, 257:9740–9744.

60 Terranova, V. P., C. N. Rao, T. Kalebic, I. M. Margulies and L. A. Liotta. 1983. "Laminin Receptor on Human Breast Carcinoma Cells," *Proc. Natl. Acad. Sci. USA*, 80:444–448.

61 Rao, C. N., S. H. Barsky, V. P. Terranova and L. A. Liotta. 1983. "Isolation of a Tumor Cell Laminin Receptor," *Biochem. Biophys. Res. Comm.*, 111:804–808.

62 Malinoff, H. L. and M. S. Wicha. 1983. "Isolation of a Cell Surface Receptor Protein for Laminin from Murine Fibrosarcoma Cells," *J. Cell. Biol.*, 96: 1475–1479.

63 Humphries, M. J., K. Olden and K. M. Yamada. 1986. "A Synthetic Peptide from Fibronectin Inhibits Experimental Metastases of Murine Melanoma Cells," *Science*, 233:467–470.

64 Kanemoto, T., R. Reich, L. Royce, D. Greatorex, S. H. Adler, N. Shiraishi, G. R. Martin, Y. Yamada and H. K. Kleinman. 1990. "Identification of an Amino Acid Sequence from the Laminin A Chain that Stimulates Metastasis and Collagenase IV Production," *Proc. Nat. Acad. Sci. USA*, 87:2279–2283.

65 Iwamoto, Y., F. A. Robey, J. Graf, M. Sasaki, H. K. Kleinman, Y. Yamada and G. R. Martin. 1987. "YIGSR, a Synthetic Laminin Pentapeptide, Inhibits Experimental Metastasis Formation," *Science*, 238:1132–1134.

66 Murata, J., I. Saiki, I. Azuma and N. Nishi. 1989. "Inhibitory Effect of a Synthetic Polypeptide, Poly(Tyr-Ile-Gly-Ser-Arg), on the Metastatic Formation of Malignant Tumour Cells," *Int. J. Macromol.*, 11:97–99.

67 Obara, M., M. S. Kang and K. M. Yamada. 1988. "Site-Directed Mutagenesis of the Cell-Binding Domain of Human Fibronectin: Separable, Synergistic Sites Mediate Adhesive Function," *Cell*, 53:649–657.

CHAPTER 13

Design of Peptide Analog Inhibitors of Proteolytic Processes

STEPHAN K. GRANT[1]
THOMAS D. MEEK[1]
BRIAN W. METCALF[1]
STEPHEN R. PETTEWAY, JR.[2]

INTRODUCTION

PROTEASES, a subset of enzymes that catalyze the hydrolysis of peptide bonds within proteins or polypeptides, play a crucial role in the maintenance and regulation of a number of biological processes. The Renin-Angiotensin System (RAS), for example, contains a cascade of proteases. In the RAS, the protein angiotensinogen is processed to the decapeptide angiotensin 1 by the proteolytic enzyme renin, and further to the octapeptide angiotensin 2 by a second protease, angiotensin-converting enzyme (Scheme 13.1). A series of later hydrolytic steps produces various other peptide products including angiotensin 3. The physiological role of the RAS both in the circulatory system and as reported recently in various tissues is quite varied [1,2]. The RAS maintains salt and volume homeostasis in the body and regulates blood pressure [3]. This hormonal system is also important for cardiovascular regulation since angiotensin 2 is a potent vasoconstrictor. The use of peptide analog inhibitors as an approach to control the RAS cascade either by blocking renin or angiotensin-converting enzyme (ACE) has had strong clinical success against several physiological disorders such as hypertension and cardiovascular diseases [4,5].

Viral infection is another biological process which is dependent upon the action of several types of enzymic reactions. Infection by the retrovirus

---

[1]Department of Medicinal Chemistry, SmithKline Beecham Pharmaceuticals, King of Prussia, PA 19406, U.S.A.
[2]Department of Antiinfectives, SmithKline Beecham Pharmaceuticals, King of Prussia, PA 19406, U.S.A.

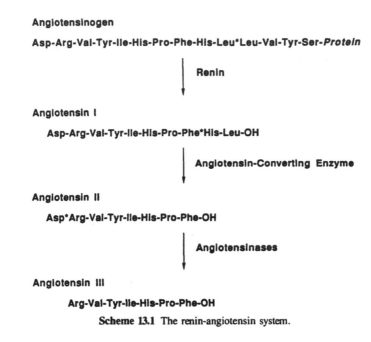

Scheme 13.1 The renin-angiotensin system.

human immunodeficiency type-1 virus (HIV-1), the causative agent of the acquired immune deficiency syndrome (AIDS) [5a], is carried out by a series of enzymatically controlled steps, each of which is a potential target for therapeutics (Scheme 13.2). The retroviral genome is composed of RNA that must be converted into DNA by virally-encoded reverse transcriptase and ribonuclease H. In turn, this DNA is incorporated into the host cell genome by the enzyme integrase to form the provirus. During subsequent steps of the life cycle of the virus the translation of the proviral mRNA produces the gag and gag-pol polyprotein precursors that contain in nascent form the structural proteins and enzymes of the virus. Processing of the polyproteins is accomplished by the virally-encoded protease (HIV-1 PR), which is autocatalytically cleaved out of the gag-pol polyprotein precursor. A variety of pathological consequences of HIV infection have been reported including depletion of white blood cell population and the eventual collapse of the host's immune system [6–8]. Blockade of the action of reverse transcriptase by azidothymidine (AZT) was the first example of an inhibitor which led to an AIDS drug targetting a specific retroviral enzyme [9]. The discovery of a virally-encoded protease, essential for the maturation of viral products, offers a target for the development of peptide analog inhibitors as anti-AIDS drugs.

In this review, we will examine in detail synthetic and naturally-occurring peptide analog inhibitors of three proteases, angiotensin-converting enzyme, renin, and human immunodeficiency virus type-1 protease.

SPECIFICITY AND CATALYTIC MECHANISMS OF PROTEASES

The action of a specific protease on an important bio-molecule, such as a regulatory peptide or an enzyme, is dependent upon the specificity of that protease for accessible cleavage sites within its substrate as well as the catalytic efficiency of the enzyme imposed by the nature of its chemical mechanism. Peptide analog inhibitors as drug candidates, are designed to specifically inhibit the target protease based on a judicious selection of the flanking amino acids in the peptide analog and structural features of the proposed mechanistic intermediates along the reaction coordinate. The description of a target protease and its rationally-derived inhibitor must therefore begin with an examination of its specificity and catalytic mechanism.

The specificity of proteases for cleavage sites within protein substrates varies widely, and depends largely on the degree of complementarity between a protein substrate and the binding site of an individual protease. The broad spectrum of substrate specificity among the proteases acts as one determinant of their individual roles in the workings of biological systems. The proteases of broad substrate specificity, such as pepsin, elastase, and chymotrypsin, are usually involved in digestion or other processes of nonspecific protein degradation. Proteases of more limited specificity such as angiotensin-converting enzyme, tissue plasminogen activa-

STEPS DURING HIV INFECTION	HIV ENZYME TARGETS
1. ADSORPTION (gp120/CD-4 receptor)	
2. REPLICATION (mRNA to cDNA)	◄——— REVERSE TRANSCRIPTASE RIBONUCLEASE H
3. INTEGRATION (provirus)	◄——— INTEGRASE
4. GENE EXPRESSION (cellular enzymes)	
5. MATURATION (processing polyproteins)	◄——— PROTEASE
6. VIRAL ASSEMBLY	
7. BUDDING & RELEASE	

Scheme 13.2 Enzyme targets in HIV infection.

tor, and renin have more narrowly-defined, regulatory metabolic functions, involved in blood pressure regulation or in fibrinolytic pathways. Other types of proteases are involved in the deactivation of biomolecules by specific proteolytic degradation. The limited proteolysis observed in these systems results primarily from structural constraints within the enzymic active sites. The accessibility of cleavage sites within these protein substrates and the temporal expression of protease genes and cellular location of the enzymes also afford a certain measure of selectivity.

Given the crucial role of proteases in metabolic processes and the potentially disastrous consequences of unchecked protein degradation to an organism, the proteases themselves are understandably subject to regulation by a variety of protease inhibitors (e.g., α_1-antitrypsin, [10]) which specifically inhibit or inactivate them. The absence of sufficient levels of these endogenous protease inhibitors can result in clinically-significant diseases and disorders, such as emphysema [11].

In addition, there exists a number of naturally-occurring protease inhibitors of low molecular weight (pepstatin A, phosphoramidon, leupeptin). These inhibitors have provided a point of departure leading to the design of synthetic, mechanism-based protease inhibitors based largely on knowledge of the catalytic mechanisms of the target proteases.

The known proteases each fall into one of four classes: serine, cysteine, metallo, and aspartic. The types of catalytic mechanisms utilized by the proteases may be divided into two categories, nucleophilic and "acid-base" catalysis, in which the serine and cysteine proteases represent the former while the metallo and aspartic proteases comprise the latter. As a result, within each of these classes of proteases there is a high degree of sequence homology found in the protein domains that constitute the catalytic and substrate binding sites.

The metallo and aspartic proteases, which are the subjects of this review, apparently utilize a general acid-base mechanism to catalyze the hydrolysis of peptide bonds. The archetypal metalloprotease is the bacterial enzyme, thermolysin. Much of the data used to derive the currently-held view of the chemical mechanism of the metalloproteases is derived from detailed structural and kinetic studies of this protease. Other proteases of this class include angiotensin-converting enzyme, collagenase, and enkephalinase. In the metalloproteases, the general acid components are the divalent zinc ion and a histidine residue, while an active site zinc ion and glutamic acid residue combine to form the general base component which binds and activates a nucleophilic water molecule. A proposed mechanism for the metalloproteases (in particular thermolysin) is shown in Scheme 13.3. Upon binding of the peptide substrate, the zinc-coordinated water molecule attacks the scissile carbonyl, which is acti-

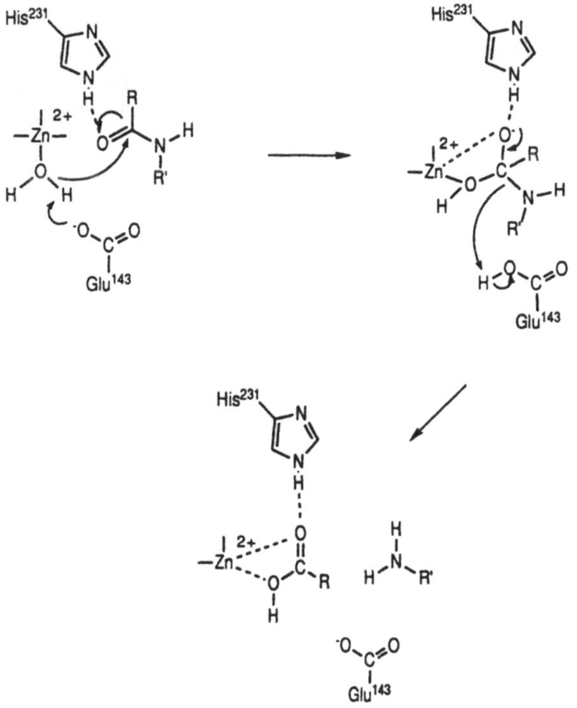

Scheme 13.3 Proposed chemical mechanism for thermolysin.

vated by general acid catalysis from the zinc ion. The zinc ion also functions, presumably, to polarize the carbonyl. Glu-143 assists as a general base by deprotonation of the water molecule in the formation of the tetrahedral intermediate, and later as a general acid in the protonation of the departing amine from this intermediate [12,13].

With the exception of the retroviral proteases, the aspartic proteases (e.g., pepsin, cathepsin D, renin, and penicillopepsin) are "pseudosymmetric" bilobal proteins composed of over 300 amino acids, in which each lobe contains one of the two catalytic aspartyl residues within a conserved sequence, Asp-Thr-Gly, at an active site found at the interface of the lobes [14,15]. In the widely-held view of the chemical mechanism of the aspartic proteases [16–18], the two proximal aspartyl residues are in opposite states of protonation and serve as both the general acid and general base components during hydrolysis (Scheme 13.4). The protonated aspartyl group effects protonation of, or hydrogen bonding to, the carbonyl oxygen of the scissile amide bond, while the unprotonated aspartyl residue deprotonates the lytic water molecule which subsequently attacks the scissile carbonyl as a hydroxide ion to form a tetrahedral adduct. The aspartyl residues are each now in states of protonation opposite to their initial status, and are thus able to reverse their roles. One aspartyl group deprotonates a hydroxyl group on the tetrahedral carbon while the other protonates the departing amine. This transfer of protons results in the formation of the carboxylic acid and unprotonated amine products, and serves to reestablish the initial protonation states of the catalytic aspartic residues.

PEPTIDE ANALOG INHIBITORS OF ACE

ACTIVE-SITE MODEL OF ACE

Since angiotensin-converting enzyme (ACE) plays a vital role in the RAS by hydrolyzing angiotensin 1 to angiotensin 2, it has received substantial interest as a therapeutic target. A major factor in the development of effective peptide analog inhibitors of ACE has been the construction of an active site model that incorporates information of apparent preference for the binding of a specific peptide sequence and knowledge of the catalytic reaction mechanism of this protease (for reviews see References [19,20]).

The sequence specificity of ACE for certain peptides was observed by Bakhle [21] who noted that ACE was inhibited by a mixture of peptides from snake venom. Structure-activity studies showed that only peptides

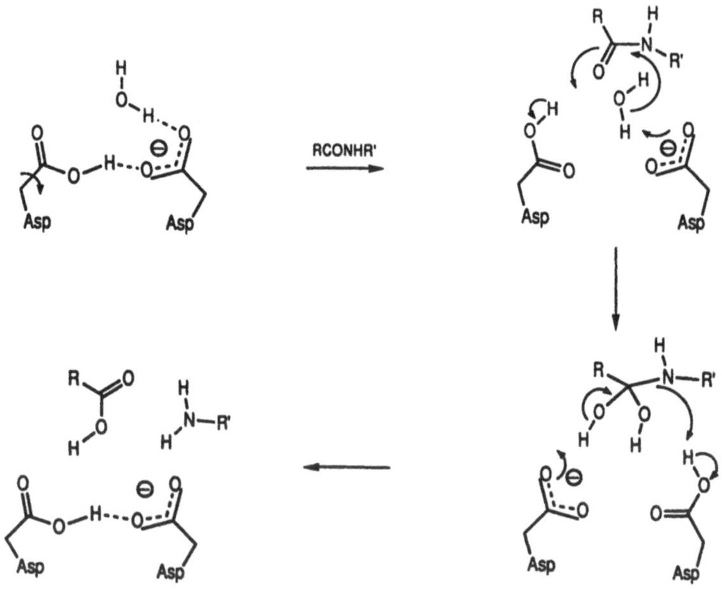

Scheme 13.4 Proposed chemical mechanism for the aspartic proteases.

with free C-terminal carboxyl groups were active. Ondetti [22] and Cushman [23] found that of these snake venom peptides, those containing the C-terminal sequence Ala-Pro were the most active inhibitors of ACE. They also determined that the potency of these naturally-occurring inhibitors was greatest with an aromatic amino acid residue located in the antepenultimate position: Phe-Ala-Pro or Trp-Ala-Pro.

Angiotensin-converting enzymes from various sources range from 140–300 kilodaltons in size and require a zinc ion for catalytic activity. Structural information of two other zinc proteases, carboxypeptidase A and thermolysin, albeit being an exoproteinase and endoproteinase, respectively, were integral in the development of the active site model of ACE. A by-product analog similar to benzylsuccinic acid (1) synthesized by Byers and Wolfenden [24] as an inhibitor for carboxypeptidase A, was proposed by Cushman and Ondetti [26] for ACE. Succinyl-L-proline (2) was designed from structure-activity studies with snake venom peptides and was found to be a moderate but specific competitive ACE inhibitor, $IC_{50} = 330$ μM [26]. This result gave strong validity to the active site model that was being formulated by structure-activity studies and comparative protein structures (Figure 13.1). The development of several potent ACE inhibitors as antihypertensive drugs has made use solely of an increasingly more detailed and sophisticated active site model that has been formed without the benefit of x-ray crystallographic or other structural information. Furthermore, the hundreds of rationally designed ACE peptide inhibitors that have been synthesized can be traced back to the three observations about the active site first reported by the early workers in this field: the requirement of a zinc metal ion, a free C-terminal Pro-CO_2^-, and a preference for an aromatic group at the antepenultimate position.

INCORPORATION OF ZINC LIGANDS

An active site model for ACE hypothesizes a similar function for the zinc ion in the active site similar to that proposed for thermolysin. The incorporation of competent zinc ligands within a peptide analog should cause it to bind more tightly to the protease, and a variety of these compounds are shown in Figure 13.2. The carboxyl group of succinyl-L-proline, for instance, was replaced by mercapto-groups to take advantage of the stronger coordination of sulfur over oxygen to zinc [26]. These mercaptoalkanoyl amino acids had an even greater inhibitory effect than succinyl-L-proline and led to the synthesis of the drug captopril (3) ($IC_{50} = 23$ nM) which is widely used in the treatment of high blood pressure. Derivatives of the free thiols also have produced a series of potent inhibitors such as the acylated thiol compound (4) ($IC_{50} = 0.5$ nM) reported by Suh et al. [27].

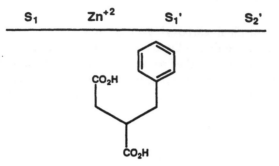

S_1 Zn^{+2} S_1' S_2'

(1) Benzylsuccinic acid

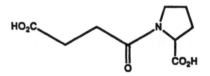

(2) Succinyl-L-proline

Figure 13.1 Active-site model of metalloproteases.

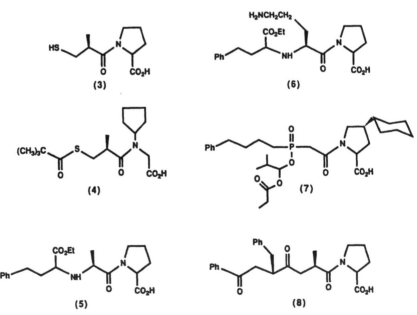

(3)

(6)

(4)

(7)

(5)

(8)

Figure 13.2 Incorporation of zinc ligands into ACE inhibitors.

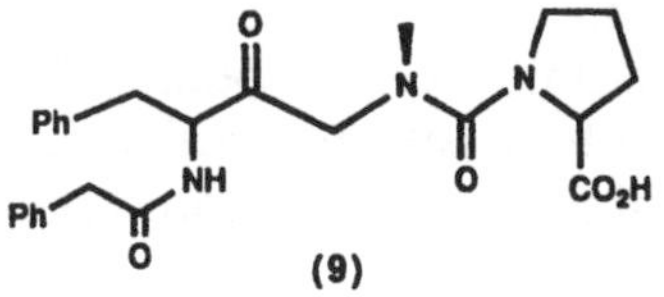

Figure 13.2 (continued) Incorporation of zinc ligands into ACE inhibitors.

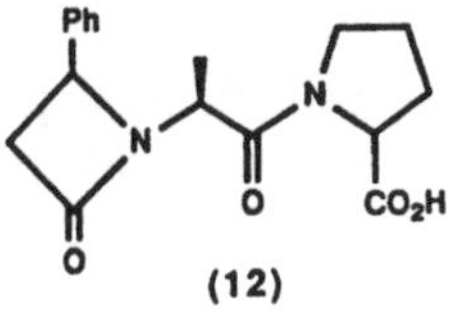

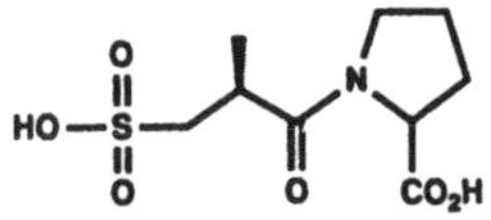

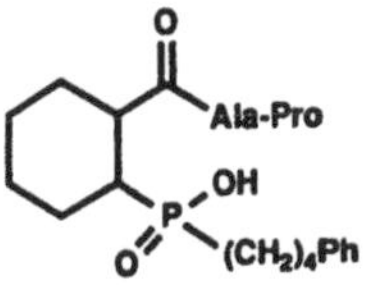

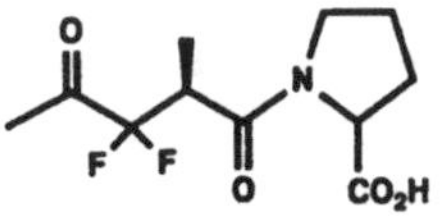

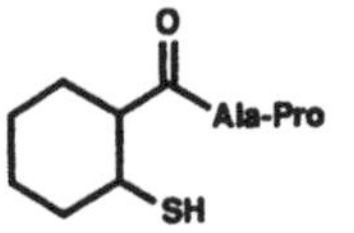

Other groups which may bind strongly to the zinc ion have been substituted for the free thiol in these mercaptoalkanoyl compounds. The incorporation of esters as prodrugs which eventuate in a carboxylate group through nonspecific hydrolysis have been successfully synthesized. Examples of the more potent ACE inhibitors of this class are enalapril (MK421, [28]) (5) (K_i = 0.2 nM, [29,30]), or enalaprilat (MK422) in its de-esterified form, and its lysyl derivative lisinopril (6) (K_i = 1–4.7 nM, [31]) which has an N-terminal, phenylethyl group for binding to the S_1 subsite.

Several functional groups have been designed in an attempt to mimic an extended and strained peptide substrate bound to the enzyme or the proposed tetrahedral oxyanion intermediate which would be coordinated to the zinc ion during substrate hydrolysis. Pauling [32] and Wolfenden [33] suggested that such transition-state mimics should have higher affinity for the enzyme. Compounds that incorporate such functional groups have been shown to be potent inhibitors of enzymes, including ACE. A large series of hydroxyphosphinyl and phosphonamidate compounds have been reported that demonstrate IC_{50} values against ACE in the nanomolar range. One of these, fosinopril (7) which also is a prodrug, has a phosphinate group as a zinc ligand with tetrahedral geometry and a cyclohexyl group appended to the prolyl moiety [34]. Several other functional groups which are transition-state analogs have been incorporated into the Ala-Pro general inhibitor structure including: ketomethylene (8) [35], ketomethylurea (9) (IC_{50} = 2 nM, [36]), sulfonoalkanoyl (10) (IC_{50} =

1.2 mM, [35]), fluoroketo (11) [37], and β-lactam groups (12) [38]. Also a series of cyclic (hydroxyphosphinyl or thiol)acyl dipeptides (13,14) (with IC_{50} = 7 nM and 3 nM, respectively) have been reported which place a constrained ring in the S_1 binding sight in order to incorporate a strong zinc ligand and a strained amide bond [39].

The S$_2'$ BINDING SITE

A major emphasis in designing ACE inhibitors has been to modify the free C-terminal proline group in the general inhibitor structure (Figure 13.3). Chemical modification of the proline ring and the introduction of larger, bulkier rings in the S$_2'$ position have produced several very potent inhibitors of ACE. Ksander et al. [40] and more recently Sawayama et al. [41] have synthesized several compounds with bicyclic and large heterocyclic groups at the C-terminus. Two very effective antihypertensive drugs contain this proline ring derivative: ramipril (15) (IC_{50} = 7.4 nM, [42]), and an enalapril analog, perindopril (S9490) (16) [43,44]. Substitution at position 4 on the proline ring with lipophilic groups was found to increase both the potency and duration of the ACE inhibitory effect. Spirapril (17) (IC_{50} = 0.8 nM, [45,46]), fosinopril (7) [47], and analogs of captopril and enalapril with a cis-4-thiophenyl group [34] are examples of these 4-substituted proline compounds.

Substitution of the proline ring by an oxoimidazolidine was described by Hayashi et al. [48] and was nearly as potent as enalapril in pharmacological activity. Six-membered ring analogs of enalapril with substitutions at

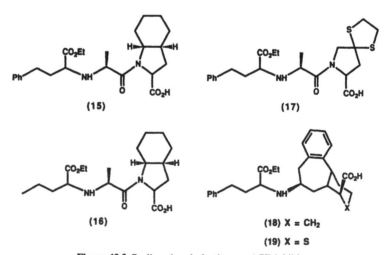

Figure 13.3 Proline ring derivatives as ACE inhibitors.

the 5 and 6 positions have also been synthesized by Yanagisawa et al. [49,50]. Within this class of proline ring substitutions are two of the most potent ACE inhibitors yet reported. These are tricyclic mimics of the tri-peptide Phe-His-Leu-CO_2^-, MDL 27,088 (18) and MDL 27,788 (19) with inhibition constants of approximately 4 pM and 46 pM, respectively [51,52].

THE S_1 BINDING SITE

The majority of ACE inhibitors that have been synthesized to date have incorporated an N-terminal aromatic group such as that found in enalapril (5). This was done in order to take advantage of the strong affinity of ACE for Phe and Trp at the antepenultimate (P_1) position that was recognized during the characterization of snake venom ACE inhibitors. Further structure-activity studies have revealed other functional groups that bind as well to the S_1 subsite. Sawayama et al. [41], for example, have determined that various amino acid substitutions, following in the order: basic > neutral > acidic > D-amino acids, bind well in the S_1 subsite. They reported that an enalapril derivative with Cbz-lysine at the N-terminus was a potent inhibitor of ACE.

PHARMACOLOGICAL PROPERTIES OF ACE PEPTIDE ANALOG INHIBITORS

ACE peptide analog inhibitors form a specific class of compounds that have two primary effects upon the RAS: blockade of the production of an-giotensin 2 and inhibition of the breakdown of bradykinin. These factors, combined with other secondary effects of ACE inhibitors, make them useful therapeutically for the treatment of several RAS-related disorders such as hypertension and congestive heart failure (for reviews see References [3,4,53,54].

Clinical data for ACE inhibitors such as captopril and enalapril when used in either monotherapy or in conjunction with diuretics demonstrate significant control of high blood pressure in 50–80% of patients with hypertension [5]. Captopril when taken orally in 25 mg recommended dosages two to three times daily reduces high blood pressure in as little as 15 minutes with a maximal effect in two hours. It has a half-life in plasma of about two hours and has shown no toxicological effects in rats at ≤ 4 g/kg [5]. Enalapril exhibits nearly identical pharmacokinetics as captopril but has a two-hour delayed time of action since it must first be de-esterified in the liver [5,55]. A number of other ACE inhibitors have demonstrated antihypertensive responses in humans, although clinical data for most of these is lacking compared to the extensive data available for captopril and enalapril. Examples of these compounds are ramipril [56], spirapril [57], cilazapril [58], and perindopril [43,59].

ACE peptide inhibitors, as hypertension drugs exhibit both primary and secondary pharmacological class effects. These effects include: increase in blood flow [5], relaxation of vascular smooth muscles [2], suppression of aldosterone levels, elevated plasma K^+ concentration [5], and elevated plasma levels of angiotensin 1, bradykinin, and prostaglandin [5,60]. As cardiovascular agents, ACE peptide analog inhibitors also exhibit hemo-dynamic effects such as reduced left ventricle hypertrophy and wall stress, reduced infarct size, induced coronary vasodilation, and an increased an-ginal threshold [2,5,61]. It has been suggested that sulfhydryl containing ACE inhibitors such as captopril have the added advantage of being oxygen scavengers and may therefore have therapeutic value in reducing cytotoxic injury in myocardial ischaema and reperfusion [62]. Recent reports have demonstrated further therapeutic value for ACE inhibitors including an anti-atherosclerotic effect by captopril in the Watanabe heritable hyper-lipididemic rabbit [63], and a reduction in proteinuria in diabetic patients [64,65].

Some side effects of ACE peptide analog inhibitors have been observed which may be attributed to their primary action on the RAS. In particular, hypotension and hyperkalemia [5] have been reported, especially in el-derly patients and those with reduced plasma renin levels. Often these complications can be treated by varying salt intake and by the use of di-uretics. Cases of persistent dry coughs and skin rashes have also accom-panied the use of captopril and enalapril [5,66]. Overall, however, ACE in-hibitors are broadly effective therapeutic agents for the treatment of RAS-related disorders and represent clear examples of the potential of modified peptides as drugs.

RENIN PEPTIDE ANALOG INHIBITORS

RENIN

Although there are multiple peptide sequences that are hydrolyzed by ACE, angiotensinogen is the only naturally-occurring substrate for renin where cleavage occurs between Leu*Leu in dog, porcine, and rat angioten-sinogen or between Leu*Val in human angiotensinogen [67,68] (and see Table 13.1). The strict substrate specificity of renin makes it an attractive candidate as a therapeutic target since it should be possible to design pep-tide analog inhibitors that would be specific toward only renin and not other human proteases. As yet there are no approved antihypertensive drugs available which target renin alone, but a number of potent inhibitors

TABLE 13.1. N-Terminal Sequence Homology of Angiotensinogens from Various Sources [68].

Source											P₁	P₁	
Dog	H-Asp	Arg	Val	Tyr	Ile	His	Pro	Phe	His	Leu	*	Leu	Val	Tyr-
Porcine	H-Asp	Arg	Val	Tyr	Ile	His	Pro	Phe	His	Leu	*	Leu	Val	Tyr-
Rat	H-Asp	Arg	Val	Tyr	Ile	His	Pro	Phe	His	Leu	*	Leu	Tyr	Tyr-
Human	H-Asp	Arg	Val	Tyr	Ile	His	Pro	Phe	His	Leu	*	Val	Ile	His-

*Indicates site of cleavage.

of this enzyme have been found (for reviews see References [69–73]. These inhibitors have been designed by using two approaches that include varying the peptide sequence or replacing the scissile bond with a transition-state or bisubstrate analog.

Whereas ACE is a zinc-containing protease, renin is an aspartic protease much like two other human proteases, pepsin and cathepsin D. There is considerable sequence and structural homology between these acid proteases which has led to a parallel development of active-site directed inhibitors based on interactions with the two aspartic acid groups within the active site. Crystallographic data of enzyme-inhibitor complexes of several fungal aspartic proteases are available from which interactions between renin and the peptide inhibitors have been modeled [71,74,75]. These models indicate that renin has a pseudosymmetrical active site composed of two carboxyl groups from the two conserved Asp-Thr-Gly sequences. Another structural feature of these proteolytic enzymes is a large flexible loop called the "flap." X-ray crystallographic studies of enzyme-inhibitor complexes indicate that the flap plays an important role in binding by forming a "lid" over the inhibitor (and by analogy substrates too) after it binds within the active site groove. Such structural information has been very useful in the rational design of human plasma renin inhibitors which have high affinity for binding and may interact with the active site carboxyl residues. Recent crystallographic data of recombinant human renin has confirmed the validity of these models [76].

STATINE-CONTAINING RENIN INHIBITORS

One of the most potent inhibitors of pepsin and other aspartic proteases is the naturally-occurring pentapeptide analog, pepstatin A (N-isovaleryl-Val-Val-Sta-Ala-Sta; Sta, statine (20) = 4S-amino-3S-hydroxy-6-methyl-heptanoic acid, Figure 13.4), a microbial metabolite [77,78]. Structural studies have shown that the hydroxyl group of the first statine residue binds between the two aspartic acid groups in the active site of aspartic pro-

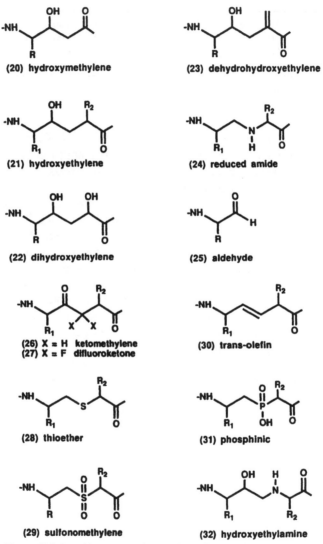

Figure 13.4 Transition-state analogs and scissile dipeptide replacements.

(20) hydroxymethylene

(23) dehydrohydroxyethylene

(21) hydroxyethylene

(24) reduced amide

(22) dihydroxyethylene

(25) aldehyde

(26) X = H ketomethylene
(27) X = F difluoroketone

(30) trans-olefin

(28) thioether

(31) phosphinic

(29) sulfonomethylene

(32) hydroxyethylamine

teases, replacing a water molecule found in the native form of the enzymes [71,74,79]. One explanation that has been proposed for pepstatin's tight binding is that it acts as a bisubstrate analog because the inhibitory functionality of the unusual amino acid statine resembles both the peptidyl portion of the substrate we well as the essential water molecule that is proposed to be integral in the hydrolytic mechanism [80]. A second explanation for the strong binding of pepstatin may also be attributed to the tetrahedral geometry of the statine group which may act as a mimic of the transition-state formed during substrate hydrolysis (see Scheme 13.4). ^{13}C NMR evidence for the binding of transition-state analogs has been reported for pepsin where binding of a potent ketomethylene-containing inhibitor (a statone) was accompanied by enzyme-catalyzed hydration of the carbonyl group [81]. The potency of pepstatin A towards renin (human kidney renin, $K_i = 13$ nM) [82] was much less than for most other aspartic proteases (e.g., pepsin, $K_1 = 0.05$ nM) [83]. This may be due to the strict peptide sequence requirements of human plasma renin.

The synthetic incorporation of statine into peptide sequences that more closely resemble angiotensinogen have been useful in producing more potent inhibitors than the natural product pepstatin A. Statine incorporation into the minimum required substrate sequence produced the potent heptapeptide renin substrate analog, isovaleryl-His-Pro-Phe-His-Sta-Leu-Phe-NH$_2$ [84] with a K_i of 0.16 nM. Alkylation of statine and shortening of the statine group (norstatine) have produced equipotent inhibitors [85]. Modifications of statine by replacement of the isopropyl group with a cyclohexyl group such as 4S-amino-5-cyclohexyl-3S-hydroxpentanoic acid [86] and a cyclohexylalanyl analog (84) have resulted in exceedingly potent inhibitors with inhibition constants approaching 10^{-11} M. A series of analogs in which the hydroxyl group is replaced by an amino group were equally as active as statine towards inhibition of renin [87].

HYDROXYETHYLENE ISOSTERES

Similar to the statine-containing peptides are the hydroxyethylene-containing dipeptide analog inhibitors which also utilize a secondary alcohol for binding within the active site of aspartic proteases. The hydroxyethylene group (21) has an additional carbon link compared to statine which is more closely isosteric with the scissile dipeptide of peptide substrates (Figure 13.4). Incorporation of dihydroxyethylene functional groups (22) as a peptide analog into inhibitors of renin were inhibitory at 200 pM [88]. These diol-containing derivatives were designed to interact directly with the carboxyl groups within the active site as well as to displace an additional water molecule at the activie site [89]. Dehydrohydroxyethylene isosteres (23) were synthesized by Kempf [90] with the thought of irreversibly inactivating the enzyme by covalently modifying an active site nucleophilic residue through Michael addition to the α,β-unsaturated ketone. Although these compounds exhibited IC_{50} values of 0.8–2 nM there was no evidence of irreversible binding after longer pre-incubation times [90].

Other functional groups such as a reduced-amide (24) or aldehyde (25) have been incorporated into effective peptide analog inhibitors of aspartic proteases. The reduced-amide peptide inhibitors should bind effectively to the enzyme since they retain the same peptide spacing as their correspond-ing substrates. These compounds were predicted to bind tightly to the en-zyme by virtue of the tetrahedral methylene group replacing the scissile carbonyl or as a bisubstrate analog. This proposal was supported by struc-tural data from complexes of protease and reduced amide inhibitor [74,79] which implicate an ionic interaction between the protonated amine of the inhibitor and the anionic active site carboxylate. Aldehydic peptides are less potent inhibitors of renin although they represent the smallest peptide analog inhibitors reported for renin (Ito et al. [79a]). Fehrentz et al. [91,92] have synthesized tripeptidic aldehydes, Boc(Cbz)-Phe(Trp)-Val(Leu)-leucinal which exhibit IC_{50} values comparable to pepstatin. Replacement of the peptide bond by other groups such as ketomethylene (26) [93], α-fluorinated ketones (27), thioether (28) [94], sulfonomethylene (29) [94], trans-olefin (30) [94], phosphinic (31) [95], and hydroxymethylenes [96–98] have also produced peptide inhibitors of renin with varying effec-tiveness. In addition, Natarajan et al. [99] have synthesized a potent renin inhibitor with an hydroxyethylamine functionality (32) and a benzyl group at the P_1, that has an $IC_{50} = 17$ nM.

ENHANCEMENT OF PEPTIDE ANALOG INHIBITOR STABILITY

Another major approach to renin inhibitor design has been to synthesize derivatives with prolonged metabolic stability. Enhancement of the stabil-ity of peptide analog inhibitors was achieved by replacing peptide bonds with functional groups that are less susceptible to hydrolysis by endog-enous proteases (e.g., chymotrypsin). Sham et al. [100] reported a series of 10-, 12-, and 14-membered ring peptide analogs that demonstrated IC_{50} values (3–70 μM) similar or slightly better to their parent compounds with human renin yet were more metabolically stable. More recently, this research group [101] synthesized compounds containing cyclic tripeptides with 14- to 16-membered rings which were not significantly degraded by chymotrypsin ($t_{1/2} > 24$ hours). Substitution of γ-lactam groups into pep-tides, however, yielded less potent renin inhibitors than their statine counterparts [102]. The incorporation of α-C-methyl and α-N-methyl backbone as a peptide analog by Thaisrivongs and co-workers [103] produced potent inhibitors of human plasma renin. Kinetic studies have indicated that compounds such as Boc-Pro-Phe-Nα-MeHis-LeuΨ [CH(OH)CH$_2$]Val-Ile-aminomethylpyridine (IC$_{50}$ = 0.26 nM) were competitive inhibitors of renin and followed a time-dependent, minimal two-step mechanism of inhibition that was attributed to a rate-limiting conformational change upon binding or by the displacement of an active site water molecule [104]. These compounds were resistant to renal degradation and demonstrated significantly longer hypotensive responses in animals. By a consideration of structure-activity studies for chymotrypsin and renin, several dipeptide analogs with phenylalanine derivatives were synthesized by Plattner et al. [105]. These compounds showed retention of renin inhibitory activity (0.7–3 nM) but were less susceptible to proteolysis by other nonspecific proteases. The replacement of peptide bonds by an hydroxyethylene group at the P$_2$/P$_3$ position [106], and a retro-inverso amide bond at the P$_3$ [85] have also produced potent inhibitors with enhanced duration of renin inhibitory activity.

PHARMACOLOGICAL PROPERTIES OF RENIN PEPTIDE ANALOG INHIBITORS

The stringent specificity of human renin compared to other aspartic proteases suggests that peptide analog inhibitors targeting this enzyme should have the advantage of being selective towards the RAS. Since ACE peptide analog inhibitors have been successfully used as antihypertensives, peptide analog inhibitors of renin should also be effective agents in the control of the RAS. Indeed, the ability of renin peptide inhibitors to reduce high blood pressure has been demonstrated in many animal models. Blood pressure and plasma renin activities were significantly reduced by the infusion of two hydroxyethylene dipeptide analogs of human renin substrates [107] into hypertensive rats [108]. Likewise, plasma renin activity and blood pressure levels were reduced in furosemide-treated cynomolgus monkeys by Boc-Pro-Phe-Nα-MeHis-LeuΨ[CH(OH)CH$_2$]Val-Ile-amino-methyl-pyridine with a 5 mg/kg dose [103]. Schaffer et al. [109] compared the responses of conscious African green and rhesus monkeys to five renin inhibitors and enalapril, an ACE inhibitor. These (3S-4S)-4-amino-5-cyclohexyl-3-hydroxypentanoic acid-containing peptides each produced significant lowering of blood pressure below the maximal value produced by enalaprilat, yet with an increase in heart rate. Sodium-depleted dogs were infused with a renin inhibitor (1.1 mg/kg per min) [110], that caused a 7-day suppression in arterial pressure with undetectable plasma renin activity. Wood et al. [111] have reported strong inhibition of renin from several subprimate and primate sources. One compound, CGP 44 099 A, lowered the blood pressure of sodium-depleted normotensive rats by 25 mm Hg.

A few studies have also found lowering of blood pressure and plasma renin activity in humans after infusion of renin peptide analog inhibitors [25,112,113]. For example, six sodium-depleted patients were injected with the Abbott renin inhibitor A-64662 which produced suppression of plasma renin activity for 24 hours and lowered angiotensin 2 and aldosterone levels [113]. Although these studies provide preliminary evidence for the efficacy of renin peptide inhibitors in controlling high blood pressure, compounds of this type exhibit poor pharmacokinetic properties. While some human clinical studies have been reported, inhibitors that have been developed for renin have been given intravenously rather than orally. Prolonged oral activity remains a goal for continued research in renin inhibition.

HIV-1 PROTEASE PEPTIDE ANALOG INHIBITORS

CHARACTERIZATION OF HIV-1 PROTEASE

Both synthetically produced [114–116] and recombinant forms of HIV-1 PR, expressed in *E. coli* [117–121] and yeast [122–124] have been reported. Debouck et al. [118] found that the protease was autocatalytically released from a bacterial expression system. Since the 99-amino acid sequence of HIV-1 PR contains the characteristic Asp-Thr-Gly triad of human and fungal aspartic proteases, it was thought that this retroviral protease might be an aspartic protease. Pearl and Taylor [125] proposed a symmetrical dimeric structure for the enzyme by molecular modeling. Recently, x-ray crystallographic data [126–128] confirmed that the tertiary structure of the protease was indeed dimeric with an active site situated at the interface between the subunits. Several conserved regions between the tertiary structure of HIV-1 PR and aspartic proteases such as pepsin and renin were recognized including the active site triad, Asp-Thr-Gly, and the two glycine-rich peptide loops which comprise the "substrate binding flaps." Crystallographic data of enzyme-inhibitor complexes also has become available recently, providing detailed structural information for the interactions between the protease and peptide analog inhibitors [129,130].

Whereas renin exhibits strict substrate specificity, there are eight different cleavage sites for HIV-1 PR within the Pr160$^{gag/pol}$ polyprotein (Table 13.2). There is limited homology between these cleavage sites, although an hydrophobic residue such as Leu, Phe, or Tyr seems to be preferred at the P_1 position. Synthetic peptides which mimic or comprise each of these sites have been shown to be substrates for the recombinant protease with K_m values between 0.1 and 10 nM [131]. The pH dependence of k_{cat}/K_m for HIV-1 PR with Ac-Arg-Ala-Ser-Gln-Asn-Tyr*Pro-Val-Val-

TABLE 13.2. Cleavage Sites for HIV-1 PR within HIV-1 gag-pol.[a]

Clevage Site	Sequence
MA/CA (p17/p24)	SQNY*PIVQ
CA/X (p24/X)	ARVL*AEAM
X/NC (X/p7)	ATIM*MQRC
NC/p6 (p7/p6)	PGNF*LQSR
TF/PR (p6/p12)	SFNF*PQIT
PR/RT (p12/p66)	TLNF*PISP
RT/ (p66/p51)	AETF*YVDE
RT/IN (p66/p32)	RKIL*FLDG

[a]CA is capsid protein, IN is integration protein, MA is matrix protein, NC is nucleocapsid protein, PR is viral protease, RT is reverse transcriptase (with RNase-H activity), TF is transframe protein, X is undefined protein, and * indicates site of cleavage [141,142].

NH$_2$ [132] gave a "bell-shaped" profile with pK_a = 3.3 and pK_b = 6.1. These pK values are in accord with the presence of two catalytically active carboxylic groups (protonated and unprotonated). The pH optimum resembles that of renin rather than the low pH values reported for the peptic and gastric acid proteases.

Inhibition studies with aspartic protease inhibitors such as pepstatin A and affinity labeling agents including the epoxide, 1,2-epoxy-3,4-nitrophenoxypropane (EPNP) and the diazomethyl ketone, N-diazo-acetyl norleucine methyl ester (DAN), further confirmed that HIV-1 PR contains an aspartic residue with catalytic activity. Pepstatin A was found to be a moderately active inhibitor (K_i = 1.4 μM). Time-dependent inactivation of the HIV-1 protease was observed with EPNP and DAN [133].

MECHANISM-BASED INHIBITORS OF HIV-1 PR

The development of peptide analog inhibitors for HIV-1 PR has proceeded in a manner similar to that for other aspartic proteases such as pepsin and renin. The identification and synthesis of these inhibitors have combined both rational design and an empirical approach to the selection of potent inhibitors of HIV-1 protease. The fact that cleavage of the Pr55^{gag} and gag/pol polyproteins occurs exclusively at eight sites (see Table 13.2) implies that specificity for the cleavage function of the enzyme must be attributable to either the primary or tertiary structures of these protein substrates. Moreover, the lack of sequence homology at each cleavage site indicates that specificity does not result from recognition of primary sequence alone. Nonetheless, three of these cleavage sites (Ser/Thr-Xaa-Yaa-Phe/Tyr*Pro) including the p17/p24 cleavage site appear to be unique to the retroviruses. Several laboratories have incorporated

TABLE 13.3. Peptide Analog Inhibitors of HIV-1 PR [134].

Inhibitor	K_i
1. Ser-Ala-Ala-PheΨ[CH$_2$N]Pro-Val-Val-NH$_2$	19 μM
2. Ser-Ala-Ala-PheΨ[PO$_2$]Gly-Val-Val-OMe	4 μM
3. Ser-Ala-Ala-PheΨ[CHOH]Val-Val-OMe	810 nM
4. Boc-Ser-Ala-Ala-PheΨ[CF$_2$CO]Val-Val-OMe	160 nM
5. Ser-Ala-Ala-PheΨ[CH(OH)CH$_2$]Gly-Val-Val-OMe	62 nM

transition-state analog motifs into the scissile dipeptide bond of peptide substrates of HIV-1 PR. Dreyer et al. [134] synthesized a series of peptide analog inhibitors (Table 13.3) having flanking sequences similar to the Tyr*Pro cleavage site between the p17 and p24 gag protein. These peptide analogs were found to be competitive inhibitors of recombinant HIV-1 PR with inhibition constants in the nanomolar to micromolar range. Their inhibitory potency followed the order (from least to greatest): reduced amide < phosphinic acid < statine isostere < difluoroketone < hydroxyethylene isostere. Rich and co-workers [135] also synthesized hydroxyethylamine derivatives based on the Tyr*Pro HIV-1 PR cleavage site. The compound Ac-Ser-Leu-Asn-PheΨ[CH(OH)CH$_2$N]Pro-Ile-Val-OMe had a dissociation constant of 0.66 nM. Structure-activity studies indicated that peptides spanning the P$_4$-P$_3'$ exhibited maximal inhibition. Analogs containing ketomethyleneamine, statine, or (3S,4S)-4-amino-3-hydroxy-5-phenylpentanoic acid groups were less active. The cleavage site between the p24 and p7 gag proteins (Met*Met) HIV-1 PR sequence was used by Miller et al. [129] for the preparation of MVT-101, a reduced amide analog, Ac-Thr-Ile-NleΨ [CH$_2$NH]Nle-Gln-Arg-amide, where Nle is the unusual amino acid norleucine. The crystal structure of a complex formed between synthetic HIV-1 PR and MVT-101 was determined to 2.3 Å resolution. The crystal structure of a symmetric inhibitor, A-74704, complexed to recombinant HIV-1 protease was also reported recently [136]. This symmetric compound, Cbz-Val-NH[S-CH(CH$_2$Ph)CH(OH)-R-CH(CH$_2$Ph)] NH-Val-Cbz, has a two-fold C$_2$ symmetry and incorporates the secondary hydroxyl-group functionality of the statine analogs into a Phe*Phe pepsin-like cleavage site. These structures further define the interactions between protease and inhibitor and should allow the design of even more potent compounds.

INHIBITION OF HIV-1 PR BY PEPTIDE ANALOG INHIBITORS IN INFECTED CELLS

At least two constraints must be imposed before the potential of this class of protease inhibitor can be realized. Unlike ACE or renin inhibitors, the target of action is intracellular, requiring that the inhibitor access the target protease within the cell and remain long enough to effect potent inhibition. Meek et al. [137] became the first group to demonstrate the inhibition of HIV-1 polyprotein processing in infected cultures by specific peptide analog inhibitors of HIV-1 protease. A key feature of HIV-1 infection that facilitated the rapid analysis of polyprotein processing in infected cells involved the measuring of processed viral proteins accumulating in chronically infected T-lymphocytes. Pulse-chase or western blot analysis was employed to measure polyprotein turnover in the chronically infected cells in order to discriminate among inhibitors capable of entering cells, accessing the target protease and sustaining inhibitory concentrations long enough to exert a potent effect over time. Four compounds (33–36) were tested in a cell-free enzyme assay and all four were found to be potent inhibitors of the enzyme (Table 13.4). However, only three were active in the pulse-chase assay, indicating that compound (36) was unable to access the protease. When these active compounds were tested in the western blot assay only two compounds (33) and (35) were able to effect a potent inhibition over time. Using this strategy the identity of specific chemical features of the peptide inhibitors that confer the properties necessary to effect a potent antiviral response should be possible. In addition to the analysis in chronically infected cells, the ability of these inhibitors to block acute or *de novo* infection and spreading of the virus in native cultures of T-lymphocytes was tested. Infection of cells in culture was blocked by either (33) or (35). Compound (35) was the most potent inhibitor of this series as determined by the lack of particle-associated reverse transcriptase activity after seven days.

Subsequent reports in the literature have confirmed the observation that synthetic peptide analog inhibitors of HIV-1 PR are capable of blocking viral protein processing in infected cells. McQuade et al. [138] demonstrated that hydroxyethylene isostere-containing inhibitors including U-81749, tert-butylacetyl-cyclohexyl-alanineΨ[CH(OH)CH$_2$]Val-Ile-aminomethylpyridine (K_i = 70 nM), blocked processing of recombinant Pr55^{gag} in a *vaccina* pseudovirion system. Roberts et al. [139] have reported that hydroxyethylamine-containing compounds based on the Tyr* Pro cleavage site which have modifications of the proline ring were sub-

TABLE 13.4. Peptide Analog Inhibitors Tested in T-Lymphocytes [137].

Inhibitor	K_i
(33) Cbz-Ala-PheΨ[CH(OH)CH$_2$]Gly-Val-Val-OCH$_3$	120 nM
(34) Ala-Ala-PheΨ[CH(OH)CH$_2$]Gly-Val-Val-OCH$_3$	18 nM
(35) Cbz-Ala-Ala-PheΨ[CH(OH)CH$_2$]Gly-Val-Val-OCH$_3$	48 nM
(36) Boc-Ser-Ala-Ala-TyrΨ[CH(OH)CH$_2$]Gly-Val-Val-OCH$_3$	180 nM

nanomolar inhibitors of HIV-1 PR. In particular, one compound which is a bicyclic prolyl derivative exhibited potent inhibition of HIV-1 protease in infected cells. The anti-HIV properties of a number of novel C_2 symmetric inhibitors of HIV-1 PR were characterized *in vitro* by Erickson and co-workers [136].

It is now clear that synthetic peptide analog inhibitors of HIV-1 PR are capable of effecting a potent inhibition of viral polyprotein processing in chronically infected T-lymphocytes. Recent results from Lambert [140] demonstrate that blockade of processing translates into a loss of infectivity by virions produced from these cells. This taken together with the ability of the peptide analogs to block acute infection provide strong evidence for the antiviral potential of this class of protease inhibitors.

Whereas, the results obtained to date are encouraging for the antiviral potential of these compounds, the pharmacology and toxicology of these compounds remains to be investigated. It will be some time before proof that this strategy leads to successful drugs like the ACE inhibitors or whether adverse pharmacological effects impede their application for treatment of HIV infection in man.

REFERENCES

1 Campbell, D. J. 1987. *J. Cardiovasc. Pharmacol. 10 (Supp. 7)*. New York: Raven Press, Ltd., pp. S1–S8.

2 Vanhoutte, P. M., W. Auch-Schwelk, M. L. Biondi, R. R. Lorenz, V. B. Schini and M. J. Vidal. 1989. *Br. J. Clin. Pharmac.*, 28:95S–104S.

3 Johnston, C. I. 1990. In *Drugs 39 (Suppl. 1)*. USA: ADIS Press Limited, pp. 21–35.

4 Burnier, M., B. Waeber, J. Nussberger and H. R. Brunner. 1990. In *Drugs 39 (Suppl. 1)*, USA: ADIS Press Limited, pp. 132–138.

5 Gavras, I. and H. Gavras. 1990. In *Adv. Inter. Med. 35*. USA: Year Book Medical Publishers, Inc., pp. 249–267.

5a Gallo, R. C. and L. Montagnier. 1988. *Scient. Am.*, 259:41–48.

6 Gottlieb, M. S., J. D. Schroff, P. T. Weisman, R. A. Wolf and A. Saxon. 1981. *New Engl. J. Med.*, 305:1424–1431.

7 Montagnier, L., J. C. Chermann, F. Barre-Sinoussi, S. Chamaret, J. Gruestk, M. T. Nugeyre, F. Rey, C. Dauguet, C. Axler-Blin, F. Vezinet-Brun, C. Rouzioux, A. G. Saimot, W. Rozenbaum, J. C. Gluckman, D. Klatzman, E. Vilmer, C. Griscelli, C. Foyer-Gazengel and J. B. Brunet. 1984. In *Human T-Cell Leukemia/Lymphoma Virus*, R. C. Gallo et al., eds., Cold Spring Harbor, New York: Cold Spring Harbor Lab., pp. 363–379.

8 Popovic, M., E. Read-Connole and R. C. Gallo. 1984. *Lancet ii*, pp. 1472–1473.

9 Mitsuya, H., K. J. Weinhold, P. A. Furman, M. H. St. Clair, S. N. Lehrman, R. C. Gallo, K. J. Bolognesi, D. W. Barry and S. Broder. 1985. *Proc. Natl. Acad. Sci. USA*, 82:7096–7100.

10 Rosenberg, S., P. J. Barr, R. C. Najarian and R. A. Hallewell. 1984. *Nature (London)*, 312:77–80.

11 Frasca, J. M., O. Auerbach, H. W. Carter and V. R. Parks. 1983. *Am. J. Pathol.*, 111:11.

12 Weaver, L. H., W. R. Kester and B. W. Matthews. 1977. *J. Mol. Biol.*, 114:119–132.

13 Hangauer, D. G., A. F. Monzingo and B. W. Matthews. 1984. *Biochemistry*, 23:5730.

14 Tang, J., M. N. G. James, I.-N. Hsu, J. A. Jenkins and T. L. Blundell. 1978. *Nature (London)*, 271:618–621.

15 Pearl, L. H. and T. L. Blundell. 1984. *FEBS Lett.*, 174:96–101.

16 James, M. N. G., I.-N. Hsu and T. J. Delbaere. 1977. *Nature*, 267:808–813.

17 James, M. N. G. and A. R. Sielecki. 1985. *Biochemistry*, 24:3701–3713.

18 Suguna, K., E. A. Padlan, C. W. Smith, W. D. Carlson and D. R. Davies. 1987. *Proc. Natl. Acad. Sci. USA*, 84:7009–7013.

19 Ondetti, M. A., D. W. Cushman, E. F. Sabo, S. Natarajan, J. Pluscec and B. Rubin. 1981. In *Molecular Basis of Drug Design*, Singer and Ondarza, eds., USA: Elsevier North Holland, Inc., pp. 235–246.

20 Bünning, P. 1983. *Clin. and Exper. Hyper-Theory and Practice*, A5(7,8): 1263–1275.

21 Bakhle, Y. S. 1968. *Nature*, 220:919.

22 Ondetti, M. A., N. J. Williams, E. F. Sabo, J. Pluscec, E. R. Weaver and O. Kocy. 1971. *Biochemistry*, 10:4033–4039.

23 Cheung, H. S. and D. W. Cushman. 1973. *Biochim. Biophys. Acta.*, 293:451–463.

24 Byers, L. D. and R. Wolfenden. 1972. *J. Biol. Chem.*, 247:606–6087.

25 Webb, D. J., P. J. O. Manheim, S. G. Ball, G. Inglis, B. J. Leckie, A. F. Lever, J. J. Morton, J. I. S. Robertson, G. D. Murray, J. Menard, A. Hallet, D. M. Jones and M. Szelke. 1985. *Hypertension*, 3:653–658.

26 Cushman, D. W. and M. A. Ondetti. 1980. In *Prog. Med. Chem. 17*, G. P. Ellis and G. B. West, eds., USA: Elsevier North Holland Biomedical Press, pp. 42–93.

27 Suh, J. T., J. W. Sliles, B. E. Williams, R. D. Youssefyeh, H. Jones, B. Loev, A. Schwab, M. S. Mann, A. Khandwala, P. S. Wolf and I. J. Weinryb. 1985. *J. Med. Chem.*, 28:57.

28 Patchett, A. A., E. Harris, E. W. Tristram, M. J. Wyvratt, M. T. Wu, D. Taub, E. R. Peterson, T. J. Ikeler, J. ten Broeke, E. R. Payne, D. L. Ondeyka, E. D. Thorsett, W. J. Greenlee, N. S. Lohr, R. D. Hoffsommer, H. Joshua, W. V. Ruyle, J. W. Rothrock, S. D. Aster, A. L. Maycock, F. M. Robinson, R. Hirschmann, C. S. Sweet, E. H. Ulm, D. M. Gross, T. C. Vassil and C. A. Stone. 1980. *Nature*, 28:280–283.

29 Greenlee, W. J., P. L. Allibone, D. S. Perlow, A. A. Patchett and E. H. Ulm. 1985. *J. Med. Chem.*, 28:434–442.

30 Borek, M., S. Charlap and W. Frishman. 1987. *Pharmacotherapy*, 7:113–148.

31 Armayor, G. M. and L. M. Lopez. 1988. *Drug Intell. Clin. Pharm.*, 22:365–372.

32 Pauling, L. 1948. *Am. Scient.*, 36:51.

33 Wolfenden, R. 1972. *Accts. Chem. Res.*, 5:10.

34 Krapcho, J., C. Turk, D. W. Cushman, J. R. Powell, J. M. Deforrest, E. R. Spitzmiller, D. S. Karanewsky, M. Duggan, G. Rovvak, J. Schwartz, S. Natarajan,

J. D. Godfrey, D. E. Ryono, R. Neubeck, K. S. Atwal and E. W. Petrillo, Jr. 1988. *J. Med. Chem.*, 31:1148–1160.

35 Almquist, R. G., W.-R. Chao, A. K. Judd, C. Mitoma, D. J. Rossi, R. E. Panasevich and R. J. Matthews. 1988. *J. Med. Chem.*, 31:561–567.

36 Natarajan, S., E. M. Gordon, E. F. Sabo, J. D. Godfrey, H. N. Weller, J. Pluscec, M. B. Rom, J. Engebrecht, D. W. Cushman, J. M. Deforrest and J. Powell. 1988. *J. Enzyme Inhibition*, 2:91–97.

37 Gelb, M. H., J. P. Svaren and R. H. Abeles. 1985. *Biochemistry*, 24:1813–1817.

38 Wharton, C. J., R. Wrigglesworth and M. Rowe. 1984. *J. Chem. Soc. Perkin Trans. I*, 1:29–39.

39 Weller, H. N. and M. B. Rom. 1988. *J. Enzyme Inhibition*, 2:183–193.

40 Ksander, G. M., A. M. Yuan, C. G. Diefenbacher and J. L. Stanton. 1985. *J. Med. Chem.*, 28:1606–1611.

41 Sawayama, T., M. Tsukamoto, T. Sasagawa, K. Nishimura, R. Yamamoto, T. Deguchi, K. Takeyama and K. Hosoki. 1989. *Chem. Pharm. Bull.*, 37:2417–2422.

42 Bünning, P., B. Holmquist and J. F. Riordan. 1983. *Biochemistry*, 22:103.

43 Vincent, M., G. Remond, B. Portevin, B. Serkiz and M. Laubie. 1982. *Tetrahedron Lett.*, 23:1677–1680.

44 Macfadyen, R. J., K. R. Lees and J. L. Reid. 1990. In *Drugs 39 (Suppl. 1)*, USA: ADIS Press Limited, pp. 49–63.

45 Smith, E. M., G. F. Swiss, B. R. Neustadt, E. H. Gold, J. A. Sommer, A. D. Brown, P. J. S. Chiu, R. Moran, E. J. Sybertz and T. Baum. 1988. *J. Med. Chem.*, 31:875–885.

46 Smith, E. M., G. F. Swiss, B. R. Neustadt, P. McNamara, E. H. Gold, E. J. Sybertz and T. Baum. 1989. *J. Med. Chem.*, 32:1600–1606.

47 Powell, J. R., J. M. Deforrest, D. W. Cushman, B. Rubin and E. W. Petrillo. 1984. *Fed. Proc. Am. Soc. Exp. Biol.*, 43:733.

48 Hayashi, K., K. Numami, J. Kato, N. Yoneda, M. Kubo, T. Ochiai and R. Ishida. 1989. *J. Med. Chem.*, 32:289–297.

49 Yanagisawa, H., S. Ishihara, A. Ando, T. Kanazaki, S. Miyamoto, H. Koike, Y. Iijima, K. Oizumi, Y. Matsushita and T. Hata. 1987. *J. Med. Chem.*, 30:1984–1991.

50 Yanagisawa, H., S. Ishihara, A. Ando, T. Kanazaki, S. Miyamoto, H. Koike, Y. Iijima, K. Oizumi, Y. Matsushita and T. Hata. 1988. *J. Med. Chem.*, 31:422–428.

51 Flynn, G. A., E. L. Giroux and R. C. Dage. 1987. *J. Am. Chem. Soc.*, 109:7914–7915.

52 Giroux, E., D. W. Beight, R. C. Dage and G. A. Flynn. 1989. *J. Enzyme Inhibition*, 2:269–277.

53 Unger, T., D. Ganten and R. E. Lang. 1983. *Clin. and Exper. Hyper-Theory and Practice*, A5(7,8):1333–1354.

54 Campanacci, L., G. Bellini, A. Cosenzi, G. Franca and A. Pieontesi. 1989. *Drugs Exptln. Clin. Res.*, 15(11,12):591–597.

55 Cushman, D. W., F. L. Wang, W. C. Fung, G. J. Grover, C. M. Harvey, R. J. Scalese, S. L. Mitch and J. M. Deforrest. 1989. *Br. J. Clin. Pharmac.*, 28:115S–131S.

56 Bünning, P. 1987. *J. Cardiovasc. Pharmacol. 10 (Suppl. 7)*, pp. S31–S35.

57 Van der Meiracker, A. H., A. J. Man in't Veld, H. J. Ritsema van Eck and A. D. H. Schalekamp. 1989. *J. Hypertension 7 (Suppl. 6)*, pp. S302–S303.

58 Kohno, M., K. Yasunari, H.-I. Murakawa, K. Yokokawa, T. Horio, N. Kurihara and T. Takeda. 1989. *J. Hypertension 7 (Suppl. 6)*, pp. S298–S299.

59 Littler, W. 1990. In *Drugs 39 (Suppl. 1)*. USA: ADIS Press Limited, pp. 43–48.

60 Pontieri, V., O. U. Lopes and S. H. Ferreira. 1990. *Hypertension*, 15:155–158.

61 Chatterjee, K. and T. De Marco. 1990. In *Drugs 39 (Suppl. 4)*. USA: ADIS Press Limited, pp. 29–40.

62 Przyklenk, K. and R. A. Kloner. 1989. *Br. J. Clin. Pharmac.*, 28:167S–175S.

63 Chobanian, A. V., C. C. Haudenschild, C. Nickerson and R. Drago. 1990. *Hypertension*, 15:327–331.

64 Stornello, M., E. V. Vlavo and L. Scapellato. 1989. *J. Hypertension 7 (Suppl. 6)*, pp. S314–S315.

65 Romanelli, G., A. Giustina, E. Agabiti-Rosei, S. Bossoni, A. Girelli, M. L. Muiesani, G. Muiesan and G. Giustina. 1989. *J. Hypertension 7 (Suppl. 6)*, pp. S312–S313.

66 Strocchi, E., G. Valtancoli and E. Ambrosioni. 1989. *J. Hypertension 7 (Suppl. 6)*, pp. S308–S309.

67 Cumin, F., D. Le-Nguyen, B. Castro, J. Menard and P. Corvol. 1987. *Biochem. Biophys. Acta*, 913:10–19.

68 Evans, D. B., J. C. Cornette, T. K. Sawyer, D. J. Staples, A. E. de Vaux and S. K. Sharma. 1990. *Biotech. Appl. Biochem.*, 12:161–175.

69 Rich, D. H., F. G. Salituro and M. W. Holladay. 1984. In *Conformationally Directed Drug Design, ACS Symposium Series 251*, J. A. Vida and M. G. Gordon, eds., Washington: American Chemical Society, pp. 211–237.

70 Wood, J. M., J. L. Stanton and K. G. Hofbauer. 1987. *J. Enzyme Inhibition*, 1:169–185.

71 Blundell, T. L., J. Cooper, S. I. Foundling, D. M. Jones, B. Atrash and M. Szelke. 1987. *Biochemistry*, 26:5585–5589.

72 Haber, E., K. Y. Hui, W. D. Carlson and M. S. Bernatowitz. 1987. *J. Cardiovasc. Pharmacol. 10 (Suppl. 7)*. New York: Raven Press, Ltd., pp. S55–S58.

73 Greenlee, W. J. 1990. In *Medicinal Research Reviews 10, No. 2*. John Wiley & Sons, Inc., pp. 173–236.

74 Foundling, S. I., J. Cooper, F. E. Watson, A. Cleasby, L. H. Pearl, B. L. Sibanda, A. Hemmings, S. P. Wood, T. L. Blundell, M. J. Valler, C. G. Norey, J. Kay, J. Boger, B. M. Dunn, B. J. Leckie, D. M. Jones, B. Atrash, A. Hallet and M. Szelke. 1987. *Nature*, 327:349–352.

75 Carlson, W. D., M. Handschumacher, N. Summers, M. Karplus and E. Haber. 1987. *J. Cardiovasc. Pharmacol. 10 (Suppl. 7)*. New York: Raven Press, Ltd., pp. S91–S93.

76 Sielecki, A. R., K. Hayakawa, M. Fujinaga, M. E. P. Murphy, M. Fraser, A. K. Muir, C. T. Carilli, J. A. Lewsicki, J. D. Baxter and M. N. N. James. 1989. *Science*, 243:1346–1351.

77 Umezawa, H., T. Aoyagi, H. Sada, M. Hamada and T. Takeuchi. 1976. *J. Antibiot.*, 29:97.

78 Rich, D. H. and E. T. O. Sun. 1980. *Biochem. Pharmacol.*, 29:2205–2212.

79 Foundling, S. I., J. Cooper, F. E. Watson, L. H. Pearl, A. Hemmings, S. P.

Wood, T. Blundell, A. Hallet, D. M. Jones, J. Sueiras, B. Atrash and M. Szelke. 1987. *J. Cardiovasc. Pharmacol. 10 (Suppl. 7).* New York: Raven Press, Ltd., pp. S59–S68.

79a Ito, A., C. Miura, H. Horikoshi, H. Miyagawa and Y. Baba. 1977. In *Peptides Chemistry, Proceedings of 15th Symposium of Peptide Chemistry,* T. Shiba, ed., Ninoh-Shi, Osaka, Japan: Protein Research Foundation, pp. 165–168.

80 Rich, D. H. 1985. *J. Med. Chem.,* 218:263–273.

81 Rich, D. H., M. S. Bernatowitz and P. G. Schmidt. 1982. *J. Am. Chem. Soc.,* 104:3535.

82 McKown, M. M., R. J. Workman and R. I. Gregerman. 1974. *J. Biol. Chem.,* 249:7770–7774.

83 Workman, R. J. and D. W. Burkett. 1979. *Arch. Biochem. Biophys.,* 194:157.

84 Boger, J., L. S. Payne, D. S. Perlow, N. S. Lohr, M. Poe, E. H. Blaine, E. H. Ulm, T. W. Schorn, B. I. LaMont, T.-Y. Lin, M. Kawai, D. H. Rich and D. F. Veber. 1985. *J. Med. Chem.,* 28:1779–1790.

85 Iizuka, K., T. Kamijo, H. Harada, K. Akahane, T. Kubota, I. Shimaoka, H. Umeyama and Y. Kiso. 1988. *Chem. Pharm. Bull.,* 36:2278–2281.

86 Nisato, D., C. Lacour, A. Roccon, R. Gayraud, C. Cazaubon, C. Carlet, C. Plouzane, J.-P. Richaud, B. Tonnerre, J.-P. Gagnol and J. Wagnon. 1987. *J Hypertension 5 (Suppl. 5),* pp. S23.

87 Thaisrivongs, S., H. J. Schostarez, D. T. Pals and S. R. Turner. 1987. *J. Med. Chem.,* 30:1837.

88 Luly, J. R., N. BaMaung, J. Soderquist, K. L. Fung, H. Stein, H. D. Kleinhert, P. A. Marcotte, D. A. Egan, B. Bopp, I. Merits, G. Bolis, J. Greer, T. J. Perun and J. J. Plattner. 1988. *J. Med. Chem.,* 31:2264–2276.

89 Hanson, G. J., J. S. Baran, T. Lindberg, G. M. Walsh, S. E. Papaioannou, M. Babler, S. E. Bittner, P.-C. Yang and M. D. Cobobbo. 1985. *Biochem. Biophys. Res. Comm.,* 132:155–161.

90 Kempf, D. J., E. de Lara, H. H. Stein, J. Cohen and J. J. Plattner. 1987. *J. Med. Chem.,* 30:1978–1983.

91 Fehrentz, J.-A., A. Heitz, B. Castro, C. Cazaubon and D. Nisato. 1984. *FEBS Lett.,* 167:273–276.

92 Fehrentz, J.-A., A. Heitz and B. Castro. 1985. *Int. J. Peptide Protein Res.,* 26:236–241.

93 Holladay, M. W., F. G. Salituro and D. H. Rich. 1987. *J. Med. Chem.,* 30:374–383.

94 Smith, C. W., H. H. Saneii, T. K. Sawyer, D. T. Pals, T. A. Scahill, B. V. Kamdar and J. A. Lawson. 1988. *J. Med. Chem.,* 31:1377–1382.

95 Allen, M. C., W. Fuhrer, B. Tuck, R. Wade and J. M. Wood. 1989. *J. Med. Chem.,* 32:1652–1661.

96 Thaisrivongs, S., D. T. Pals, W. H. Kati, S. R. Turner and L. M. Thomasco. 1985. *J. Med. Chem.,* 28:1555–1558.

97 Thaisrivongs, S., D. T. Pals, W. M. Kati, S. R. Turner, L. M. Thomasco and W. Watt. 1986. *J. Med. Chem.,* 29:2080–2087.

98 Fearon, K., A. Spaltenstein, P. B. Hopkins and M. H. Gelb. 1987. *J. Med. Chem.,* 30:1617–1622.

99 Natarajan, S., C. A. Free, E. F. Sabo, J. Lin, E. R. Spitzmiller, S. G. Samaniego,

S. A. Smith and L. M. Zanoni. 1988. In *Peptides, Chemistry and Biology, Proceedings of the Tenth American Peptide Symposium*, G. R. Marshall, ed., Leiden: ESCOM, p. 131.

100 Sham, H. I., G. Bolis, H. H. Stein, S. W. Fesik, P. A. Marcotte, J. J. Plattner, C. A. Rempel and J. Greer. 1988. *J. Med. Chem.*, 31:284–295.

101 Sham, H. L., C. A. Rempel, H. Stein and J. Cohen. 1990. *J. Chem. Soc. Chem. Commun.*, 9:666–667.

102 Thaisrivongs, S., D. T. Pals, S. R. Turner and L. Kroll. 1988. *J. Med. Chem.*, 31:1369–1376.

103 Thaisrivongs, S., D. T. Pals, D. W. Harris, W. H. Kati and S. R. Turner. 1986. *J. Med. Chem.*, 29:2088–2093.

104 Kati, W. M., D. T. Pals and S. Thaisrivongs. 1987. *Biochemistry*, 26:7621–7626.

105 Plattner, J. J., P. A. Marcotte, H. D. Kleinert, H. H. Stein, J. Greer, G. Bolis, A. K. L. Fung, B. Bopp, J. R. Luly, H. L. Sham, D. J. Kempf, S. H. Rosenberg, J. F. Dellaria, B. De, I. Merits and T. J. Perun. 1988. *J. Med. Chem.*, 31:2277–2288.

106 Kempf, D. J., E. de Lara, H. H. Stein, J. Cohen, D. A. Egan and J. J. Plattner. 1990. *J. Med. Chem.*, 33:371–374.

107 Szelke, M., B. Leckie, A. Hallett, D. M. Jones, J. Sueiras, B. Atrash and A. F. Lever. 1982. *Nature*, 229:555–557.

108 Beattie, E. C., J. J. Morton, B. J. Leckie, J. Sueiras-Diaz, D. M. Jones and M. Szelke. 1989. *J. Hypertension 7 (Suppl. 6)*, pp. S220–S221.

109 Schaffer, L. W., T. W. Schorn, R. J. Winquist, J. F. Strouse, L. Payne, P. K. Chakravarty, S. E. de Laszlo, J. ten Broeke, D. F. Veber, W. L. Greenlee and P. K. S. Siegl. 1990. *J. Hypertension*, 8:251–259.

110 Hall, J. E. and H. L. Mizelle. 1990. *J. Hypertension*, 8:351–359.

111 Wood, J. M., S. C. Mah, H. P. Baum, M. de Gasparo, F. Cumin, H. Rueger and J. Nussberger. 1990. *J. Pharm. Exp. Ther.*, 253:513–517.

112 Haber, E. 1984. *J. Hypertension*, 2:223–230.

113 Bursztyn, M., I. Gavras, C. P. Tifft, J. H. Bauer, J. C. Melby and H. Gavras. 1989. *J. Hypertension 7 (Suppl. 6)*, pp. S306–S307.

114 Schneider, J. and S. Kent. 1988. *Cell*, 54:363–368.

115 Nutt, R. F., S. F. Brady, P. L. Darke, T. M. Ciccarone, C. D. Colton, E. M. Nutt, J. A. Rodkey, C. D. Bennett, L. H. Waxman, I. S. Sigal, P. S. Anderson and D. F. Veber. 1988. *Proc. Natl. Acad. Sci. USA*, 85:7129–7133.

116 Copeland, T. D. and S. Oroszlan. 1988. *Gene Anal. Tech.*, 5:109–115.

117 Farmerie, W. G., D. D. Loeb, N. C. Casavant, C. A. Hutchinson, III and R. Swanstrom. 1987. *Science*, 236:305–308.

118 Debouck, C., J. G. Gorniak, J. E. Strickler, T. D. Meek, B. W. Metcalf and M. Rosenberg. 1987. *Proc. Natl. Acad. Sci. USA*, 84:8903–8906.

119 Graves, M. C., J. J. Lim, E. P. Heimer and R. A. Kramer. 1988. *Proc. Natl. Acad. Sci. USA*, 85:2449–2453.

120 Kohl, N. E., E. A. Emini, W. A. Schleif, L. J. Davis, J. C. Heimbach, R. A. F. Dixon, E. M. Scolnick and I. S. Sigal. 1988. *Proc. Natl. Acad. Sci. USA*, 85:4686–4690.

121 Darke, P. L., C.-T. Leu, L. J. Davis, J. C. Heimbach, R. E. Diehl, W. S. Hill, R. A. F. Dixon and I. S. Sigal. 1989. *J. Biol. Chem.*, 264:2307–2312.

122 Kramer, R. A., M. D. Schaber, A. M. Skalka, K. Ganguly, F. Wong-Staal and E. P. Reddy. 1986. *Science*, 231:1580-1585.

123 Barr, P. J., M. D. Power, C. T. Lee-Ng, H. L. Gibson and P. Luciw. 1987. *Biotechnology*, 5:486-489.

124 Pichuantes, S., L. M. Babe, P. J. Barr and C. S. Craik. 1989. *Proteins*, 6: 324-337.

125 Pearl, L. H. and W. R. Taylor. 1987. *Nature*, 329:351-354.

126 Navia, M. A., P. M. D. Fitzgerald, B. M. McKeever, C.-T. Leu, J. C. Heimbach, W. K. Herber, I. S. Sigal, P. L. Darke and J. P. Springer. 1989. *Nature*, 337:615-620.

127 Wlodawer, A., M. Miller, M. Jaskolski, B. K. Sathyanarayana, E. Baldwin, I. T. Weber, L. M. Selk, L. Clawson, J. Schneider and S. B. H. Kent. 1989. *Science*, 245:616-621.

128 Lapatto, R., T. Blundell, A. Hemmings, J. Overington, A. Wilderspin, S. Wood, J. R. Merson, P. J. Whittle, D. E. Danley, K. F. Geoghegan, S. J. Hawrylik, S. E. Lee, K. G. Scheld and P. M. Hobart. 1989. *Nature*, 342:299-302.

129 Miller, M., J. Schneider, B. K. Sathyanarayana, M. V. Toth, G. R. Marshall, L. Clawson, L. Selk, S. B. H. Kent and A. Wlodawer. 1989. *Science*, 246:1149-1152.

130 Fitzgerald, P. M. D., B. M. McKeever, J. F. VanMiddlesworth, J. P. Springer, J. C. Heimbach, C.-T. Leu, W. K. Herber, R. A. F. Dixon and P. L. Darke. 1990. *J. Biol. Chem.*, 265:14209-14219.

131 Moore, M. L., W. M. Bryan, S. A. Fakhoury, V. W. Magaard, W. F. Huffman, B. D. Dayton, T. D. Meek, L. H. Hyland, G. B. Dreyer, B. W. Metcalf, J. E. Strickler, J. G. Gorniak and C. Debouck. 1989. *Biochem. Biophys. Res. Comm.*, 159:420-425.

132 Hyland, L. J., B. D. Dayton, M. L. Moore, A. Y. L. Shu, J. R. Heys and T. D. Meek. 1990. *Anal. Biochem.*, 188:408-415.

133 Meek, T. D., B. D. Dayton, B. W. Metcalf, G. B. Dreyer, J. E. Strickler, J. G. Gorniak, M. Rosenberg, M. L. Moore, V. W. Magaard and C. Debouck. 1989. *Proc. Natl. Acad. Sci. USA*, 86:1841-1845.

134 Dreyer, G. B., B. W. Metcalf, T. A. Tomaszek, Jr., T. J. Carr, A. C. Chandler, III, L. Hyland, S. A. Fakhoury, V. A. Magaard, M. L. Moore, J. E. Strickler, C. Debouck and T. D. Meek. 1989. *Proc. Natl. Acad. Sci. USA*, 86:9752-9756.

135 Rich, D. H., J. Green, M. V. Toth, G. R. Marshall and S. B. H. Kent. 1990. *J. Med. Chem.*, 33:1285-1288.

136 Erickson, J., D. J. Neidhart, J. VanDrie, D. J. Kempf, X. C. Wang, D. W. Norbeck, J. J. Plattner, J. W. Rittenhouse, M. Turon, N. Wideburg, W. E. Kohlbrenner, R. Simmer, R. Helfrich, D. A. Paul and M. Knigge. 1990. *Science*, 249:527-533.

137 Meek, T. D., D. M. Lambert, G. B. Dreyer, T. J. Carr, T. A. Tomaszek, Jr., M. L. Moore, J. E. Strickler, C. Debouck, L. J. Hyland, T. J. Matthews, B. W. Metcalf and S. R. Petteway. 1990. *Nature*, 343:90-92.

138 McQuade, T. J., A. G. Tomasselli, L. Liu, V. Karacostas, B. Moss, T. K. Sawyer, R. L. Heinrikson and W. G. Tarpley. 1990. *Science*, 247:454-456.

139 Roberts, N. A., J. A. Martin, D. Kinchington, A. V. Broadhurst, J. C. Craig, I. B. Duncan, S. A. Galpin, B. K. Handa, J. Kay, A. Krohn, R. W. Lambert, J. H. Merrett, J. S. Mills, K. E. B. Parkes, S. Redshaw, A. J. Ritchie, D. L. Taylor, G. J. Thomas and P. J. Machin. 1990. *Science*, 248:358-361.

140 Lambert, D. M. 1990. Personal communication.

141 Leis, J., D. Baltimore, J. M. Bishop, J. Coffin, E. Fleissner, S. P. Groff, S. Oroszlan, H. Robinson, A. M. Skalka, H. M. Temin and V. Vogt. 1988. *J. Virol.*, 62(5):1808–1809.

142 Oroszlan, S. and R. B. Luftig. 1990. In *Current Topics in Microbiology and Immunology, Vol. 157*. Berlin-Heidelburg: Springer-Verlag, pp. 152–185.

Index

355